Crohn's & Colitis

FOR DUMMIES®

A Wiley Brand

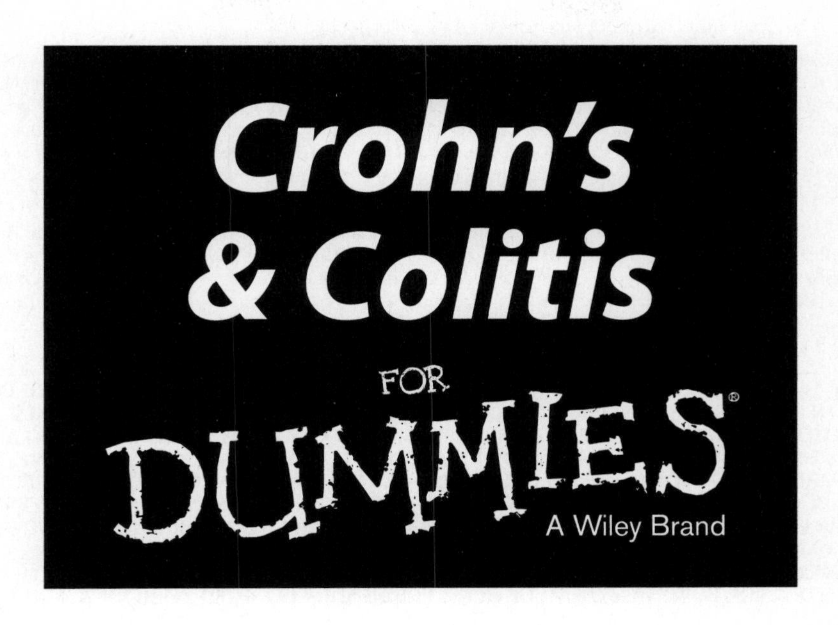

by Tauseef Ali, MD

Foreword by David T. Rubin, MD
Professor of Medicine and Co-Director of the Inflammatory Bowel Disease Center, The University of Chicago Medicine

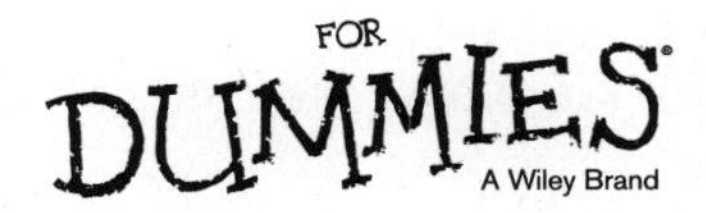

Crohn's & Colitis For Dummies®

Published by
John Wiley & Sons Canada, Ltd.
6045 Freemont Blvd.
Mississauga, ON L5R 4J3
www.wiley.com

For general information on John Wiley & Sons Canada, Ltd., including all books published by Wiley, please call our warehouse, Tel 1-800-567-4797. For reseller information, including discounts and premium sales, please call our sales department, Tel 416-646-7992. For press review copies, author interviews, or other publicity information, please contact our marketing department, Tel 416-646-4584, Fax 416-236-4448.

For technical support, please visit www.wiley.com/techsupport.

Wiley publishes in a variety of print and electronic formats and by print-on-demand. Some material included with standard print versions of this book may not be included in e-books or in print-on-demand. If this book refers to media such as a CD or DVD that is not included in the version you purchased, you may download this material at http://booksupport.wiley.com. For more information about Wiley products, visit www.wiley.com.

Library and Archives Canada Cataloguing in Publication Data

Ali, Tauseef

Crohn's and colitis for dummies / Tauseef Ali.

Includes index.

ISBN 978-1-118-43959-3 (pbk); ISBN 978-1-118-43964-7 (ebk); ISBN 978-1-118-43966-1 (ebk);
ISBN 978-1-118-43970-8 (ebk)

1. Crohn's disease. 2. Colitis. I. Title.

RC862.E52A45 2013 616.3'44 C2013-901739-9

Printed in the United States

1 2 3 4 5 RRD 17 16 15 14 13

About the Author

Dr. Tauseef Ali serves as a faculty member in the Department of Medicine, Section of Digestive Diseases and Nutrition, at the University of Oklahoma College of Medicine. He is the director of the department's comprehensive Inflammatory Bowel Disease Program and a staff gastroenterologist at OU Medical Center and St. Anthony Hospital, Oklahoma City. Dr. Ali graduated from Pakistan's King Edward Medical University, one of the most prestigious medical universities in Asia, established in 1860. He finished his internal medicine residency and gastroenterology subspecialty fellowship at the OU College of Medicine. During his training, Dr. Ali spent some time at the University of Chicago to learn about inflammatory bowel disease and received direct mentoring from Dr. David T. Rubin, an internationally renowned authority in Crohn's and colitis.

Dr. Ali has a great passion for inflammatory bowel disease and has presented many papers on the topic at the regional, national, and international levels. He has published many research and review articles on Crohn's and colitis. His areas of interest include the effect of sleep problems on inflammatory bowel disease and the impact of health literacy on disease outcomes.

As a member of the American College of Physicians, the American College of Gastroenterology, the American Gastroenterology Association, the American Society of Parenteral and Enteral Nutrition, the Southern Society of Clinical Investigators, and the Crohn's and Colitis Foundation of America, Dr. Ali is actively involved in many educational and scholarly activities. He has served as the academic editor-in-chief of *World Journal of Gastroenterology* and has been a reviewer in many gastroenterology journals.

Dr. Ali regularly tweets the latest research in Crohn's and colitis. You can find him at www.twitter.com/ibdtweets.

Dedication

To my wonderful parents, Rizwana and Asghar; my beautiful wife, Ammara; and my lovely kids, Mohid, Moiz, and Anaya, who were a constant support and source of fun and inspiration while I was working on this book.

Author's Acknowledgments

First, I would like to thank God for giving me the capability to write this book. I would like to thank Anam Ahmad, my acquisitions editor, who thought I had what it takes to put Crohn's and colitis in plain English. I thoroughly enjoyed working with Elizabeth Kuball, my project editor, who took great care of my words while patiently guiding me through the *For Dummies* process. I greatly appreciate the support of the entire editorial staff at John Wiley & Sons Canada, Ltd.; you were a great help in my endeavor to write this book. I also want to extend my thanks to Dr. Raymond Cross from the University of Maryland, who served as the book's technical editor and provided valuable suggestions to make this book the best resource guide for patients, as well as their friends and family members.

I would like to specially acknowledge my mentor, Dr. David T. Rubin, who is a source of inspiration and motivation for me. I would like to thank Dr. William Tierney, who throughout my training and during my time as a faculty member, taught me the art of medical ethics. Special thanks go to Amber Crosby, Belinda Frost, and Theresa Rush, not only for their support and valuable suggestions, but also for the way that each, in her own way, encourage and inspire me. I would like to thank Sameera Omar for her comments and suggestions, especially on the chapters related to pregnancy and childhood issues. I also want to thank my brilliant medical student Joshua Wadlin, who helped me collect medical information that I drew upon in writing the book. A special feeling of gratitude to my loving parents, Muhammad Asghar and Rizwana Asghar, and to my parents-in-law, Dr. Janbaz Ahmad and Jawairia Ahmad, and other family members who have always supported and encouraged me. I would like to express extreme gratitude to my wife, Ammara, whose support and appreciation was more invaluable to me while I was writing this book than she could ever know.

Last but not least, I would like to extend my gratitude to all my patients, who in their efforts to find relief from their condition have given me the gift of learning.

Publisher's Acknowledgments

We're proud of this book; please send us your comments at http://dummies.custhelp.com. For other comments, please contact our Customer Care Department within the U.S. at 877-762-2974, outside the U.S. at 317-572-3993, or fax 317-572-4002.

Some of the people who helped bring this book to market include the following:

Acquisitions and Editorial

Project Editor: Elizabeth Kuball

Acquiring Editor: Anam Ahmed

Copy Editor: Elizabeth Kuball

Technical Editor: Raymond Cross, MD

Production Editor: Lindsay Humphreys

Editorial Assistant: Kathy Deady

Cover Photos: © Iuliya Sunagatova / iStockphoto

Cartoons: Rich Tennant (www.the5thwave.com)

Composition Services

Senior Project Coordinator: Kristie Rees

Layout and Graphics: Carrie A. Cesavice, Joyce Haughey, Andrea Hornberger

Proofreaders: Melissa D. Buddenbeck, John Greenough

Indexer: Ty Koontz

Illustrator: Kathryn Born

John Wiley & Sons Canada, Ltd.

Deborah Barton, Vice President and Director of Operations

Jennifer Smith, Publisher, Professional Development

Alison Maclean, Managing Editor, Professional Development

Publishing and Editorial for Consumer Dummies

Kathleen Nebenhaus, Vice President and Executive Publisher

David Palmer, Associate Publisher

Kristin Ferguson-Wagstaffe, Product Development Director

Publishing for Technology Dummies

Andy Cummings, Vice President and Publisher

Composition Services

Debbie Stailey, Director of Composition Services

Contents at a Glance

Table of Contents

Part IV: Living and Coping with Crohn's and Colitis 195

Foreword

When I started my training in gastroenterology, most people I met had never heard of Crohn's disease or ulcerative colitis. Today, I rarely meet anyone who hasn't heard of these conditions, and most people today know someone who suffers from them. This is due, in part, to the fact that the number of new cases of Crohn's disease and ulcerative colitis is rising in North America and around the world, and we don't yet know why. In addition, most inflammatory bowel disease (IBD) patients have no family history of IBD and no idea why this mysterious illness is affecting them. IBD is a substantial source of physical suffering and psychological distress, and until recently, it was often thought to be uncontrollable.

Today, we no longer think of IBD as uncontrollable. In the last decade, unprecedented advances have been made in the diagnosis and treatment of Crohn's disease and ulcerative colitis. We have made substantial progress in the understanding of the genetic, environmental, and immunological causes of these conditions, have created new technologies that aid in accurate diagnosis and disease assessment, and most important, have developed many new therapies that are effective at controlling bowel inflammation and improving patients' quality of life. In fact, IBD has moved from a dreaded and life-threatening disease of "crisis management" to a chronic, manageable condition whose management is now focused on prevention of complications and long-term, stable control.

Unfortunately, many patients are still misinformed or do not have access to expert care. The Internet is full of misinformation, and many physicians have had difficulty keeping up with the latest developments in the field. In *Crohn's & Colitis For Dummies*, Dr. Tauseef Ali skillfully addresses these unmet needs. As an IBD expert, he provides some of the latest theories and advice about disease management. And as a caring and experienced physician, he addresses the educational needs of patients and their family members.

Dr. Ali applies the tried-and-true formula of the *For Dummies* series to Crohn's disease and ulcerative colitis, and succeeds in breaking down complex and confusing symptoms and concepts into easy-to-understand chapters, well-defined terms, and myth-busting explanations. When you read this book, you feel Dr. Ali's calming and compassionate presence, gently guiding you and providing straightforward advice and information. It's obvious why having a dedicated physician like him in your corner can make a huge difference in your disease management and good health.

So, until we have cures for Crohn's disease and ulcerative colitis, all patients and their family members should have a copy of *Crohn's & Colitis For Dummies!*

David T. Rubin, MD
Professor of Medicine
Co-Director, Inflammatory Bowel Disease Center
The University of Chicago Medicine

Introduction

Millions of people suffer from inflammatory bowel disease (IBD) around the world: more than 1 million in the United States, nearly 200,000 in Canada, and approximately 2 million in Europe. The incidence of this disease is on the rise. Some recent studies suggest that more than 30,000 people are diagnosed with IBD every year in the United States alone. Crohn's disease and ulcerative colitis, the two major types of IBD, are chronic inflammatory diseases of the intestine. They're thought to occur because of a malfunctioning of the immune system, genetic defects, or exposure to certain environmental factors — or perhaps a combination of all three. Crohn's disease and ulcerative colitis mostly affect younger people. There is no miracle drug to cure IBD, but many treatment options can provide relief.

About This Book

In this book, I don't tell you everything there is to know about Crohn's disease and ulcerative colitis. Instead, I give you the information you need in order to make the right decisions about your treatment. I've also made sure that the information I provide is clear and easy to understand — not a bunch of medical mumbo-jumbo. In this book, you find out what happens in Crohn's disease and ulcerative colitis — the symptoms they can cause, how they can affect your life at home and at work, what you can do to feel good and function normally, and how you can protect yourself and your family against the long-term unpredictability of the disease. I also offer useful tips, introduce you to the members of your healthcare team, and point you in the direction of other useful resources.

There's nothing wrong with reading this book from beginning to end, but you don't have to do that to get the most out of this book. Instead, you can use this book as a reference, drawing on the Table of Contents and Index to locate the information you need.

Conventions Used in This Book

I don't use many special conventions throughout this book, but I do use a few that you should be aware of:

- When I mention a drug, I list the generic name first, followed by the brand name(s) in parentheses.
- When I refer to Crohn's disease, sometimes I just call it *Crohn's*. And when I refer to ulcerative colitis, sometimes I just call it *colitis*. Anytime I refer just to *colitis*, know that I'm talking about ulcerative colitis. (Other types of colitis exist; see Chapter 2 for more information.)
- When I introduce a new term, I use *italics* and define the term shortly thereafter, often in parentheses.
- All web addresses appear in `monofont`.

Note: When this book was printed, some web addresses may have needed to break across two lines of text. If that happened, rest assured that we haven't put in any extra characters (such as hyphens) to indicate the break. So, when using one of these web addresses, just type in exactly what you see in this book, pretending as though the line break doesn't exist.

What You're Not to Read

You can skip two types of text without missing crucial information:

- **Sidebars:** These shaded gray boxes include information that may interest you but isn't critical to your understanding of the subject at hand.
- **Anything marked by the Technical Stuff icon:** For more information on the Technical Stuff icon, see "Icons Used in This Book," later in this Introduction.

Foolish Assumptions

Every book is written with a specific audience in mind, and this one is no different. As I wrote this book, I made some basic assumptions about who you are. One or more of the following likely applies to you:

- You have Crohn's or colitis, think that you may have it, or have a friend or family member who has it.
- You want information that can help you or a loved one manage Crohn's or colitis more effectively.
- You want information on the latest treatment for Crohn's or colitis.
- You want to work with your doctor to obtain the best possible care — and, yes, you sort of want to impress her with your knowledge.
- You want to take charge of your own body.
- You like books with black-and-yellow covers.

How This Book Is Organized

I've divided this book into six parts, so you can skip directly to the ones that pique your interest. Here's a brief overview of each part.

Part I: The Who, What, and Why of Crohn's and Colitis

Your doctor may have delivered the news that you or a loved one has Crohn's or colitis. Or maybe he said you *might* have this disease or *probably* have this disease. You may be wondering and trying to figure out what it means to you and your loved ones. This part gives you the big picture. Chapter 1 describes how this illness can affect your daily living and how to cope and live with this disease. Chapter 2 gives you the details about Crohn's and colitis, defining and explaining various signs and symptoms, as well as organ systems involved with the diseases. Chapter 3 takes you on a tour of the wonderful and amazing human digestive system and introduces you to the different parts of your digestive organs. Chapter 4 sheds light on how and why people get Crohn's or colitis, explaining various factors such as diet, environment, genes, and the immune system and their roles in causing Crohn's and colitis.

Part II: Getting Medical Help

Developing a long-lasting relationship with your doctor is critical in dealing with Crohn's or colitis. In Chapter 5, I help you find the right doctor and assemble your healthcare team to manage your Crohn's and colitis. I also guide you on what questions to ask your doctor and how to manage your health records and keep them straight for your and your doctor's ease. In Chapter 6, I explain the different tests and investigations that are commonly performed to diagnose Crohn's and colitis. Chapter 7 covers the different medications used to treat these diseases, how they work, and their common side effects. When medications fail to control the disease, surgery is the next step; Chapter 8 describes various surgeries, when they may be right for you, and potential complications they bring.

Part III: Healing and Dealing with the Disease

In this part, I aim to give you power over your Crohn's and colitis. Chapter 9 covers nutrition, which plays an important part in your well-being. Although Crohn's and colitis put you at risk for malnutrition, deficiency of nutrients can also adversely affect your immune system and healing process. I fill you in on the importance of nutrients and provide details about their functions, how to get them, and their importance in the management of Crohn's and colitis.

Prevention is better than cure, and in Chapter 10 I discuss important preventive steps that are important to keep you healthy as a person with Crohn's or colitis. I also talk about vaccinations, bone scans, and skin care in this chapter.

Chapter 11 deals with alternative and complementary therapies, including the role of different herbs in treating these diseases. I also tell you about worm therapy, the latest hype in the management of Crohn's and colitis.

Part IV: Living and Coping with Crohn's and Colitis

Having Crohn's or colitis can make you feel isolated, embarrassed, and afraid. It can greatly affect how you interact with your family, your co-workers, your friends, and the world at large. Chapter 12 helps you face the diagnosis and live a happy life, despite your disease. Chapter 13 describes different triggers that you can avoid to prevent flares. Chapter 14 offers tips and techniques for working and traveling with Crohn's or colitis.

Part V: Considering Special Populations with Crohn's and Colitis

In Chapter 15, I describe various issues related to kids and teens who've been diagnosed with Crohn's or colitis. I also provide tips for surviving school and college — at least when it comes to these diseases. (I can't offer any advice on getting a date to the prom or making it to that 8 a.m. class.)

Getting pregnant with Crohn's and colitis is an important issue, and I devote Chapter 16 to this topic. In this chapter, I also fill you in on which Crohn's and colitis drugs are safe to take during pregnancy and while breastfeeding.

Part VI: The Part of Tens

Could there be a *For Dummies* book without a Part of Tens? Not a chance. In this part, I give you some pearls of wisdom — they're small, but worth a fortune. In Chapter 17, I fill you in on ten myths about Crohn's and colitis and give you a better and more accurate picture of the facts. In Chapter 18, I tell you about ten great resources for more information about Crohn's and colitis.

Icons Used in This Book

Icons are a handy *For Dummies* way to catch your attention as you slide your eyes down the page. They can help you pick out the key ideas and points of information throughout the book. The icons come in several varieties, each with its own special meaning:

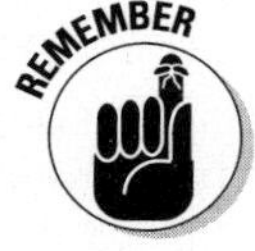

The Remember icon marks information you'll want to, well, remember.

When my inner geek comes out, I mark the information with the Technical Stuff icon. Text marked with this icon provides information that's interesting but not critical to your understanding of the topic at hand.

The Tip icon marks time-saving and stress-saving information that you can use to improve your life when you have Crohn's or colitis.

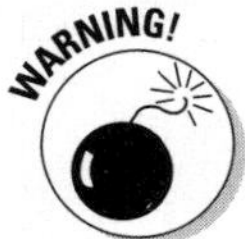

The Warning icon alerts you to some pitfalls. I save this icon for critical issues, material important enough that could bring harm your way if you don't heed it.

Where to Go from Here

You can dive in anywhere that interests you and get valuable information. Use the Table of Contents and Index to find the information you need. If you aren't sure where to start, you can't go wrong with Part I.

No matter where you choose to begin, begin now! In your hands, you hold the information you need to live well with Crohn's and colitis.

Part I

The Who, What, and Why of Crohn's and Colitis

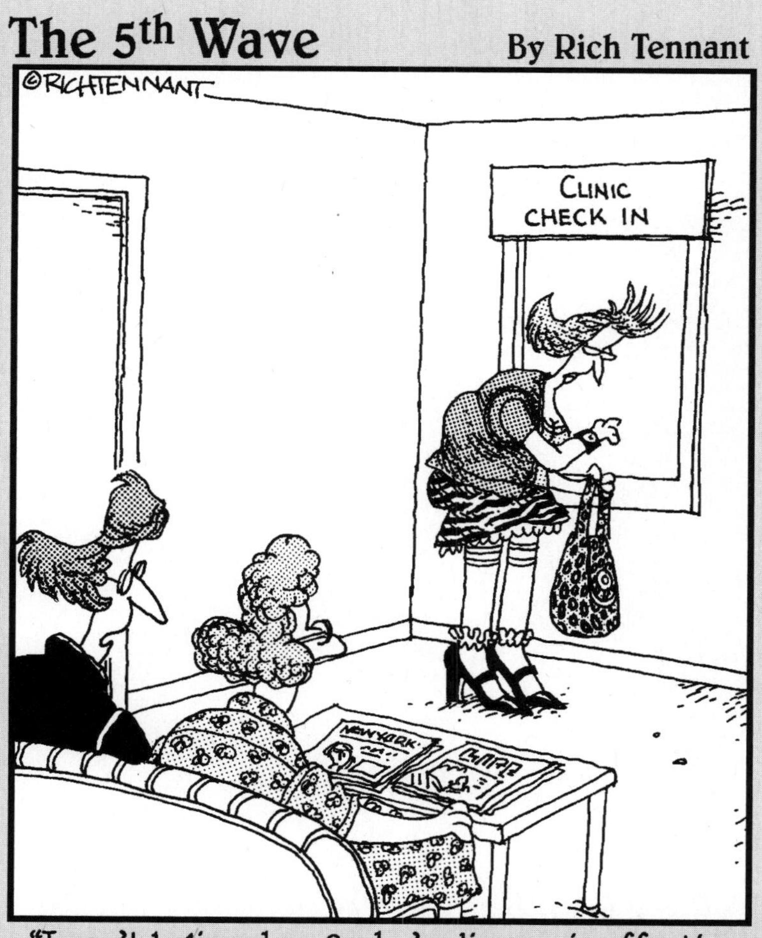

"I can't believe her Crohn's disease is affecting her body any worse than her sense of style is."

In this part . . .

When you're new to Crohn's and colitis — either your own diagnosis or the diagnosis of a loved one — you may be overwhelmed. Your head is spinning with questions. And this part is for you. Here you find out what Crohn's and colitis are, how your digestive system works, and who gets these diseases and why.

Chapter 1

Crohn's and Colitis One Step at a Time

In This Chapter

- Finding out about Crohn's disease and ulcerative colitis
- Reviewing the treatment options
- Taking control of your quality of life
- Living a full life with Crohn's and colitis
- Looking at issues specific to pregnancy and kids

Knowing your disease is key to your quality of life. Knowledge is power! While I was writing this book, I thought about the questions I hear most often from my patients and their family members. I answered those questions just as I do for my patients. This chapter is an overview of the book as a whole — it gives you a taste of what I elaborate on in the chapters that follow.

Knowing Crohn's and Colitis

Crohn's and colitis are chronic inflammatory diseases of the intestines. Together, these illnesses are also known as *inflammatory bowel disease.* So, what exactly are Crohn's and colitis?

When you get a cut to your skin, it hurts, bleeds, swells, and eventually forms a scar. Similarly, Crohn's and colitis cause cuts inside your intestinal wall; these cuts are called *ulcers.* Pain, bleeding, and swelling occur with ulcers, too — they just happen inside your intestinal wall where you can't see them. Eventually, scars form (just as you might have a scar from a bad cut on your skin), leading to the formation of *strictures* (abnormal narrowing) and causing obstruction. This happens more frequently in Crohn's disease and rarely in ulcerative colitis. In Chapter 2, I offer even more information on what Crohn's and colitis are.

The signs and symptoms of Crohn's and colitis (also covered in Chapter 2) depend on the part of the intestines involved:

- **Crohn's disease:** Crohn's disease most commonly involves the last part of the small intestine and the beginning of the large intestine. The common symptoms of Crohn's disease are abdominal pain, especially on the right lower side of the abdomen, diarrhea, and weight loss.
- **Colitis:** Colitis can involve the whole large intestine or a part of it. The process of inflammation usually starts in the rectum and moves upward to involve other parts of the colon. Bloody diarrhea is a common symptom of colitis. *Urgency* (the sudden feeling of needing to have a bowel movement) and *tenesmus* (the feeling of incomplete relief after the bowel movement) are also common symptoms and are caused by the inflammation of the rectum, also known as *proctitis.*

In both diseases, the process of inflammation can also cause fever, loss of appetite, weight loss, night sweats, and fatigue. Your nutritional status is usually compromised and if you don't pay attention to your diet and calorie intake, you can easily become malnourished.

If it's been a while since you took a biology class and you need a refresher course on the digestive system, check out Chapter 3.

Who gets Crohn's and colitis? We still don't have the exact answer to this question. Scientists believe that different factors may play a role in causing these illnesses — including malfunctioning of the immune system, genetic defects, or exposure to certain environmental factors. For more information on who gets Crohn's and colitis, turn to Chapter 4.

Getting the Treatment You Need

The first part of getting treated for Crohn's disease is assembling your healthcare team. Crohn's and colitis are lifelong diseases, so you want to choose a doctor you can trust and with whom you can develop a long-term relationship. You also need to be familiar with other key players of your healthcare team, such as nurses, nutritionists, psychiatrists, and surgeons. For more information on assembling your team, turn to Chapter 5.

When it comes to getting diagnosed with Crohn's or colitis, most of the time it's symptoms of diarrhea, abdominal pain, and blood in stools that prompts people to go to the doctor's office. Your doctor will run a battery of tests to rule out (or rule in) the diagnosis of Crohn's or colitis. These tests may include blood tests, stool tests, endoscopic exams, and radiology tests. The different tests used to confirm the diagnosis of Crohn's or colitis are covered in Chapter 6.

There is no cure for Crohn's or colitis, but medications work in the majority of patients. Many drugs are available for the treatment of these diseases. The drugs help to control symptoms and bring the disease under control. You'll have to take these medications long term (until your doctor changes your prescription or you require surgery). For more information on the various medications used to treat Crohn's and colitis, turn to Chapter 7.

In some patients, medications may stop working or patients may be unable to tolerate the medications because of side effects. In these cases, your doctor will talk to you about surgery. Colitis is cured after surgery, but Crohn's disease comes back even after surgery and may require further medications or surgeries. For more on the surgical options for treating Crohn's and colitis, check out Chapter 8.

Recognizing That You're Not Powerless

Some people with chronic conditions like Crohn's or colitis get discouraged — you don't want to have to cope with a disease that has the potential to disrupt your life and cause pain. But the good news is, you can take all kinds of steps to improve your quality of life when you have Crohn's or colitis.

A key part of your health as a person who has Crohn's or colitis is your diet. Eating a well-balanced diet and avoiding trigger foods are very important steps when it comes to managing these illnesses. Good nutrition is important for your immune system and your body's ability to heal from the inflammation. Nutrition is also important for kids and pregnant women suffering from Crohn's and colitis because they have increasingly higher demands for calories and because malnutrition can really affect growth and worsen the process of inflammation. On the other hand, your body may not be able to handle sugar, high-fiber foods, and fatty foods, especially during periods of active disease, and you may want to avoid them. For more information on the role diet has in Crohn's and colitis, check out Chapter 9.

Crohn's and colitis can affect your whole body, not just your digestive system. For example, you may be more prone to a variety of skin conditions, including skin cancer. In addition, Crohn's and colitis can impact the balance of calcium and vitamin D in your body, which can lead to osteoporosis or osteopenia (a precursor to osteoporosis). For more information on whole-body health for people with Crohn's and colitis, turn to Chapter 10.

When you have Crohn's or colitis, you don't have to rely solely on conventional medicine. You can try a variety of alternative and complementary therapies, from exercise and physical therapy to herbal therapy and homeopathy to traditional Chinese medicine and more. Chapter 11 has the lowdown on a variety of options that may improve your quality of life.

Living a Full Life with the Disease

When you first get diagnosed with Crohn's or colitis, handling the diagnosis is a challenge. Then you have to figure out a way to talk about it to your family and friends — because they'll be affected by your diagnosis, too (after all, you're a big part of their lives). In Chapter 12, I offer advice on these subjects and more, including planning for the holidays. Chapter 12 is also for you if you're not the one with Crohn's or colitis, but your family member or friend has the disease.

Part of living and coping with Crohn's and colitis is figuring out how to avoid triggers that cause flares. Common triggers include different drugs or foods, smoking, stress, and lack of sleep. Chapter 13 is all about how to reduce triggers in your life so you can focus on what you'd rather be doing — living!

Work and travel are two big parts of life for many people, and when you have Crohn's or colitis, you need to know how to manage your disease while you do one or both. You may need to talk about your diagnosis with your employer — something that can cause stress in and of itself, depending on your relationship with your boss and how secure you feel in your job. And anxiety can increase if you're on the road and find yourself needing a bathroom fast. Chapter 14 covers work and travel, offering useful tips for doing both when you have Crohn's or colitis.

Special Advice for Pregnant Women and Kids

Twenty-five percent of Crohn's and colitis patients are under the age of 20, and the number of kids suffering from these diseases is increasing. The goal for treating kids is all about controlling symptoms while causing minimal disruption to their lives, from school to sports to hanging out with friends. In Chapter 15, I offer advice to parents of kids with Crohn's and colitis.

Finally, if you have Crohn's or colitis and you want to get pregnant (or don't want to get pregnant), Chapter 16 is for you. There, I discuss everything from libido and sex to fertility. I also fill you in on the impact of your disease on the life of your baby.

Chapter 2

Defining Crohn's and Colitis

In This Chapter

- Getting clear on Crohn's and colitis
- Identifying the symptoms of Crohn's and colitis
- Exploring the other organs involved in Crohn's and colitis
- Taking a peek at the complications

You've heard of Crohn's and colitis — maybe you've even been diagnosed with one of these diseases — but you may not know exactly what they are. If so, you've come to the right place. In this chapter, I explain what Crohn's and colitis are and introduce you to inflammatory bowel disease (IBD) in general. I fill you in on the symptoms of Crohn's and colitis and tell you which organs in the body can be affected by these diseases. Finally, I explain the complications that can occur because of Crohn's and colitis — from intestinal complications to nutritional complications to cancer.

Information is power, and the information you find in this chapter will empower you to talk with your doctor about your condition and get the best possible treatment so you can live a long, happy, and healthy life.

What Crohn's and Colitis Are

Crohn's disease and ulcerative colitis are closely related to each other — I usually call them "cousins" because they have a lot in common. But recognizing these diseases as two separate entities is important, because their symptoms and treatments could be different.

Looking at the big picture: Inflammatory bowel disease

Inflammatory bowel disease is a chronic inflammation of the gastrointestinal tract, usually involving the small and large intestines (see Figure 2-1). Doctors still aren't sure what causes IBD, but various factors — from defects in the immune system to genetic abnormalities to environmental factors — are thought to play a role.

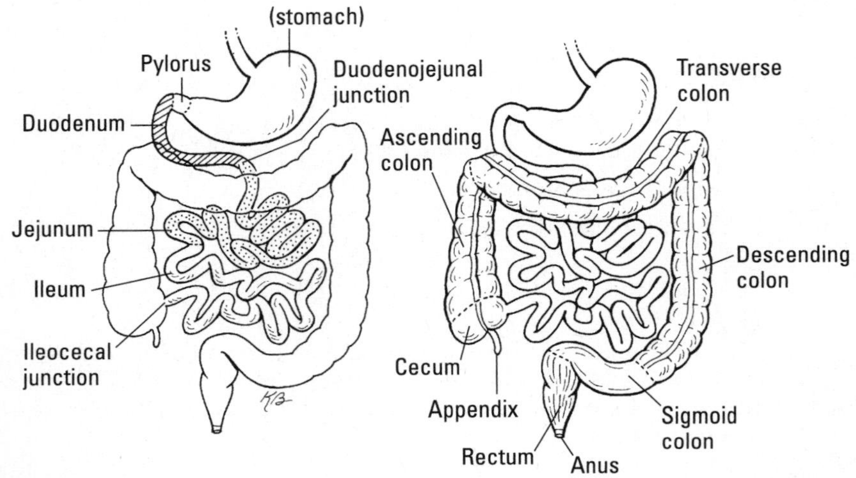

Figure 2-1: The small intestine and large intestine.

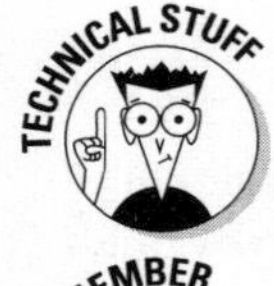

IBD is actually a group of conditions. The two main types of IBD are Crohn's disease and ulcerative colitis, but other conditions also fall under the IBD umbrella, including microscopic colitis (which includes collagenous colitis and lymphocytic colitis) and indeterminate colitis.

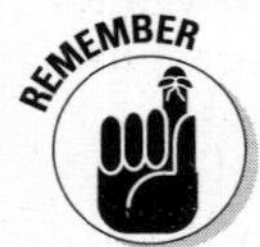

Throughout this book, when I refer to *colitis,* I'm talking about ulcerative colitis. If I'm referring to another type of colitis, I use the more specific term.

Zeroing in on Crohn's and colitis

Crohn's and colitis are the two main types of IBD. In this section, I define these two conditions and explain how they differ from each other. First, though, you need just a little info on the intestinal tract.

The intestinal tract is made up of several layers, one on top of the other, kind of like an onion (see Figure 2-2). The innermost layer of the intestinal tract, called the *mucosa,* helps in the absorption of food and secretes digestive enzymes. This layer is wrapped in another layer, called the *submucosa,* followed by a layer of muscle, called *muscularis.* The outermost layer is called the *serosa.*

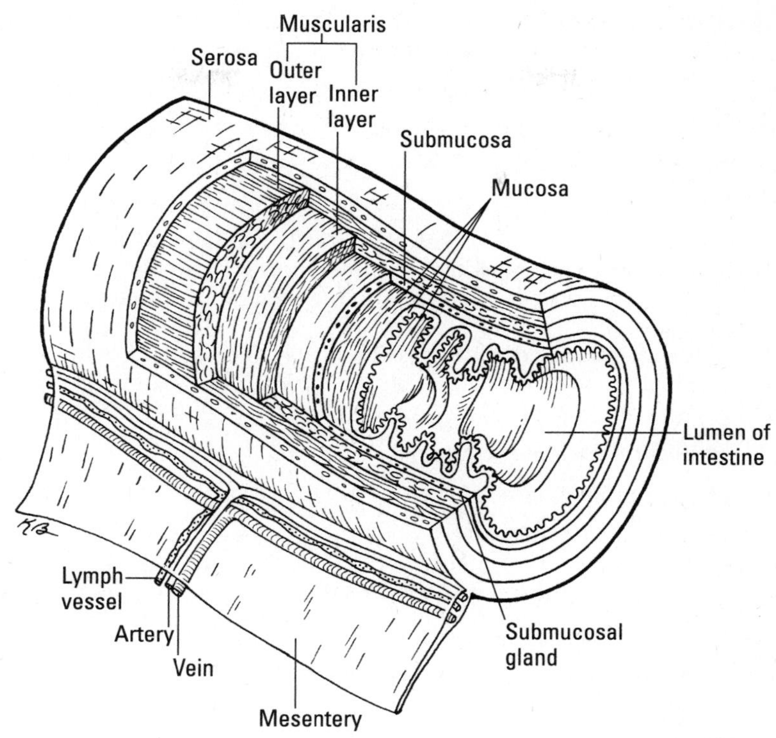

Figure 2-2: The layers of the intestinal tract.

Illustration by Kathryn Born

Defining Crohn's disease

In Crohn's disease, the inflammation begins in the mucosa but can eventually involve all the layers of the intestine (refer to Figure 2-2). In medical terminology, this inflammation is called *transmural inflammation.* Crohn's disease can involve any part of the gastrointestinal tract, from the mouth to the anus. However, the most common site of inflammation is the last part of the small intestine (the *terminal ileum*) along with the large intestine.

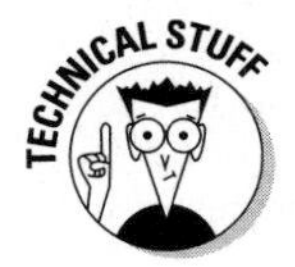

You may hear your doctor call Crohn's disease by other names, including the following:

- Crohn's colitis
- Crohn's disease of the colon
- Granulomatous enteritis
- Ileitis
- Ileocolitis

- Regional enteritis
- Regional ileitis
- Terminal ileitis

Defining colitis

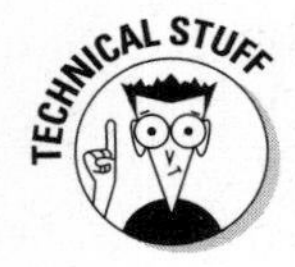

In ulcerative colitis, the inflammation is mostly confined to the mucosa (refer to Figure 2-2). In severe cases of colitis, the inflammation can sometimes trickle down to other layers. The inflammation usually starts in the *rectum* (the last part of the intestines) and may spread throughout the colon.

You may hear your doctor call ulcerative colitis by a number of other names:

- Colitis ulcerosa
- Idiopathic proctocolitis
- Idiopathic ulcerative colitis
- Nonspecific ulcerative colitis

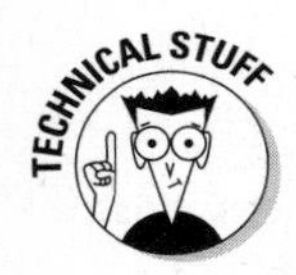

There are other forms of colitis, but the one I talk about in this book is ulcerative colitis. Here's a brief rundown of the other types of colitis:

- **Infectious colitis:** Inflammation of the colon due to an infection, such as virus or bacteria
- **Ischemic colitis:** Inflammation of the colon that occurs when the intestines don't get enough blood, such as with extremely low blood pressure and shock
- **Neutropenic colitis:** Inflammation of the colon that happens in cancer patients undergoing chemotherapy
- **Radiation colitis:** Inflammation of the colon caused by radiation therapy in cancer patients

When patients are first diagnosed with ulcerative colitis, approximately 45 percent of them have a form of the disease limited to the rectum and *sigmoid* (the last part of the colon), 35 percent have the disease extending beyond the sigmoid but not involving the entire colon, and 20 percent have involvement of the entire colon.

In some patients, the inner lining of the last few inches of the ileum becomes mildly inflamed. This is called *backwash ileitis.* Doctors don't know the exact cause of this phenomenon yet.

The history of Crohn's disease

Medical historians suggest that Crohn's disease was first described as early as the 9th century A.D. Alfred the Great (849–899 A.D.) suffered from a painful illness for much of his life. Records described his illness as abdominal pain, discomfort, diarrhea, and rectal problems beginning at the age of 20. Now we know that this was probably Crohn's disease. In 1913, Sir Kennedy Dalziel published an article in the *British Medical Journal* describing patients having transmural inflammation of the small and large intestines, a characteristic finding of Crohn's disease.

In 1932, Dr. Burrill Bernard Crohn and his two colleagues, Dr. Leon Ginzburg and Dr. Gordon Oppenheimer, published an important paper describing similar conditions in 14 patients; they called it "terminal ileitis." This paper was presented to a large medical audience in New York and, as a result, was given a large amount of recognition and publicity. Because Crohn was the first author on the paper, the disease was subsequently called Crohn's disease.

Seeing how Crohn's and colitis are different

Crohn's disease and ulcerative colitis, the two major types of IBD, can be treated very differently. However, the two diseases also share many common symptoms, and sometimes it's hard to distinguish the two types, especially in the early years. It's estimated that approximately 9 percent of patients initially diagnosed with one of these diseases has a change in diagnosis within two years.

Sometimes even experienced physicians have difficulty differentiating these two types of IBD. The term *indeterminate colitis* has been coined to describe such cases.

Location of the disease

Crohn's disease can affect any part of the digestive tract, from the mouth to the anus; most commonly, it occurs in the last section of the small intestine and the beginning of the colon. Colitis affects only the colon. See Figure 2-3 for an illustration of where these two diseases occur.

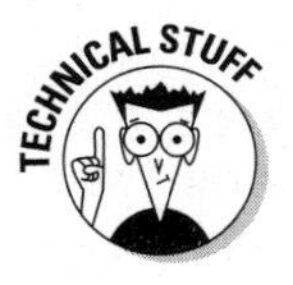

The terminal ileum is the last part of the small intestine. This part may show some mild inflammation in ulcerative colitis. This condition is referred to as *backwash ileitis.*

The history of colitis

Ulcerative colitis is even older than Crohn's disease. The first description of ulcerative colitis dates back to ancient Greece. Many physicians from this period, including Hippocrates (ca. 460–377 B.C.), described a condition of chronic diarrhea associated with blood and ulceration of the large intestines. In the late 1600s, Thomas Sydenham (1624–1689) coined the term *bloody flux* to describe this type of diarrheal disease. Historians have speculated that Bonnie Prince Charles, The Young Pretender (1720–1788), suffered from ulcerative colitis and cured himself by adopting a milk-free diet in 1745. Sir Samuel Wilks (1824–1911) described "ulcerative colitis" as a specific disease for the first time in 1859 and recognized it as distinct from the then more common infectious diarrhea. In 1909, around 300 cases of ulcerative colitis were collected from various London hospitals and presented at a symposium of the Royal Society of Medicine.

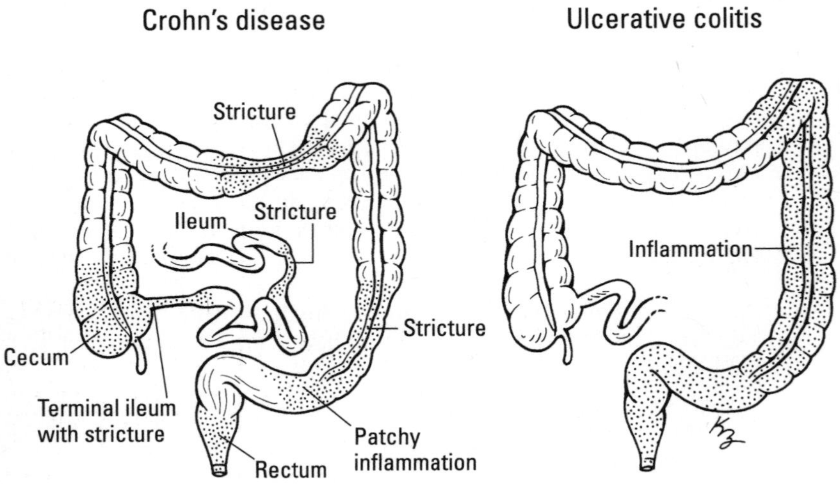

Figure 2-3: The location of Crohn's disease and ulcerative colitis in the gut.

Illustration by Kathryn Born

Pattern of inflammation

Crohn's disease is a patchy one; it can involve different segments of the intestines at the same time, and the segment of the intestine between the two diseased areas may appear normal. Colitis, on the other hand, tends to be continuous; it begins in the rectum and spreads up through the colon.

In Crohn's disease, the entire wall of the intestine can get inflamed. The term *transmural inflammation* often is used to describe the type of inflammation in Crohn's disease. Because of this involvement of multiple layers of the intestinal wall, patients are more prone to deep ulceration, perforation, and stricture and fistula formation. On the other hand, only the innermost lining of the intestinal wall is involved in the majority of colitis patients; this type of inflammation is called *mucosal inflammation.*

Appearance of the intestine

During a colonoscopy, the physician can view the mucosa of the colon and the terminal ileum. In Crohn's disease, the mucosa shows deep ulcers and may show areas that appear normal.

In colitis, the mucosa shows continuous inflammation, characterized by redness and superficial ulcers in the mucosa. There are no patches of healthy tissue in the diseased section.

The effect of smoking

In Crohn's disease, smoking makes the disease worse and increases the risk of flares and surgery. Studies also have shown that the outcomes of surgery are poorer in smokers and that Crohn's disease recurs early in patients who smoke.

For some unclear (and surprising) reasons, smoking has a protective effect in colitis. Therefore, colitis is sometimes called a "disease of nonsmokers."

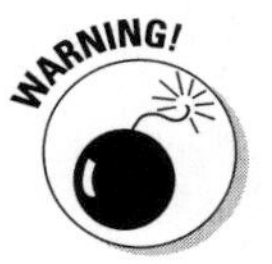

Even though smoking has a protective effect in colitis, smoking is *not* recommended because of its other significant health risks. If you smoke, you should quit — regardless of whether you have colitis.

Treatment

The drugs used to treat Crohn's disease and colitis are similar in many cases. The mainstays of treatment — mesalamine, corticosteroids, and other immunosuppressant drugs — are used to treat both conditions. (I discuss the different treatment options in detail in Chapter 7.) When medical therapy fails to control symptoms and inflammation in Crohn's disease, surgery often is required to remove the diseased part of the bowel (see Chapter 8). However, Crohn's disease eventually comes back after surgery. For some patients, it may take a few months for the disease to recur; in other cases, Crohn's disease may not come back for a few years. In ulcerative colitis, removal of the colon, also called *colectomy,* is considered a cure.

The Signs and Symptoms

Crohn's and colitis have a way of interfering with your quality of life — work, sleep, travel, diet, social life, and even sex all can be affected. Some people with Crohn's and colitis don't realize just how bad they've been feeling (and for how long) until they've been diagnosed and treated and the signs and symptoms have started to ease. In this section, I discuss various common and not-so-common signs and symptoms of Crohn's and colitis.

A *sign* is something objective that you or your doctor observes or that your doctor finds on a physical exam (for example, being pale, having a rash, or passing blood in the stool). A *symptom* is something that you can feel and tell your doctor about (for example, nausea or abdominal pain).

Inflammation, flare, and remission: Medical jargon 101

Your doctor will use the terms *inflammation, flare,* and *remission* when discussing and managing your symptoms. It helps if you know what the terms mean:

- **Inflammation:** Have you ever gotten a paper cut on your finger, and noticed how your finger swelled up around the cut? That's inflammation. The ability of your body to get rid of damaged tissue and foreign invaders such as microbes is essential to your very survival. The mechanism by which your body accomplishes this is called *inflammation.* Inflammation is a protective response to get rid of the agents that cause initial injury and also the consequences of the injury (such as dead tissue). Without inflammation, infections would go unchecked and wounds would never heal.

  However, inflammation may become harmful in some situations. The same mechanism designed to destroy foreign invaders and dead tissues also has the ability to injure normal tissues. When inflammation is inappropriately directed against your own body tissues or isn't appropriately controlled, it becomes the cause of chronic injury. This happens in many diseases such as rheumatoid arthritis, lupus, and asthma. IBD is an illness involving chronic inflammation of the digestive tract. This inflammation of the digestive tract, leading to ulcer formation and bleeding, is the cause of many symptoms in patients suffering from the disease.

- **Flare:** A flare (sometimes called a *flare-up* or *disease flare*) is the active state of IBD, including Crohn's and colitis. IBD is a chronic disease characterized by intermittent periods of active disease (flares) and periods of little or no disease activity (remission). The duration and severity of the flares vary widely from person to person. During flares, patients have symptoms of abdominal pain, diarrhea, fever, or blood in the stool (depending upon the type and location of IBD). People with colitis usually have increased diarrhea and blood in the stool, requiring frequent (and sometimes embarrassing) visits to the bathroom. People with Crohn's disease may have increased abdominal pain, fever, and diarrhea.

  One of the goals of IBD therapy is to prevent these flares. Taking medications regularly and avoiding missing medications prevents flares. Stress, depression, foods, drugs, and infections also can trigger a flare. During a flare, physicians may order some blood tests and stool studies to assess the severity of inflammation and rule out other causes, like infections.

- **Remission:** When you get an illness, your doctor treats you to end the illness. When you feel better and the medical condition is completely gone, you are said to have been "cured." Unfortunately, although researchers are working hard to find a medical cure, there is no cure for Crohn's and colitis. Current medical therapy can temporarily reduce or end signs and symptoms of IBD. This is called *remission.*

Before I get into listing all the various signs and symptoms of Crohn's and colitis, I want to start with a list of red flags — signs and symptoms that could mean something is wrong and that you should consult your doctor right away.

- **Intolerable abdominal pain:** If you develop intolerable abdominal pain, it may point toward intestinal obstruction, perforation, or severe inflammation. You may also notice other signs like nausea, vomiting, and abdominal distension.
- **Weight loss:** When you have Crohn's or colitis and you're losing weight, that's a sign that inflammation is still active. Most of your body energy is being diverted to control inflammation, and your nutrition is not keeping up with the amount of energy your body is expending.

  If you've had colitis for many years and you're now starting to lose weight, this could be worrisome. Longstanding colitis puts you at risk for cancer, so be sure to notify your doctor immediately about any weight loss you experience.
- **Fever and chills:** If you develop any fever with or without chills, this may point toward worsening inflammation or infection in your intestines or an intestinal *abscess* (collection of pus).
- **Severe bleeding:** If you notice blood in your stool every time you go to the bathroom, it may be a sign of severe inflammation.

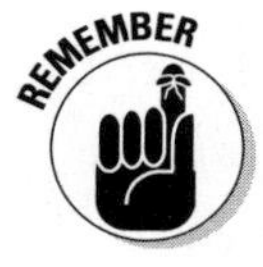

If you experience any of the preceding signs or symptoms, consult your doctor right away.

In the following sections, I cover the various signs and symptoms of Crohn's and colitis in detail.

Blood in stool

One of the most common symptoms of Crohn's and colitis is the presence of blood in the stool. Blood in the stool doesn't always look like the bright red blood you're used to seeing when you cut yourself, though. When you have Crohn's or colitis, you need to pay closer attention to your stool than the average person does.

The normal color of stool varies from light brown to dark brown. The color of blood in the stool varies depending on the site of bleeding and the transit time (how long it takes for the stool to get out of your body). If the bleeding is higher up in the gastrointestinal tract, the blood is black. If the bleeding is in the lower part of the gastrointestinal tract, the blood is bright red.

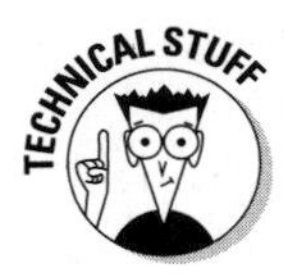

Two medical terms are used to describe blood in stool:

- **Hematochezia:** Passage of fresh blood from the anus, usually with or in the stool. Hematochezia is a common symptom in colitis. In Crohn's disease, it happens only when the colon and/or rectum are involved.
- **Melena:** Passage of dark, tarry stools from the anus. Melena indicates bleeding from the upper gastrointestinal tract such as the stomach and small intestines. Stomach and small intestinal ulcers occur in Crohn's disease and can be the source of this kind of bleeding.

Regardless of which type of bleeding you're experiencing, if the bleeding occurs for a long period of time, it can lead to iron-deficiency anemia due to loss of iron in the blood. Massive bleeding can lead to a decrease in blood volume and shock in some cases. Always contact your doctor if you continue to have bleeding or experience a massive increase in blood in your stool.

Keep in mind that certain foods with natural or artificial coloring may cause stools to be red. For example, Kool-Aid, red gelatin, tomato juice, or large amounts of beets can lead people to think they're bleeding. Similarly, iron supplements, Pepto-Bismol, blood swallowed as a result of a nosebleed, and blood ingested as part of the diet (as with the traditional African Massai diet, which includes a lot of blood drained from cattle) all can cause the stool to be dark and tarry.

Diarrhea

Diarrhea is the frequent passage of watery or semi-formed stools. All people — whether they have Crohn's and colitis or not — get diarrhea from time to time, often from stomach flu. But diarrhea also is a common symptom of Crohn's and colitis.

You may get diarrhea for different reasons:

- Inflammation of the intestines leads to release of different chemicals, enzymes, and hormones from your intestines that, in turn, stimulate the cells of the mucosa to secrete more fluids and mucus.
- Poor absorption of food leads to diarrhea.
- When the terminal ileum is involved, bile acid may not get absorbed and can enter the colon. Bile acid is an irritant, and your colon cells secrete lots of mucus and water to get rid of it. This leads to what your doctor may call *bile acid diarrhea.* This also happens after surgical removal of the terminal ileum.

Abdominal pain

Abdominal pain is a common symptom of Crohn's and colitis. The pain can be anywhere in your abdomen. The terminal ileum and right colon are in the lower-right side of the abdomen and are commonly involved in Crohn's disease. So, the pain in Crohn's disease is usually on the lower-right side. The pain is usually because of inflammation, but narrowing of the *lumen* (inside space of your intestines) if you develop stricture also can cause pain. This type of pain is usually colicky (severe pain due to spasm, distention, or narrowing of the intestines that starts and stops abruptly) in nature.

Colitis also can produce generalized abdominal pain because of the colonic inflammation. Because the most common site for colitis is the rectum and sigmoid, you may feel lower-left abdominal pain in colitis.

Urgency

Urgency is the sudden need to have a bowel movement. In Crohn's and colitis, urgency usually happens secondary to inflammation of the rectum. Diarrhea itself can cause urgency in some patients. Treatment of the underlying inflammation with anti-inflammatory medications leads to relief of the symptom of urgency.

Tenesmus

Tenesmus is a constant sensation of fullness and incomplete relief during bowel movement. You may feel an urgent desire to defecate without being able to produce much feces. Tenesmus can produce abdominal or rectal pain.

Infection and inflammation of the rectum (called *proctitis*) are the major causes of tenesmus. Scientists have found that anxiety can worsen the symptom. Treatment of inflammation with medical therapy controls tenesmus. Sometimes physicians have to use local therapy, such as suppositories or enemas, to control the symptom faster and more effectively.

Other symptoms

Aside from the common signs and symptoms of Crohn's and colitis, some people also experience the following:

- **Excessive gas:** Gas is not life threatening (despite what your family and friends may think). Most gas has no smell and consists of oxygen and a mixture of other gases, such as nitrogen, hydrogen, sulfur, and methane. Some of these gases are produced by bad bacteria residing inside your intestines.
- **Fatigue:** Who *wouldn't* feel tired when suffering from chronic abdominal pain, frequent bouts of diarrhea, and lack of nutrition? It's no big surprise if you complain of fatigue with Crohn's and colitis. But don't ignore this symptom because there could be other causes for your tiredness. Be sure to talk to your doctor about your fatigue.
- **Anemia:** People with Crohn's and colitis may have different types of anemia, such as iron-deficiency anemia and B12-deficiency anemia. Anemia is one of the common causes of fatigue. Your doctor can check for anemia with a simple blood test.
- **Depression:** Crohn's and colitis may make you feel depressed. Recent studies have shown that depression also has a negative impact on Crohn's and colitis. To add insult to injury, people suffering from depression often feel fatigue.

Measuring the severity of your disease

Scientists use different scales to determine how severe your Crohn's and colitis are. Most of these scales are used in research studies. Here are two examples:

- **Truelove and Witts classification of severity of ulcerative colitis:** Under this system of classification, *mild disease* is defined as fewer than four stools per day, no fever, no increased heart rate, and mild anemia; *severe disease* is defined as more than six stools per day (with blood), fever, increased heart rate, and severe anemia; and *moderate disease* is somewhere between mild and severe.
- **Harvey-Bradshaw Index for Crohn's disease:** The Harvey Bradshaw Index uses abdominal pain, the number of stools, abdominal mass, joint pains, and a few other signs and symptoms. Each sign or symptom is assigned a number. If your total score exceeds 4, you have active disease; if you have a score of 16 or more, you have severe disease.

You also may hear or read about the Crohn's Disease Activity Index (CDAI) and the Mayo scoring system for ulcerative colitis. These systems have been used in clinical trials of different medications when scientists have tried to assess the effectiveness of the drugs.

Other Parts of the Body Involved in Crohn's and Colitis

When your gut is sick, your whole body may suffer. Crohn's and colitis aren't just diseases of your intestines; they also can affect your other body systems. In fact, up to 25 percent of Crohn's and colitis patients have other organs involved besides their intestines.

The mutation in the genes or changes in the immune functions that are thought to cause Crohn's and colitis can affect other parts of the body, and some organs are affected by the drugs you take for the treatment (see Chapter 7). In this section, I cover the different parts of the body affected by Crohn's and colitis.

Bones and joints

Bones and joints are the most common parts of the body affected in Crohn's and colitis.

Bones

It is generally estimated that one in seven people suffering from Crohn's and colitis have *osteoporosis* (thin and brittle bones) and nearly half of Crohn's and colitis patients have *osteopenia* (bones on the way to becoming weak). Osteoporosis increases your risk of bone fractures and it is estimated that Crohn's and colitis patients are at a 40 percent higher risk of fractures than the general population. Sophisticated tests (including the DEXA scan) can detect whether you have osteoporosis.

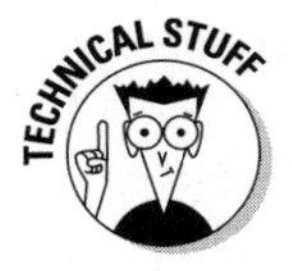

The results of the DEXA scan are given in T scores. When your T score on the DEXA scan is less than –2.5, you have osteoporosis; a score between –2.5 and –1.0 means you have osteopenia.

There are different risk factors for weak bones in Crohn's and colitis:

- **Inflammation:** Inflammation is a hallmark of Crohn's and colitis. Different chemicals released during inflammation (such as TNF-α) can have a direct effect on the bones, making them weak.
- **Steroids:** People with Crohn's and colitis often are treated with steroids, and steroids are notorious for weakening the bones. If you take more than 5 mg of prednisone for more than three months, your bones will start becoming thin and brittle.

- **Low calcium and vitamin D:** People with Crohn's and colitis aren't able to absorb calcium and vitamin D very well through the inflamed intestines. In addition, eating a diet that doesn't have enough calcium and vitamin D, as well as not getting enough exposure to sunlight, lead to low levels of calcium and vitamin D. Calcium and vitamin D are very important for bone health. Their deficiency causes osteoporosis.
- **Smoking:** Smoking has a direct negative effect on bone health. It's also known to cause flares of Crohn's disease and increase inflammation, thus indirectly affecting bones.

In Chapter 10, I explain how you can prevent and treat bone problems in Crohn's and colitis.

Joints

Approximately one in five Crohn's and colitis patients suffer from joint pain (with or without signs of active Crohn's or colitis). Crohn's patients have a greater chance of getting arthritis than colitis patients do. Joint pain caused by inflammation (known as *arthritis*) can occur with the flare of your intestinal inflammation (or even without intestinal inflammation). Knees, ankles, shoulders, and wrists are the most common joints involved, but any other joint can be affected. The joints become painful and swell to different degrees. They also become stiff and warm to the touch.

Aching or pain in your joints can occur even without inflammation; this condition is known as *arthralgia.* Arthralgia is different from arthritis. A person with arthritis also has arthralgia, but many patients with arthralgia don't have arthritis.

There are two types of arthritis in Crohn's and colitis:

- **Peripheral arthritis:** Affects the joints of the arms and legs. The discomfort may be *migratory,* moving from one joint to another. This type of arthritis is more common with inflammation of the colon. Fortunately, peripheral arthritis doesn't cause joint damage or deformity.

  There are two main types of peripheral arthritis in Crohn's and colitis:

  - Type 1 (also called pauciarticular arthropathy): This type affects four or fewer joints. Large joints, such as the knees and ankles, are the main ones involved.
  - Type 2 (also called polyarticular arthropathy): This type affects five or more joints. Small joints, such as the fingers and wrists, are the main ones involved.
- **Axial arthritis (also known as spondylitis or spondyloarthropathy):** Affects the joints of the backbone and hips. If the backbones fuse together, this condition can cause permanent damage. Because your ribs are attached to your backbone, the condition can restrict your breathing in advanced cases.

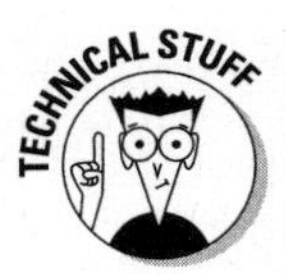

A rare but severe form of axial arthritis, known as *ankylosing spondylitis,* causes inflammation of the spinal joints and produces pain and stiffness in your lower back. It occurs more commonly in Crohn's disease than colitis. Men are affected more than women, and it typically strikes people under the age of 30. There may be a genetic component to ankylosing spondylitis. In this type of arthritis, your vertebrae slowly begin to fuse together, causing fusion of the spine and deformity of your backbone. It also may produce inflammation of the eyes, lungs, and heart valves. Your doctor may send you to a rheumatologist for further assessment. Regular exercise helps to keep the joints happy and improves stiffness.

Steroids can shut down the blood supply to bones. Without blood, the bone tissue dies and the bone collapses. This condition usually occurs in the bones of large joints such as the shoulder, hip, and knee. If this happens, your joint stops working and you suffer from extremely severe pain; if it happens in your hip joint, you can't walk. In the medical terminology, this is called *aseptic necrosis* or *avascular necrosis of a joint.* Treatment is usually pain medications and physical therapy; in some cases, replacement with an artificial joint may be needed.

If you're experiencing joint pain, your doctor will examine the joint to check for swelling and deformities and order X-rays to rule out osteoporosis or breaks in the bones. Your doctor may suggest some topical creams and gels you can apply to the skin, warm compresses, or heating pads to relieve the pain. If the pain persists, your doctor may send you to a rheumatologist and physical therapist.

Non-steroidal anti-inflammatory drugs (NSAIDs), such as ibuprofen (Advil) and naproxen (Aleve), are generally *not* considered safe in Crohn's and colitis; some studies show that these drugs may cause flares of the disease. Talk to your doctor before taking these medications.

Skin

The skin is commonly affected in Crohn's and colitis because of an inflammation process affecting the skin or because of deficiencies of important nutrients.

Two common skin problems affect Crohn's and colitis patients:

- **Erythema nodosum:** This skin condition results in small, round, painful, red nodules on the skin. They're most commonly seen on the shins and ankles. The nodules appear with increased inflammation of the intestines and disappear with treatment of the disease. Women are affected more than men.

- **Pyoderma gangrenosum:** This skin condition occurs more commonly in patients with colitis. It starts as a small blister (which may look like a bug bite) and then slowly progresses to a large, painful ulcer. Treatment of this skin condition can be difficult. You may have to apply topical cream to treat the ulcer; in some cases, oral immunosuppression medications such as steroids or anti-TNF drugs may be required. When the ulcer heals, it usually leaves a scar.

See Chapter 10 for more information on skin conditions affecting people with Crohn's and colitis.

Liver and gallbladder

The liver is an important organ. It functions like a refinery in your body, taking up all the digested food, medicines, and other chemicals you absorb from the intestines. Further processing and packaging occurs in your liver, and then the materials are sent to different parts of your body via blood. The liver also filters out harmful and toxic substances from the blood.

The liver produces *bile,* which is a digestive juice that helps in the digestion of fat. After bile is produced in the liver, it's stored in the gallbladder, which is located just underneath your liver. Bile is transported to the gallbladder and then to the intestines via bile ducts.

Your liver, gallbladder, and bile ducts can be affected in Crohn's and colitis. In the following sections, I cover some of the related conditions that can occur.

Hepatitis

Hepatitis (inflammation of the liver cells) can occur as a result of the autoimmune process or viral infections. Hepatitis A, B, and C are common viral forms of hepatitis. Taking medications that suppress your immune system increases your risk of viral infections, so your doctor will check for viral hepatitis before putting you on these therapies (specifically biologic therapies, such as anti-TNF therapy).

Checking for hepatitis B before starting biologic therapy is extremely important. If you have undiagnosed hepatitis B and biologic therapy activates the virus, it can lead to acute liver failure and even death.

Autoimmune hepatitis is not very common. In Crohn's and colitis, your immune system attacks your intestines; similarly, in autoimmune hepatitis, your immune system attacks your liver cells.

Gallstones

The bile from the gallbladder is secreted into the intestines via bile ducts to help with fat digestion and absorption. After the bile has done its job, it's reabsorbed from the last part of the ileum back into the liver and then back to the gallbladder.

If your ileum is inflamed, as it is in Crohn's disease, bile absorption suffers and there will be less bile in the gallbladder. Salts and cholesterol in the gallbladder begin to crystallize and turn into stones. About one-quarter of Crohn's patients develop gallstones. These stones can get stuck in the gallbladder or the bile duct, producing severe abdominal pain. The pain is usually on the upper-right side of the abdomen and colicky in nature — in other words, there is severe pain due to spasm, distention, or narrowing of the intestines that starts and stops abruptly. Fatty food worsens the pain.

If you're experiencing these symptoms, your doctor may order an ultrasound of the gallbladder to look for gallstones. If you have gallstones, surgery is usually the next step.

Primary sclerosing cholangitis

Primary sclerosing cholangitis (PSC) is inflammation of the bile ducts inside the liver, as well as outside the liver. It causes narrowing and blockage of the ducts. After a long period of time, PSC causes scarring of the liver called *cirrhosis.* PSC happens more with colitis than with Crohn's disease. It doesn't produce any symptoms in the beginning; instead, it's usually detected by blood tests that show abnormalities in liver enzymes. Later on, when the scarring in the liver blocks the pathway for bile and waste matter, the bile backs up in the liver, causing *jaundice* (yellow skin), weight loss, nausea, and itching.

Your doctor may suggest an MRI of the liver or injecting dye into the bile ducts via an endoscope to see the narrowing. She may even order a liver biopsy to rule out cirrhosis.

Occasionally, PSC may lead to liver cancer or cancer of the bile ducts, called *cholangiocarcinoma.*

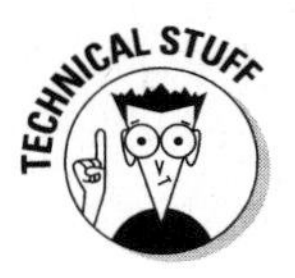

If you've been diagnosed with PSC, there is about a 70 percent chance you may have colitis. You're also at an increased risk for colon cancer. Your doctor will suggest regular colonoscopies to screen for colon cancer.

Doctors can't predict who will get PSC, and effective treatment doesn't exist. Some doctors use a medicine called ursodiol (Actigall, Urso) to control inflammation in the liver and bile ducts. If the disease advances to cirrhosis, you doctor may send you to a liver transplant specialist for further examination and management.

Kidneys and bladder

Your intestines are in very close proximity to the kidneys and bladder, and the inflammation in your intestines can sometimes spill over to these organs.

You can develop inflammation of the bladder, as well as an abnormal connection between the intestines and bladder called *fistula.* The feces can then travel to your bladder through the fistula instead of just coming out of the anus. This can cause you to pass foul-smelling, frothy urine. Some patients also notice passing gas while they urinate or even seeing vegetable matter in their urine. This can also be the cause of frequent urinary tract infections in people with Crohn's disease.

People with Crohn's or colitis also are at risk for kidney stones. Oxalate and uric acid stones are common types of kidney stones in Crohn's and colitis. Too much oxalates can cause oxalate stones in the kidney. In healthy intestines, calcium binds the extra oxalates in the intestines to prevent its absorption. In Crohn's disease, fat isn't absorbed from the intestines correctly, and the body uses calcium to bind the unabsorbed fat. This allows more oxalates to be absorbed because calcium is busy doing another job. Deficiency of calcium also produces a similar condition.

Your doctor may ask you to increase calcium in your diet and cut down on oxalate-containing foods (such as spinach, sweet potatoes, peanuts, and beans) to prevent oxalate stones.

Eyes

Although it's not very common, the eyes can become inflamed in Crohn's and colitis. Like the intestines, the eyeball is covered with different protective layers; inflammation can happen in any of these layers. The common eye conditions are

- **Episclertis and scleritis:** Inflammation of the outermost layer of the eyes. It can cause redness in the eyes, eye pain, and excessive tears.
- **Uveitis:** Inflammation of the entire middle layer of the eye. It usually causes headaches, deep eye pain, and sensitivity to bright light. If untreated, it can lead to blindness.

Certain drugs also can cause eye problems. For example when you take steroids for a long period, you can get infections such as conjunctivitis (commonly known as pinkeye) and even cataracts.

Complications of Crohn's and Colitis

Persistent inflammation of the intestines brings different complications. Some of these complications are directly related to inflammation and happen in the intestines. Other complications are indirect, such as a nutritional deficiencies and effects on other organs that you may suffer because of disturbances in the process of digestion and absorption.

Intestinal complications

If the inflammation in your intestines persists, you may suffer from a variety of intestinal complications. I cover these complications in this section.

Toxic megacolon

Toxic megacolon is severe inflammation of the colon leading to dilation of the colon and making the patient acutely ill with high fever, abdominal distension, and severe pain. It happens in about 5 percent of patients suffering from severe colitis.

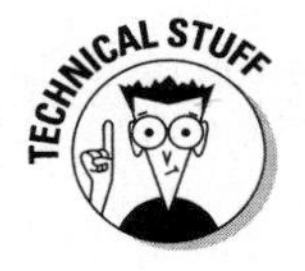

A human colon is divided into different parts, including the sigmoid colon, descending colon, transverse colon, ascending colon, and cecum. A normal cecum is usually less than 9 centimeters in diameter. In toxic megacolon, the diameter of the cecum becomes greater than 12 centimeters.

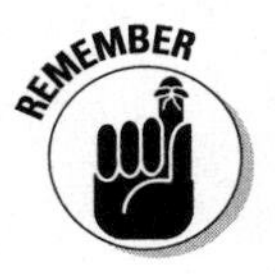

Toxic megacolon can happen spontaneously in patients with Crohn's disease of the colon and ulcerative colitis — in other words, it can happen without any specific cause. However, pain medications such as narcotic drugs and antidiarrheal drugs can slow down the intestine and lead to accumulation of toxic materials. This increases the risk of developing toxic megacolon. For this reason, Crohn's and colitis patients shouldn't take narcotics and over-the-counter antidiarrheal medications without getting the green light from their doctors.

Although rare, toxic megacolon is a dreaded complication. The diagnosis is usually made with X-rays in which the radiologist finds an abnormally dilated colon. If your doctor suspects that you have toxic megacolon, you'll be admitted to the intensive care unit (ICU) with resuscitation with intravenous fluids, antibiotics, and very close monitoring. A surgeon will be involved. Doctors will keep a very close eye on you, and if there is no improvement within 24 to 48 hours, you may require surgery. If untreated, toxic megacolon leads to perforation of the intestinal wall, sepsis, and death.

Strictures

When you get a cut on your skin, the swelling and redness that occur are the process of inflammation. After the healing occurs, you may have a scar. Similarly, when inflammation of your intestines is present for a long time, it can cause scarring. Scar tissue isn't as flexible as healthy tissue, so the scar can narrow the lumen of your intestine. This narrowed lumen is called a *stricture.* Strictures can be mild or severe, depending on how much they block the intestine.

Crohn's disease is characterized by inflammation that involves the deeper layers of your intestines, so strictures are much more common in Crohn's disease than they are in colitis.

If a stricture is very narrow it can cause blockage of food, which results in abdominal pain, cramps, and distention. Intestinal strictures of the small intestine usually are diagnosed with a small bowel follow-through (SBFT) X-ray or CT scan.

The bowel must increase the strength of its contractions to push the intestinal contents through the stricture. So, the contracting segment of the intestine *above* the stricture may experience an increased pressure. This pressure sometimes weakens the bowel wall in that area, causing the intestines to become abnormally wide. If the pressure becomes too high, the bowel wall may rupture. This perforation can result in *peritonitis* (severe infection of the abdominal cavity), *abscesses* (collections of infection and pus), and *fistulas* (tubular passageways originating from the bowel wall and connecting to other organs or the skin). Strictures of the small bowel also can lead to bacterial overgrowth, which is another intestinal complication of Crohn's and colitis.

Long-standing inflammation in ulcerative colitis increases your risk of colon cancer that sometimes can present as stricture of the colon.

Fistulas

The gastrointestinal tract starts from the mouth and ends at the anus. It's like a hollow tube covered with multiple layers of tissue. These tissue layers, which are wrapped around each other like layers of onion, get inflamed in IBD. The persistent inflammation can create a hole in the intestine, and the tissue layers can get connected to the other part of the intestines or to the skin through this hole, leading to a formation of an abnormal tunnel. This causes food to bypass parts of the intestine or waste matter to come out to the skin near the anus. This abnormal connection is a *fistula.*

Fistulas are common in Crohn's disease. Approximately one-quarter of people with Crohn's disease develop fistulas. Fistulas can be diagnosed during endoscopy and/or radiology tests, such as SBFT X-ray or CT scan. Immunosuppressive therapy such as anti-TNF drugs are frequently used to treat fistulas. If medical therapy fails to close the fistula, surgery is often required. Sometimes, a combination of both medical and surgical therapy is needed to treat a fistula.

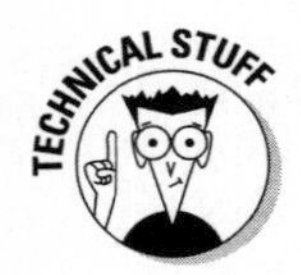

There are different types of fistulas, depending on the connection between the two body cavities. Here are some common fistulas in patients suffering from IBD:

- **Enterocutaneous fistula:** This type of fistula connects the intestines to the skin.
- **Perianal fistula:** This type of fistula connects the rectum to the perianal skin (the skin around the anal opening).

- **Enteroenteric fistula:** This type of fistula abnormally connects the two intestines together.
- **Enterovesical fistula:** This type of fistula goes from the intestines to the bladder. It may result in frequent urinary tract infections or the passage of gas when you urinate.

These four types of fistulas are illustrated in Figure 2-4. There are other types of fistulas as well, including the *rectovaginal fistula* (connecting the rectum to the vagina, leading to passage of feces through the vagina).

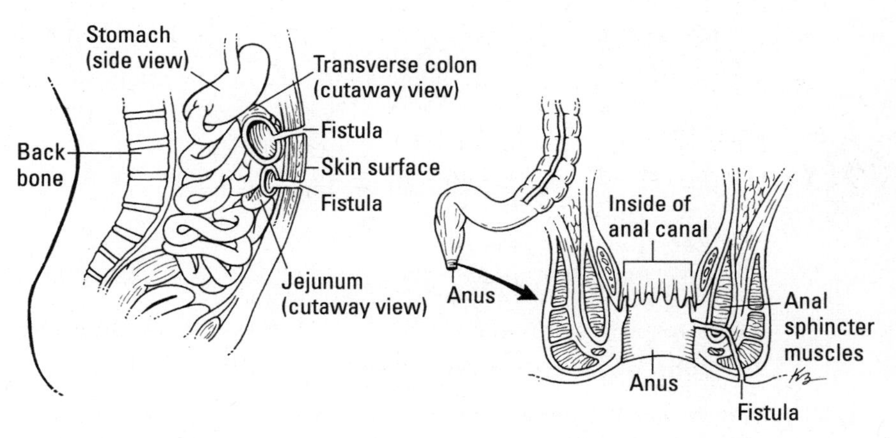

Enterocutaneous fistula

Perianal fistula

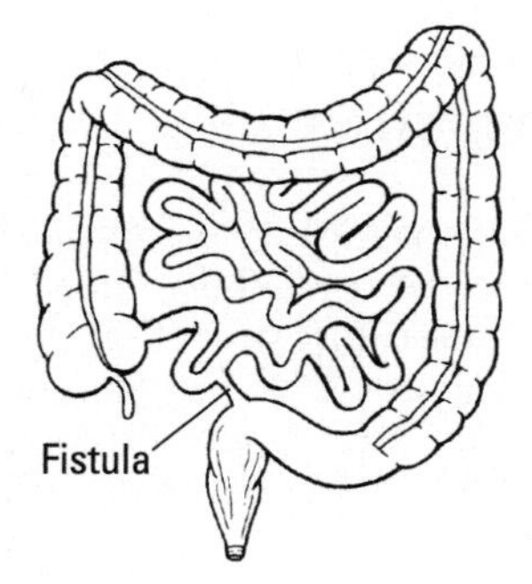

Enteroenteric fistula

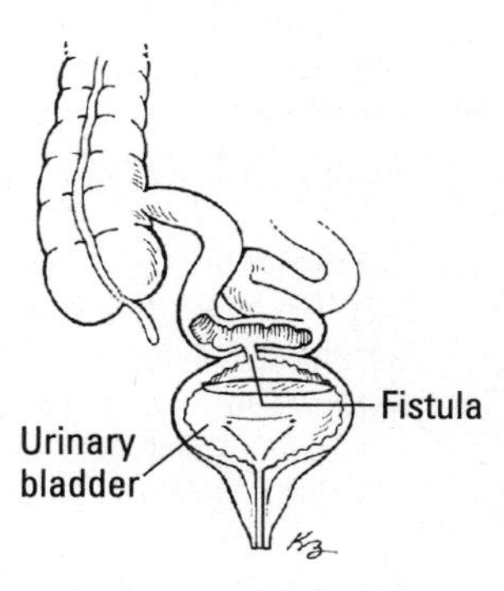

Enterovesical fistula

Illustration by Kathryn Born

Figure 2-4: Different types of intestinal fistulas in IBD.

Anal fissures

An *anal fissure* is a small tear in the lining of the anus. Fissures occur when the lining of the anal canal is stretched to its limit. General causes of fissures include large, hard stools; prolonged diarrhea; childbirth; and anal sex. In people with Crohn's and colitis, the inflammation of the anal canal and persistent diarrhea are usually the cause of anal fissures.

Anal fissures cause painful bowel movements and rectal bleeding. They may produce severe pain that feels like passing razor blades or cut glass. These symptoms can last for a few minutes to hours.

Increasing your fluid intake and taking a sitz bath are very helpful. If symptoms don't improve with these measures, your doctor may use medical therapy such as a nitroglycerin suppository or calcium channel blocker. These drugs relax the internal anal sphincter and help with the symptoms and healing of the fissure.

To prevent anal fissures, follow these recommendations:

- Keep the anal area dry.
- Avoid straining during bowel movements.
- Wipe with soft materials or a moistened cloth or cotton pad.
- Drink plenty of fluids to prevent constipation.
- Promptly treat any constipation or diarrhea.
- Exercise regularly to promote regular bowel movements.
- Avoid anal sex — it can cause irritation or trauma.

Nutritional complications

Your body needs energy to build and strengthen your muscles, bones, and other organs. You also need energy to perform daily chores and to stay active and free from illnesses. Your gastrointestinal (GI) tract is the gateway to this energy. After the food is broken down into small pieces in your stomach and intestines, important nutrients such as carbohydrates, proteins, fats, and vitamins are released and absorbed through the intestines. These nutrients produce calories and generate energy. If your intestines aren't working properly, your body will be deprived of these important nutrients and complications will develop as a result of nutritional deficiencies.

In this section, I cover some of the nutritional complications that can occur as a result of Crohn's and colitis.

Malnutrition

Malnutrition is an imbalance of nutritional supply and demand. This imbalance affects the functions of your organs. IBD is a double-edged sword: You can't absorb nutrients because of inflamed intestines (a decrease in supply). But the different chemicals and hormones released during inflammation increase your body's energy expenditure (an increase in demand). This puts your body at high risk for malnutrition. Malnutrition is extremely important in children because it can jeopardize their growth and development.

Malnutrition affects almost every organ of your body except the brain, which is usually spared. These effects can be reversed by providing appropriate nutrition. Here are some of the important organ functions that are affected by malnutrition:

- **Heart:** Your heart is a muscle, so it's affected by malnutrition just as your other muscles are. In malnutrition, the heart becomes weak and doesn't pump out blood with good force, which leads to a slow heart rate and low blood pressure.
- **Lungs:** In malnutrition, the muscles of your diaphragm can become weak. As a result, you can have trouble breathing and getting enough oxygen in your blood.
- **Skin and wound healing:** Malnutrition causes the skin to become dry and wrinkled. In addition, wounds don't heal as well in a malnourished person. When you're well nourished, you have more collagen at the site of your surgery wound, which helps with good healing, so your doctors will pay extra attention to your nutrition prior to surgery.
- **Hair:** If you're malnourished, your hair can become thin and sparse and be easily pulled out (for example, when you brush your hair).
- **Bone marrow:** Your bone marrow is a factory for blood cells. Red blood cells carry oxygen to different parts of the body, and white blood cells play an important role in fighting infections. White blood cells are also important in Crohn's and colitis, keeping bacteria away from inflammation sites. In severe malnutrition, your bone-marrow factory slows down and you get *leukopenia* (deficiency of white blood cells) and *anemia* (deficiency of red blood cells).
- **Immune system:** Your immune system is vulnerable to malnutrition. In people with Crohn's and colitis, the immune system is already malfunctioning and under stress because of inflammation. Malnutrition is another hit to the immune system. The important cells of the immune system, such as white blood cells, become weak, which in turn leads to more infections and more malnutrition.

You can assess your nutrition in several ways:

- If you're losing weight without trying, that can be a sign of malnutrition.
- *Body mass index* (BMI), a measure of body fat based on height and weight, is another way to check your nourishment status. A BMI lower than 18.5 is considered malnourished; a BMI lower than 16 is considered severely malnourished. You can check your BMI at `www.nhlbisupport.com/bmi`.
- Your doctor may check certain protein levels in your body, such as your albumin level, with a blood test to check your nutritional status. A low albumin level indicates lower nutritional status.

Vitamin and mineral deficiency

Vitamins and minerals play an important role in the functions of the different organs. Crohn's and colitis patients are particularly vulnerable to vitamin and mineral deficiencies. Here are the vitamins and minerals that are most likely to be deficient in people with Crohn's and colitis:

- **Vitamin B12:** Vitamin B12 is absorbed in the *terminal ileum* (the last part of the small intestine before it joins the large intestine). When the terminal ileum is inflamed (as it is in Crohn's disease), vitamin B12 absorption is reduced, putting you at risk for the deficiency of this vitamin. The deficiency of this vitamin can result in anemia and affect the growth of nerves, which can cause numbness and tingling in your hands and feet.
- **Vitamin A:** Vitamin A, which is absorbed in the small intestine, is a fat-soluble vitamin, which means it requires fat for absorption. If you have Crohn's disease involving the ileum or you've had the ileum removed, you may become deficient in bile, a necessary chemical for fat absorption. Fat malabsorption then leads to deficiency of fat-soluble vitamins such as vitamin A. Not getting enough vitamin A in the diet and inflammation of the small intestine are other causes of vitamin A deficiency. Vitamin A is important for vision and skin, and its deficiency leads to night blindness and dry skin.
- **Vitamin D:** Vitamin D is absorbed in the small intestine. You also make vitamin D in your skin through sunlight. Vitamin A is another fat-soluble vitamin. Fat malabsorption, not getting enough vitamin D in the diet, inflammation of the small intestines, and poor sunlight exposure can put you at risk of vitamin D deficiency. Vitamin D is critical to bone health and immune system function. The deficiency of vitamin D causes weakening of the bones, putting them at risk for fractures.
- **Vitamin E:** Vitamin E is absorbed in the small intestine. It's also a fat-soluble vitamin, so fat malabsorption and inflammation of the small intestine can cause a deficiency. Vitamin E is a powerful antioxidant and is also important to muscle and nerve function. Its deficiency can lead to neurological problems and muscle weakness.
- **Vitamin K:** Vitamin K is absorbed — you guessed it! — in the small intestine. It's another fat-soluble vitamin. Inflammation of the small intestine

and fat malabsorption are the usual causes of vitamin K deficiency in people with Crohn's disease. Vitamin K is important for proper blood clotting, as well as for bone health. A vitamin K deficiency leads to bleeding (such as gum bleeding, heavy menstrual bleeding, and easy bruising) and weakening of bones.

- **Iron:** There are two types of important cells in the blood: white blood cells and red blood cells. White blood cells fight infection, and red blood cells carry oxygen. Red blood cells do their work with the help of iron, which holds the oxygen tightly until it's time to deliver it to the organs.

  There are three ways you can have iron deficiency.

  - Low iron intake: You may not be getting enough iron in your diet. This isn't common, but it can happen if you don't eat red meat (which is rich in iron).
  - Decreased iron absorption: Even if you're getting enough iron, you may not be able to absorb it. Iron is mostly absorbed in the small intestine, particularly in the duodenum. Inflammation of the duodenum (which happens in Crohn's disease) leads to decreased iron absorption and can cause iron deficiency.
  - Increased iron loss: Even if you're getting enough iron and absorbing it well, you can have iron deficiency if you lose more iron than you take in. In Crohn's and colitis, inflammation of the intestines produces ulcers and bleeding. You may lose a significant amount of blood and the iron stored in it.

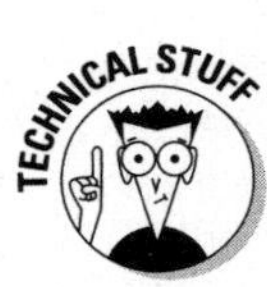

    You can lose up to 1 1⁄2 ounces of blood per day in your stools without seeing anything. Losing small amounts of blood on a daily basis leads to iron deficiency.

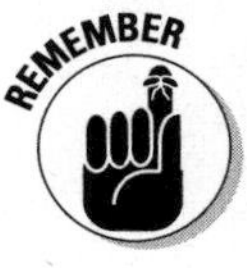

  Iron deficiency produces symptoms of extreme fatigue, pale skin, weakness, shortness of breath, brittle nails, and poor appetite. It can also cause cravings for ice and dirt, as well as an uncomfortable tingling and crawling feeling in your legs called *restless leg syndrome.* Be sure to tell your doctor if you develop these symptoms so that you can be checked for iron deficiency.

- **Zinc:** Zinc is needed for proper immune system functioning, for the senses of smell and taste, and for wound healing. During pregnancy and childhood, the body needs zinc to grow and develop properly. You can lose zinc with diarrhea, so Crohn's and colitis patients are at increased risk of being zinc deficient. Symptoms of zinc deficiency include slow wound healing, weakness, white flecks in the fingernails, and impaired senses of taste and smell. Zinc deficiency also can cause a skin problem known as *acrodermatitis enteropathica,* which causes inflammation of the skin on the elbows, knees, mouth, and *perineum* (the area between the genitals and anus).

  If your doctor suspects zinc deficiency, she may suggest that you eat high-protein foods, which contain a lot of zinc. Beef, pork, and lamb are rich in zinc.

The cancer connection

People with Crohn's and colitis have an increased risk of various cancers. If you have inflammation in your body for a long time, that can put you at an increased risk for developing cancer in the inflamed area. Immunosuppression medications used in the treatment of Crohn's and colitis also increase the risk of cancer by suppressing your immune system. I review the cancers that are more common in Crohn's and colitis patients in the following sections. Turn to Chapter 10 for more on cancer screening.

Although it's important to be aware of the increased risk of cancer if you have Crohn's or colitis, don't stress out about it. Cancer still isn't common, even if you have Crohn's and colitis. In Crohn's and colitis patients, there is only about a 7 percent chance of developing colon cancer even after 30 years. In people taking immunosuppressive medications (such as azathioprine and anti-TNF drugs), the risk of lymphoma is about 0.04 percent to 0.06 percent (in order words, 4 to 6 people per 10,000), as compared to 0.02 percent in the general population (2 per 10,000).

Colon cancer

The colon is the last part of your GI tract. The main function of the colon is to absorb water and salts and give the waste matter its final shape and form (see Chapter 3 for more on the function of the colon). The inside of the colon is lined by a layer of cells called *mucosa.* The cells present in the mucosa are under a lot of stress because of the persistent inflammation. Sometimes these cells start growing abnormally and develop into precancerous and cancerous cells. Persistent inflammation, gene mutation, and defects in the immune system promote this abnormal growth and cancer development.

If you have inflammation of the colon lasting eight to ten years, you're at risk for colon cancer. Your doctor is aware of the risk of colon cancer in people who've had Crohn's and colitis long term, so you'll undergo regular colonoscopies to watch for cancerous or precancerous lesions.

Cervical cancer

Human papillomavirus (HPV) is a type of virus that has been linked to cervical cancer. Certain medications, such as the immunosuppressive drugs given to people with Crohn's and colitis, may increase the risk of cervical cancer. One possibility is that these drugs weaken the immune system and let HPV run free.

Women with Crohn's and colitis should have regular Pap smears (which test for cervical cancer), especially when they're on immunosuppressive medications.

Lymphoma

People with Crohn's and colitis are at an increased risk for *lymphoma* (cancer of the lymphatic system) after taking certain immunosuppressive medications (like azathioprine or anti-TNF drugs such as infliximab). The risk increases further if you take more than one immunosuppressive drug and for a longer period of time. There is some controversy about whether Crohn's disease or colitis itself increases the risk of lymphoma.

The risk of lymphoma is highest in male patients under the age of 35 who are getting azathioprine and anti-TNF therapy. However, sometimes the benefits of the medical therapy outweigh the risks. Be sure to discuss this risk with your doctor.

Skin cancer

Crohn's and colitis patients are at increased risk of skin cancers. The same immunosuppressive drugs that increase the risk of lymphoma also increase the risk of skin cancer. There are different types of skin cancers; melanoma is the most dangerous and aggressive one, but immunosuppressive drugs don't cause melanoma (although some newer data does suggest that they may increase the risk). Other types of skin cancers are basal cell and squamous cell cancers. Immunosuppressive medication such as azathioprine increase the risk of non-melanoma skin cancers by making your skin sensitive to UV light from the sun. If caught early, your dermatologist can treat skin cancer with minor surgery to remove the cancer tissue or burning the tissue with liquid nitrogen spray.

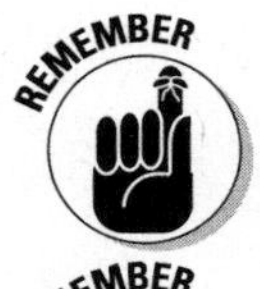

Patients taking thiopurine drugs, such as azathioprine (Imuran) or 6-MP, have three times the risk of developing skin cancer compared to patients not taking these drugs.

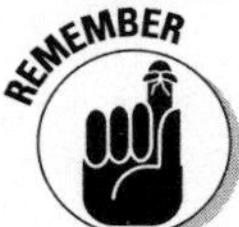

To prevent skin cancer, follow these suggestions:

- Seek shade during midday hours (11 a.m. to 4 p.m.), when the sun's UV rays are the strongest.
- Wear clothing to protect exposed skin.
- Use sunscreen with a sun protective factor (SPF) of 15 or higher. It should have both UVA and UVB protection. Apply the sunscreen 15 to 30 minutes before going outside.
- Examine your moles and freckles every month to check for any changes. See a dermatologist if you notice any of the following:
    - A mole or discoloration that appears suddenly or begins to change
    - A sore that isn't healing
    - An area of skin that is red and bumpy

Chapter 3

How the Digestive System Works

In This Chapter

- Following the path of your digestive tract
- Knowing the functions of different parts of the digestive tract
- Getting familiar with the liver, pancreas, and gallbladder
- Understanding the effects of inflammation on your digestive system

The food you eat contains important nutrients that provide energy and nourishment to your body. These nutrients in your food are contained in large molecules that are chemically glued together. *Digestion* is the mechanical and chemical process in which these molecules are broken down into smaller pieces. This process occurs in the 20- to 30-foot-long structure called the *gastrointestinal tract* (also known as the *alimentary canal*). This pipelike structure extends all the way from your mouth to your anus. Special enzymes and chemicals are secreted inside the digestive tract to help the process of digestion.

The process of *absorption* occurs after the food is digested and broken down into basic nutrients like carbohydrates, proteins, and fats. These nutrients then enter your bloodstream after being transported across the intestinal wall and circulate to different tissues to provide energy and support growth and function. Any unabsorbed food and waste matter are handled by the process of *excretion* and expelled out in the form of stool.

In this chapter, I lead you through the gastrointestinal (GI) tract because, in Crohn's and colitis, this is where the trouble lies. Knowing how your GI tract should work gives you some insight into what's going on when it doesn't work exactly as it should. I also introduce you to the liver, pancreas, and gallbladder, which play important roles in your digestive system. Finally, I explain how inflammation mucks things up and spell out the different kinds of inflammation.

Tracking the Journey of Food inside the Gastrointestinal Tract

The GI tract (shown in Figure 3-1) consists of the oral cavity (the mouth), the esophagus, the stomach, the small intestine, the large intestine, and the anus. Each of these parts plays an important role in breaking down the food you eat and transporting it across the intestinal wall so that your body gets the nutrients it needs.

The oral cavity (or mouth)

The starting point of the GI tract is the *oral cavity* (more commonly known as the mouth). The inside of the mouth is lined by a pink and moist layer called the *mucosa.* The tongue and 32 teeth also reside in the mouth; the teeth break down food by the process of chewing and the tongue rolls the food down into a long pipe called the *esophagus.*

Saliva is a clear, watery solution that the salivary glands produce constantly in your mouth. The average person produces 2 to 4 pints of saliva every day. Saliva moistens food and makes it easier for you to swallow. Enzymes present in saliva help in the digestion of carbohydrates. Saliva also cleans the inside of your mouth and teeth, helping to prevent infections. *Amylase enzymes* are then secreted in the saliva to digest carbohydrates.

Chewing is an important process. Nutrition experts advise to chew your food properly (20 to 30 chews per bite). If you chew properly, you can accomplish almost one-third of digestion in your mouth. You'll also enjoy the taste of the food better and longer. The downside to *not* chewing your food properly is that the stomach has to work overtime to break down food that falls into the stomach in lumps. And if your stomach is inflamed, as it is in Crohn's disease, valuable nutrients locked inside the food may not be available to be absorbed into the bloodstream.

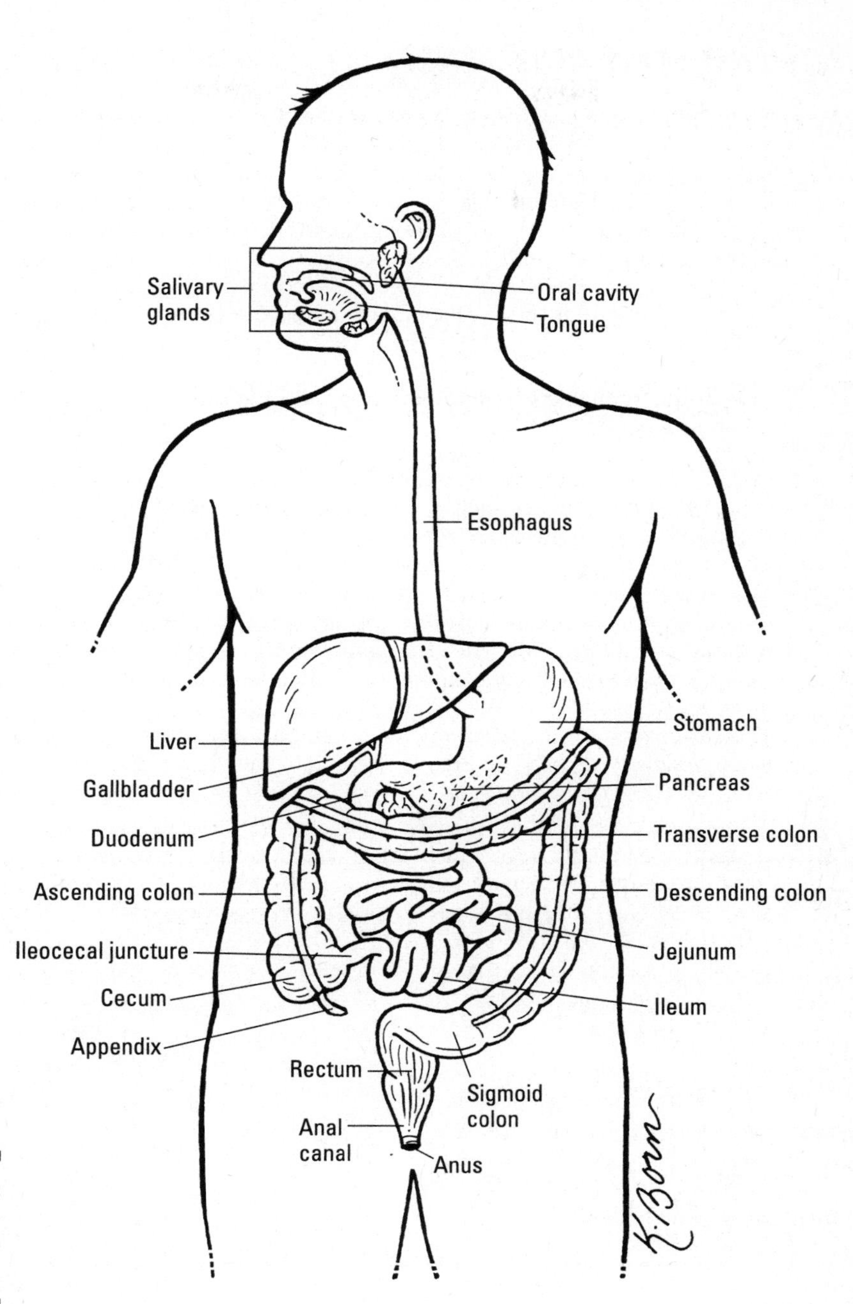

Figure 3-1: The anatomy of the GI tract.

Illustration by Kathryn Born

The stomach

The *stomach* is a large, sacklike organ that functions like a grinding machine. The stomach is wrapped in five layers. The innermost layer is called the *mucosa.* The next layer is called the *submucosa.* The submucosa is surrounded by three muscle layers that help move and mix the stomach contents. The outermost layer of the stomach is called the *serosa.* The mucosa of the stomach has cells that secrete stomach acid and certain enzymes to digest the food. The stomach mixes the food with the acid and other enzymes to break the food into smaller particles and then propels the food into the small intestine.

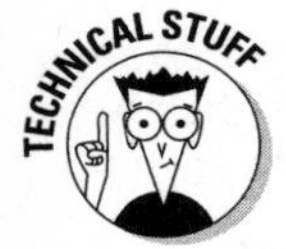

The stomach normally expands to hold about a liter of food, but it can hold as much as a gallon!

Because of its acidic environment, the stomach also acts as a decontamination chamber for bacteria and other toxic substances that may have gained entry along with your food.

You may be wondering how the stomach is protected from its own acid. The mucosa of the stomach secretes a thin layer of bicarbonate that coats the internal lining to protect the stomach from the acid. If there's a breakdown in this protective layer, a stomach ulcer may form.

The processed food, called *chyme,* resembles an oatmeal-like paste. Chyme slowly passes through a narrow opening in the stomach called the *pylorus* and into the small intestine.

How fast are foods digested?

Different foods are digested at different rates in the stomach. Here are some examples:

- **Liquids:** A few minutes
- **Fruits and vegetables:** 30 to 45 minutes
- **Whole grains:** One and a half to two hours
- **Dairy products:** One and a half to three hours
- **Meat:** Three to four hours

Tea and coffee speed up the digestive process and can push foods out of the stomach before they're completely broken down. They can also irritate the lining of the esophagus (causing heartburn) or stimulate the intestines (causing diarrhea).

The small intestine

When the stomach has finished its work, it pushes the partially digested food into the first part of small intestine, called the *duodenum.* The lining of the duodenum has special cells that squirt a lot of mucus onto the wall of the intestine to protect it from stomach acid. The enzymes from the liver, pancreas, and gallbladder enter the duodenum through small ducts and mix with the food. These enzymes help break down the food even more.

Iron in food is most efficiently absorbed in your duodenum. People with inflammatory bowel disease (IBD) can develop iron-deficiency anemia because they lose blood (and red blood cells are big stores of iron in the body). People with IBD also can become iron deficient if they can't absorb iron — for example, because of *duodenitis* (inflammation of the duodenum). This condition can happen in Crohn's disease.

After food leaves the duodenum, it travels to the second part of the small intestine, called the *jejunum.* Most of the absorption of food occurs in the jejunum. Carbohydrates, proteins, and fats are broken down to simple sugars, amino acids, and fatty acids. At this point, they're small enough to be absorbed or transported through the lining of the small intestine to enter the cells and the bloodstream. The blood takes these elements to different parts of the body to provide fuel so they can perform their respective jobs.

The process of absorption continues in the third part of the small intestine, called the *ileum.* Vitamin B12, which plays a key role in normal brain functioning and in the formation of blood, is absorbed in the ileum. Bile salts, which enter the intestine via the bile duct in the duodenum (helping in the process of fat digestion and absorption), are also absorbed in the ileum and travel back to the liver to be excreted again through the bile duct. In addition to the majority of the other nutrients, around 8 to 10 liters of fluid are also absorbed in the small intestine every day.

The large intestine

Undigested and unabsorbed waste material enters the large intestine via the *ileocecal valve,* which is located at the junction of the small and large intestines. The ileocecal valve is one of the most common sites for Crohn's disease to occur.

The colon is divided into the following segments: cecum, hepatic flexure, ascending colon, transverse colon, splenic flexure, descending colon, sigmoid colon, and rectum. The absorption of extra water and salts occurs in the colon, and waste material takes the form of feces.

Billions of bacteria reside in the colon. They perform the process of fermentation on food material, especially fiber. The products of fermentation (such as acetate and butyrate) serve as a fuel to colon cells to keep them healthy. The friendly bacteria that are involved in the fermentation process are called *probiotics* (see Chapter 9). Along with providing beneficial fermentation products, probiotics keep bad bacteria from colonizing in your colon.

Feces are stored in the rectum until you're ready to go the bathroom.

The anus

The journey comes to an end when feces are excreted out through the anus. The anus is surrounded by two different types of muscles that form rings around it — the internal and external anal sphincter muscles. These muscles relax during the act of defecation.

Getting Help from the Liver, Pancreas, and Gallbladder

The liver, pancreas, and gallbladder are important organs of the GI tract, even though the bulk of the food you eat doesn't actually pass through them. These three organs play key roles in helping the process of digestion and absorption.

Liver

The liver is the largest and heaviest organ of the body. It's located in the upper-right side of the belly, just below the ribs. The liver performs more than 500 different jobs every day! The main functions of the liver are as follows:

- **Processing food:** When food is broken down into smaller particles by the process of digestion, it's absorbed through the intestinal wall. From there, these smaller food particles are transported to the liver via a big vein called the *portal vein.* Further processing occurs in the liver where glucose (from carbohydrates), amino acids (from proteins), and fatty acids (from fat) are supplied to different organs according to your body's needs. Some of these nutrients are stored within the liver to be used later.
- **Removing toxins:** Your liver removes toxin and waste matter from the blood. It acts like a filter. After the food is processed in the liver, the

waste matter and toxic substances are extracted and sent back to the intestines or to the kidneys to be removed from the body. When you take medications, they undergo further breakdown in the liver and are converted into useful chemicals to help your body. Some of the toxic and harmful substances that you may have ingested and absorbed are also deactivated in the liver.

- **Making bile:** *Bile* is a yellow-green fluid that's made by the liver to help in the digestion of fat. Fat usually doesn't mix easily with other food substances and isn't easily digested. Bile contains bile salts that allow fats to mix better with other substances, which improves absorption. Bile is secreted into the *lumen* (hollow space) of the intestines.

Pancreas

The pancreas produces important enzymes and hormones that help in the process of digestion. The enzymes are secreted into the intestines and help in the breakdown of carbohydrates, proteins, and fats. The hormones are secreted directly into the blood; the pancreas produces an important hormone called *insulin* that regulates your blood sugar levels.

Table 3-1 lists the important pancreatic enzymes and their target nutrients.

Table 3-1 Pancreatic Enzymes

Enzyme	*Target Nutrient*	*Breakdown Products*
Trypsin	Protein	Amino acids
Peptidase	Protein	Amino acids
Lipase	Fat	Fatty acids and glycerol
Amylase	Carbohydrate	Glucose and fructose

Gallbladder

The gallbladder is a pear-shaped sack that is present just under the liver. When you eat fatty food, your gallbladder contracts, squeezing bile into the intestines. Bile has two important functions:

- It breaks down the fat to help in the digestion and absorption of fat.
- It carries toxic materials from the liver to the intestines to be excreted in the stool.

There are two bladders in your body: The urinary bladder holds urine (which is made in the kidneys), and the gallbladder holds bile (which is made in the liver). Just as the urinary bladder stores urine before it's excreted, the gallbladder stores bile before it's delivered to the intestines. The key difference: Urine is a waste liquid and is of no use to the body, whereas bile is extremely important for the process of digestion.

Understanding How Inflammation Affects the Digestive Process

The previous sections explain how the GI tract works. In this section, I fill you in on what happens when inflammation takes the stage. Inflammation is a process through which the body tries to get rid of damaged tissue and foreign invaders, such as bacteria. When you cut your finger, you see swelling, redness, and bleeding — all of which are features of inflammation, and all of which serve an important purpose. But when inflammation is inappropriately directed against your own body tissues or isn't appropriately controlled, it becomes the cause of chronic injury. Inflammation of the GI tract — which is seen in Crohn's and colitis — causes similar features. In Crohn's disease, any part of the GI tract — from the oral cavity to the anus — can be involved; in colitis, only the colon and rectum are involved.

The inflammation in Crohn's can involve all the layers of the GI tract including the mucosa, submucosa, muscularis, and serosa. In colitis, only the mucosa is involved.

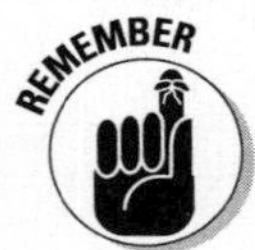

Your GI tract is also home to the largest part of your body's immune system. Special immune cells in the GI tract protect you from harmful invaders like bacteria and toxic substances.

Gastritis: Inflammation of the stomach

Inflammation of the stomach lining is called *gastritis.* The most common causes for gastritis include

- A bacterial infection called *Helicobacter pylori*
- Use of non-steroidal anti-inflammatory drugs (NSAIDs), such as aspirin, ibuprofen (Advil, Motrin), and naproxen (Aleve)
- Excessive alcohol consumption
- Severe illness

Although uncommon, Crohn's disease also can affect the stomach. The inflammation leads to swelling and redness of the mucosa and formation of ulcers.

Common signs and symptoms of gastritis include

- Upper abdominal pain or burning
- Nausea
- Vomiting
- Loss of appetite
- Feeling of fullness after a few bites of food

A diagnosis of gastritis from Crohn's is usually made with an upper endoscopy that enables your doctor to take biopsies. When it's confirmed by biopsy, the treatment of IBD along with acid-suppression therapy lead to symptom relief and healing of the mucosa.

Enteritis: Inflammation of the small intestine

Inflammation of the small intestine is called *enteritis.* The small bowel, especially the last part of the ileum, is a very common site of involvement in Crohn's disease. Enteritis results in swelling, redness, and ulcer formation in the small intestine. This affects the process of digestion and absorption of food and water, leading to malabsorption, malnutrition, and dehydration.

Depending on its location, enteritis is also known as

- **Duodenitis:** Inflammation of the duodenum
- **Jejunitis:** Inflammation of the jejunum
- **Ileitis:** Inflammation of the ileum
- **Terminal ileitis:** Inflammation of the last part of the ileum

Terminal ileitis is the most common for Crohn's disease. For this reason, Crohn's disease is also known as terminal ileitis.

The common signs and symptoms of enteritis include

- Abdominal pain
- Cramping

- Diarrhea
- Blood in the stool
- Anemia
- Weight loss

Crohn's disease of the duodenum can be diagnosed with upper endoscopy and biopsies of the inflamed tissue. However, the upper endoscope can't go beyond the duodenum. Capsule endoscopy, small bowel follow-through, CT scan, and MRI are usually done to look for Crohn's disease in the jejunum and ileum. Treatment of Crohn's disease with appropriate medications helps improve the mucosal inflammation and reverses the malabsorption and malnutrition.

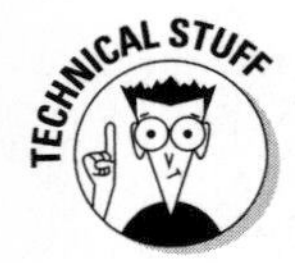

Vitamin B12 is absorbed in the ileum. When the terminal ileum is inflamed or has been removed by surgery, you suffer from vitamin B12 deficiency. Your physician may check your B12 levels (through a simple blood test) to help determine whether inflammation is healing.

Colitis: Inflammation of the large intestine

Inflammation of the lining of the colon is called *colitis.* Both Crohn's disease and ulcerative colitis can involve the colon. If colitis is due to Crohn's disease, it's called *Crohn's colitis.* The inflammation of Crohn's colitis is usually patchy in nature, which means there are areas of normal mucosa in between the inflamed mucosa. Ulcerative colitis is a continuous inflammation that starts from the rectum and spreads upward.

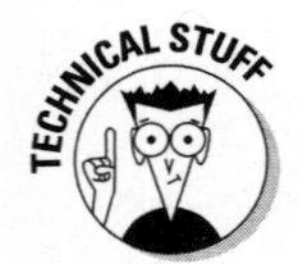

In 10 percent to 15 percent of patients, it may not be easy to distinguish Crohn's colitis from ulcerative colitis. This entity has been given a separate name of *IBD, type undetermined* or *indeterminate colitis.*

Inflammation of the colon produces similar signs of swelling, redness, and ulcers as described in the preceding section. Because the colon is involved in the absorption of water and salts, inflammation of the colon often results in loose stools.

Common signs and symptoms of colitis are

- Diarrhea
- Blood in the stool
- Abdominal pain or cramping
- Urgency to move your bowels
- Fatigue

The diagnosis of colitis is made by colonoscopy. In ulcerative colitis, your doctor may see redness, bleeding, and ulceration of the lining of the colon. Despite its name, the ulcers in ulcerative colitis are usually small and superficial. On the contrary, the ulcers in Crohn's disease are often irregularly shaped and can be quite deep.

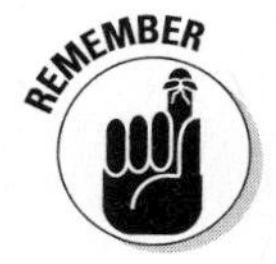

Scientists believe that long-standing inflammation of the colon, especially if left untreated, can lead to colon cancer. The risk of colon cancer increases significantly after eight to ten years of colitis. Your doctor will send you for a colonoscopy at regular intervals to rule out colon cancer or catch it at an earlier stage.

Proctitis: Inflammation of the rectum

Inflammation of the lining of the rectum is called *proctitis.* This condition commonly happens in colitis where your rectum is the starting point of the inflammation. Proctitis can also happen in Crohn's, where it may also be associated with other findings, such as *fistulas* (abnormal connection between the intestines or between the intestine and the skin) and *fissures* (tears in the lining of the anal canal).

There are other reasons for proctitis in patients with Crohn's and colitis, such as infection with various bacteria and viruses. The risk of certain types of infections are higher if you're on immunosuppressive medications such as steroids. Besides Crohn's and colitis, certain sexually transmitted diseases (especially in men who have sex with men) also present as proctitis.

Common signs and symptoms of proctitis are

- Urgency to move your bowels
- *Tenesmus* (the sensation of incomplete relief during bowel movement)
- Diarrhea
- Blood in the stool
- Mucus discharge
- Pain during a bowel movement
- Soreness in the rectal area

Frequent bowel movements and accidents can also cause irritation and rash on the skin surrounding the anus.

There are different types of *proctitis* and colitis depending on the location of the inflammation in the rectum and colon, as shown in Figure 3-2. When colitis is limited to only the rectum and sigmoid colon, it is known as *proctosigmoiditis.* When it involves your rectum, sigmoid colon, and descending colon, it is referred to as *left-sided colitis.* When the colitis has spread into the transverse colon and beyond, it is called *pancolitis.*

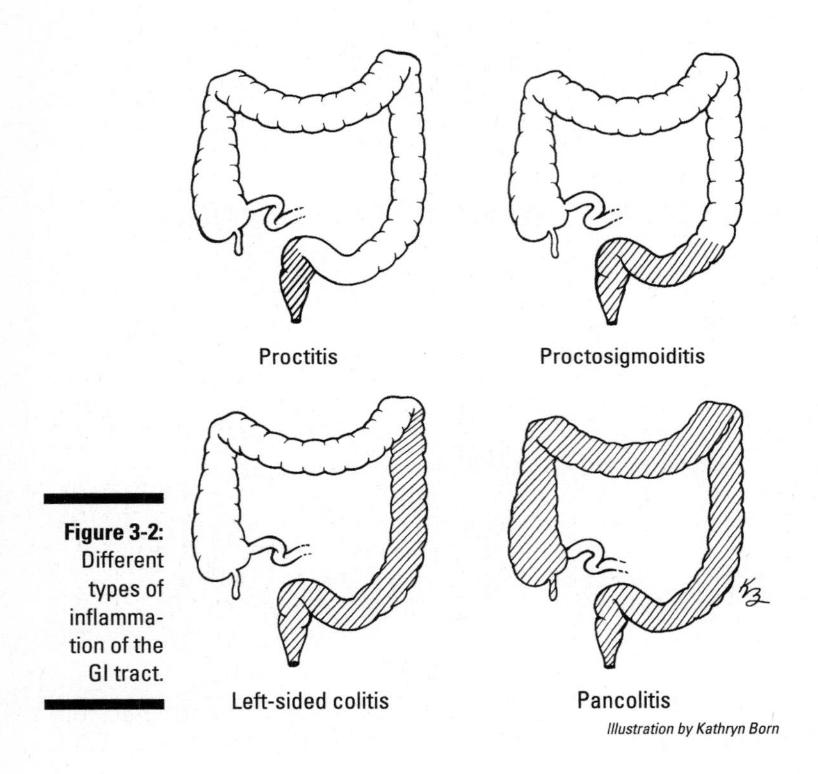

Figure 3-2: Different types of inflammation of the GI tract.

Chapter 4

Who Gets Crohn's and Colitis and Why

In This Chapter

- Looking at age, gender, and geography as they relate to Crohn's and colitis
- Recognizing the role of immune system and genes in Crohn's and colitis

Around the world, millions of people suffer from Crohn's and colitis, and the diseases are on the rise. So, if you've been diagnosed with Crohn's or colitis, you're definitely not alone. Even so, you may be asking, "Why me?"

The causes of Crohn's and colitis are still not known, but researchers have found abnormalities in the immune systems of people suffering from the diseases. In addition, about 15 percent to 30 percent of people with Crohn's or colitis have a relative with the disease, so scientists believe that genetic factors are also involved. In addition, medical research is showing that certain environmental factors — such as the food you eat or the air you breathe — can cause or trigger the diseases.

In this chapter, I review the different factors that can cause Crohn's and colitis. I also discuss certain characteristics of patients that put them at a higher risk of getting the diseases.

Who Gets Crohn's and Colitis

Anyone can get Crohn's or colitis, but the diseases are more common among certain groups than others. Here are some key factors to keep in mind:

- **Age:** The most common age for diagnosis of Crohn's and colitis is around 15 to 30 years. However, there is also a rising increase in the elderly population, above the age of 60, who are being diagnosed with Crohn's or colitis for the first time.

- **Gender:** Some studies have shown that Crohn's disease is slightly more common in adult women than in adult men. But the reverse is found in kids — boys get Crohn's disease more often than girls. Colitis occurs equally often in men as it does in women.
- **Geography:** Crohn's and colitis are more common in some parts of the world than in others. For example, residents of Europe and North America are at higher risk of getting Crohn's and colitis. In addition, northern areas of Europe and North America have more people diagnosed with Crohn's and colitis than southern parts of the continents do. Finally, Crohn's and colitis are more common in urban areas than in nonurban areas. Scientists have proposed different reasons for these variations; difference in diet, environment, sunlight exposure, industrialization, exposure to pollutants and chemicals, and hygiene may contribute to this variation.

I cover some of these factors in greater detail later in this chapter.

The Role of the Immune System in Crohn's and Colitis

The immune system is your body's defense against invaders such as infectious organisms. When you a get a skin cut, different kinds of bacteria and viruses may enter your body through the break in your skin. Your immune system responds and eliminates these invaders while the skin heals itself and seals the puncture. The immune system is made up of a network of cells and organs that work together to protect your body.

An immune system primer

The immune system is made of different cells, tissues, and organs. In this section, I walk you through the various components of the immune system, so you understand how things go wrong.

The function of the immune system is summarized in Figure 4-1.

Bone marrow

Bone marrow is a special spongelike tissue that's present inside your large bones. It produces your white blood cells (called *leukocytes*) and red blood cells (called *erythrocytes*). White blood cells are an important component of the immune system.

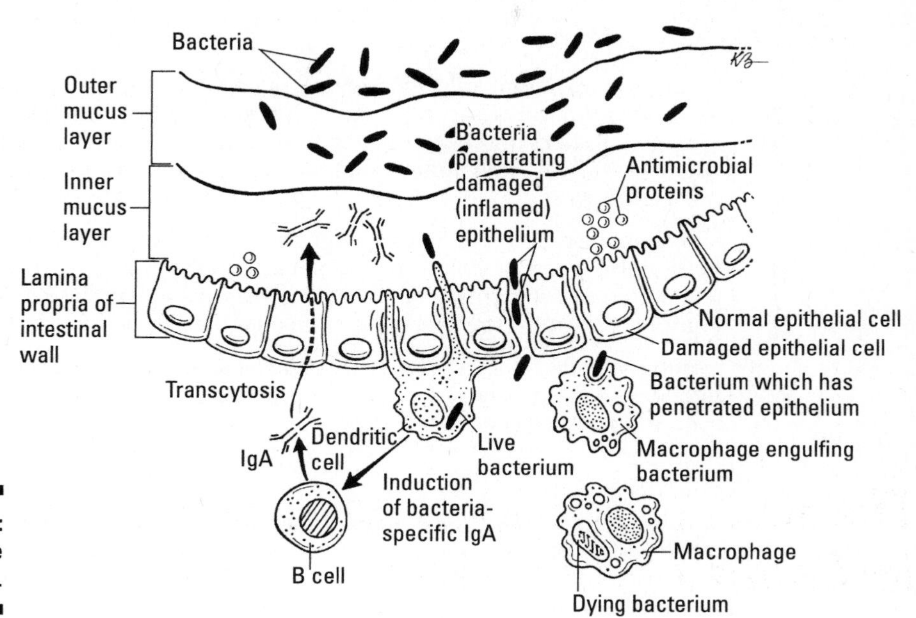

Figure 4-1: The immune system.

Spleen

The spleen is an important organ located on the left side of your abdomen, just below the ribs. It acts like a filter to remove bacteria and viruses from your blood. It also removes old blood cells that aren't able to carry out their functions anymore.

Complements

One of the first parts of the immune system that meet invaders such as bacteria or viruses is a group of proteins called the *complements.* This system is composed of approximately 26 different proteins. The proteins flow freely in the blood and can quickly reach the site of an invasion. When activated, the complement proteins can trigger inflammation and send signals to other immune cells.

The important functions of the complement proteins include

- Directly killing some bacteria and foreign cells
- Producing molecules that attract other immune cells and proteins
- Making bacteria more susceptible to killing

Phagocytes

The *phagocytes* are a group of white blood cells that are specialized in finding and eating bad bugs and dead tissue. Phagocytes come in three different types:

- **Granulocytes:** Think of granulocytes as small soldiers that often take the first stand during an infection or intrusion. They attack any invader in large numbers and keep on attacking until the invader dies. The pus you see in an infected wound is chiefly made of granulocytes, which die during this process.
- **Macrophages:** Think of macrophages as big soldiers that are lined up behind the granulocytes. They're more powerful than granulocytes when it comes to fighting an infection. They also alert the rest of the immune system to the presence of an invader.
- **Dendritic cells:** Think of dendritic cells as special soldiers that devour intruders. Like macrophages, they send signals to the rest of immune system to activate.

Lymphocytes

Lymphocytes are another type of white blood cells. These cells have special units attached to their surfaces called *receptors.* Receptors are very specialized parts of the lymphocytes. Each receptor can match only one specific *antigen* (a part of the intruder body).

To understand the receptors, think of a hand that can pick only one particular type of item — for example, bad apples — but nothing else. If you had a hand like this, you'd be a true bad-apple-picking champion, but you'd have a hard time doing much of anything else. In your body, each receptor on a lymphocyte equals a hand in search of a bad apple. The lymphocytes patrol your body until they find antigens of the right size and shape to match their specific receptors. It may seem limiting that the receptors of each lymphocyte cell can match only one specific type of antigen, but your body makes up for this by producing so many different lymphocytes that your immune system can recognize nearly all invaders.

There are two main types of lymphocytes: T cells and B cells.

T cells

There are two types of T cells: helper T cells and killer T cells. Helper T cells are the major regulating authority of your immune system. Their primary job is to activate killer T cells and B cells. Helper T cells are themselves activated when a phagocyte comes close to it and presents a fragment of captured antigen (bacteria) to the receptor of the helper T cell. When the receptor of the helper T cell recognizes the invader, it activates the T and B cells to start the fight against the invaders. The killer T cells then release chemicals to kill the invader and eat it out.

Types of immunity

All the specialized cells and proteins of the immune system offer your body protection against different diseases. This protection is called *immunity.* You have three different types of immunity:

- **Innate immunity:** This is the natural immunity you're born with. Innate immunity is present in your skin and in the mucosa of your digestive tract. If there is invasion, such as bacteria breaking into the mucosa, your body tries to heal the break quickly, and special immune cells present in the mucosa attack the invading agent.
- **Adaptive immunity:** The next level of protection is adaptive immunity. This is an active immunity that develops throughout your life. It involves your white blood cells (such as lymphocytes) and develops as you're exposed to diseases and are immunized against a disease through vaccines.
- **Passive immunity:** You get passive immunity from other sources. Passive immunity lasts for a short time. For example, antibodies in a mother's breast milk provide her baby with temporary immunity until the baby develops its own immune system.

B cells

B cells, when they're activated by helper T cells, produce specific proteins called *antibodies.* Antibodies also help your body destroy the intruders such as bacteria. B cells produce antibodies at an amazing rate and can release thousands of antibodies in seconds.

Antibodies

Antibodies (also called immunoglobulin, or Ig) are a special type of large, Y-shaped, sticky protein made by B cells. When antibodies find the right invader, they attach to it. The attached antibody serves as an appetizing coating for eater cells, such as macrophages. Antibodies also neutralize toxins and incapacitate viruses, preventing them from infecting new cells.

The healthy human body has thousands and thousands of antibodies, each specific to one special target (antigen). The body is capable of producing large quantities of some antibodies on demand.

Antibodies come in five classes: IgA, IgD, IgE, IgM, and IgG. IgG antibodies are the most important class. They circulate in the blood and other body parts and directly attach to viruses and bacterial toxins.

When your gut's immune system goes awry

Your intestinal tract is lined up with the first line of defense, innate immunity, as well as with other reserve soldiers in the form of adaptive immunity. Your immune system is always alert and active. That's why most of the bacteria, viruses, or parasites that are present everywhere — in the air you breathe and in the food you eat — cannot harm you. Your immune system hunts them down, destroys them, and wraps their remains for elimination from the body.

If the immune system isn't working properly, these invaders can cause damage to the body, such as your intestinal wall, and the process of inflammation goes on without anything there to keep it in check. One of the theories behind Crohn's and colitis is that it's caused by a defect in the immune system that can let the bad bacteria invade your intestinal mucosal wall. Usually, the innate immunity is able to act as a first line of defense; your white blood cells (granulocytes and macrophages) attack these invaders and kill them. If the invaders survive these soldiers (because the soldiers are dysfunctional), the next level of defense, including lymphocytes, are there for your protection. Any defect in function and regulation of these defenders (white blood cells) will cause damage to your mucosa. This will lead to ulcer formation, bleeding from the mucosa, and a chronic inflammation process, all of which are hallmarks of Crohn's and colitis.

Environmental Factors

Scientists have identified a number of factors in the environment that may be the cause or trigger of Crohn's and colitis. In this section, I walk you through all these factors, telling you what we know today.

Food

Inflammatory bowel disease (IBD) was thought to be rare in certain parts of the world, such as Asia and South America, but there has been a recent increase in the number of people diagnosed with it in these parts of the world. Scientists have proposed the introduction of a "Western diet" as the possible culprit in these countries. The Western diet is rich in fats and refined sugars and low in fruits and vegetables. This type of diet may change the normal balance of good and bad bacteria living inside the intestines. It may even lead to production of certain chemicals that can cause inflammation of the gut.

Here's what we know about specific components of diet, and how they may contribute to Crohn's and colitis:

- **Fat:** A high intake of total fat in our diet has been shown to increase the risk of Crohn's and colitis. Omega-3 fatty acids (which are present in fish) are anti-inflammatory; in some small studies, omega-3s have been shown to protect you from Crohn's and colitis. Larger studies have not shown this beneficial effect, however, so the jury is still out on omega-3s (at least when it comes to Crohn's and colitis — they're beneficial for your health in other ways, including boosting heart health).

  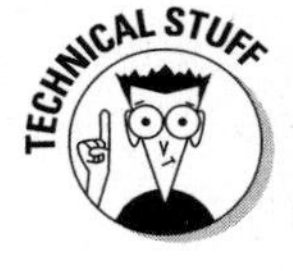

  In an interesting study from the Harvard Medical School about fat and its association with intestinal inflammation, the scientists used genetically altered mice as a model of human Crohn's and colitis. These mice can't produce anti-inflammatory chemicals naturally produced in the human body to protect from inflammation. Some of the mice were fed a low-fat diet, and others were fed a diet with saturated fat or a diet with polyunsaturated fat. Over the next six months, mice fed saturated fat were twice as likely to develop inflammation in the intestines compared to those fed polyunsaturated fat. In the high-fat diets, 37 percent of total calories came from the fat, which is very similar to the typical Western diet. Scientists think that the inflammation in these mice came from an uncontrolled growth of bad bacteria residing inside the intestine. These bad bacteria grow quickly when they're exposed to food rich in saturated fat. Recently, some other studies have also found a similar association between high fat intake and development of Crohn's or colitis in humans.

- **Carbohydrate:** Higher intake of refined sugars such as table sugar (sucrose) has been shown to increase the risk of developing Crohn's disease.

  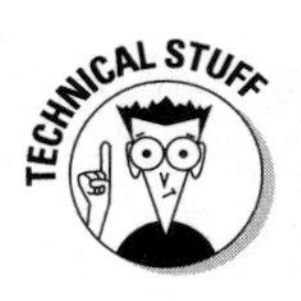

  Some smaller clinical studies have shown some association between the rising incidence of Crohn's and colitis and the increasing consumption of artificial sweeteners. Scientists have proposed that a change in the pH of the intestines and bacteria residing inside the intestines as the possible cause leading to development of inflammation. However, this association has not been confirmed in any large clinical trial.

- **Protein:** Some studies show that a higher intake of protein, especially protein from animal sources, increases the risk of Crohn's and, even more so, colitis. Studies have also found an increased risk of both Crohn's and colitis with increased consumption of red meat.

  Researchers have found that animal proteins, including fish, can increase the risk of developing Crohn's and colitis. Although not confirmed, the hypothesis is that a diet high in protein can damage the digestive tract by producing toxic substances such as ammonia and hydrogen sulfide. A high-protein diet is also thought to alter the natural balance of good and bad bacteria in your colon.

- **Fiber, fruits, and vegetables:** A higher intake of fiber (at least 22 g per day), fruits (at least two servings per day), and vegetables (at least two servings per day) seems to protect against Crohn's and colitis.

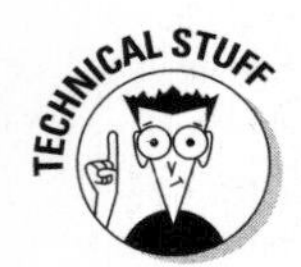

When the bacteria present in the colon break down complex carbohydrates (such as fibers), they produce chemical compounds known as *short-chain fatty acids.* These fatty acids are very important food for the colon cells. If you deprive the colon of such nutrients, the mucosa becomes inflamed. Scientists think that deficiency of such nutritional elements may contribute to the cause of colitis.

Air

As I mention earlier in this chapter, Crohn's and colitis are more common in people living in urbanized and industrialized areas. Researchers also think that the content of nitrogen and sulfur in the air may play an important role in causing Crohn's and colitis. Coal and automobile industries have increased the contents of these gases in the air. Scientists think these gases are somehow causing changes in the intestinal immune system and leading to development of inflammation and illnesses such as Crohn's and colitis.

The air you breathe isn't entirely beyond your control. Smokers are at an increased risk of having Crohn's. Smoking also increases the severity of the disease and puts you at risk for severe Crohn's requiring surgery. Smokers who continue to smoke after surgery are more likely to have a recurrence of the disease and need further surgery.

Strangely enough, smoking protects against colitis. How this happens is still a mystery. But don't use this strange fact as a reason to continue smoking or take up smoking! Smoking causes a host of health problems, and whatever protection it offers against colitis doesn't outweigh all the harm smoking causes.

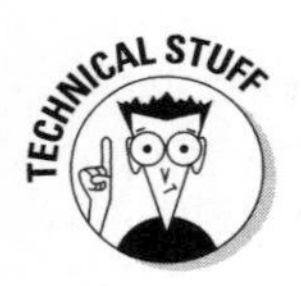

Scientists have discovered nicotine receptors on the internal lining of the intestines, but therapy with nicotine-containing drugs hasn't shown very good results in research studies. So, there must be other chemicals in the smoke that protect against developing colitis.

Hygiene

Western countries are becoming super-clean. They've developed a cleaner lifestyle, and because of this, people no longer need to fight germs as much as they did in the past. As a result, the immune system has shifted away from fighting infection to developing more allergic diseases and autoimmune diseases such as asthma, eczema, and Crohn's and colitis.

A scientist named David Strachan proposed the hygiene hypothesis in 1989 when he observed that children from larger families have less chance of having allergic diseases such as hay fever or eczema. He thought that this was because of exposure to more infectious agents through their brothers and sisters.

The hygiene hypothesis is based on the possibility that a child could be overprotected from the exposure to common germs because of improved hygiene. As a result, the body fails to make the standard immune response. If the child then comes into contact with bad bugs later in life, the immune system could respond inappropriately, causing an abnormal inflammatory process such as IBD.

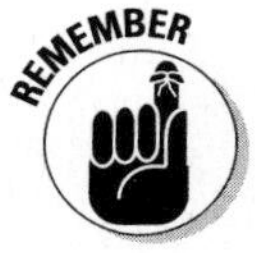

Exposure to bacteria early in life is important in programming the immune system of the digestive tract so that when you come in contact with these bacteria as an adult, the appropriate inflammatory response happens.

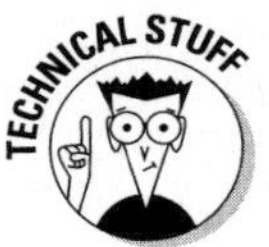

Studies have shown than young kids who are exposed to antibiotics at an early age have increased risk of developing Crohn's and colitis. This is probably because antibiotics have killed even good bacteria in their intestines. So, these medications should be used carefully and only on your doctor's advice.

Other environmental factors

In addition to the food you eat, the air you breathe, and your exposure (or lack of exposure) to bacteria as a child, the following environmental factors may play a role in Crohn's and colitis:

- **Worms:** Recent studies have found that certain worms called *helminthes* are very important in regulating the immune system of the intestines. These worms may have anti-inflammatory properties as well and may prevent you from developing Crohn's and colitis. A higher rate of helminth infections may be one of the reasons we don't see much Crohn's and colitis in underdeveloped countries. Scientists are looking at worm therapy as a cure to IBD (see Chapter 11).
- **Drugs:** Several drugs may increase your risk of developing IBD:
    - **Oral contraceptives:** Research on oral contraceptives causing Crohn's and colitis is still inconclusive. Some, but not all, studies have shown that oral contraceptive pills increase the risk of having Crohn's and colitis.

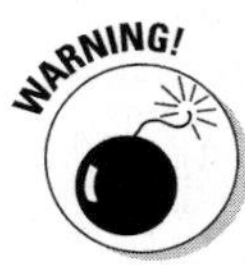

      Carefully consider the potential benefits and risks of stopping oral contraceptive pills. Talk with your doctor about the pros and cons.

    - **Isotretinoin (Accutane, Amnesteem, Claravis, and Sotret):** Isotretinoin is used for the treatment of acne. Recently research has shown that taking this drug may increase your risk of having Crohn's and colitis. Not all studies have shown this link, and some scientists believe that there is just an association between acne and Crohn's and colitis, and drugs used to treat acne may not be the culprit.

- **Tetracycline-class antibiotics such as Doxycycline (Doryx, Monodox, Vibramycin, and Vibra-Tabs):** This class of antibiotics is frequently used in the treatment of acne. New studies have shown that taking tetracycline such as doxycycline may increase the risk of getting Crohn's and colitis.

A recent study from Finland showed that kids taking antibiotics such as cephalosporin, a sister drug of penicillin, are three times more likely to get Crohn's disease. Similarly, another study from Canada showed that kids have an increased risk of getting Crohn's and colitis if they received antibiotics as early as the first year of their lives. These studies don't necessarily prove that antibiotics are the definite cause of Crohn's or colitis, but antibiotics may contribute to the development of these diseases by changing the balance of good and bad bacteria inside the intestines. ***Remember:*** Not all the patients who take antibiotics develop the disease.

The mystery of the appendix

Your appendix is a small, closed tube about the size of your finger. It attaches to the beginning of your large intestine (the *cecum*), where the small and large intestines meet. The appendix is open at the end that connects to the cecum and closed at the other end. If the open end of the appendix gets plugged for some reason — either because of swelling or because something from the large intestine gets stuck in the opening — the appendix starts to swell. The swelling shuts off the blood supply, and the appendix tissue dies. An operation to remove the swollen appendix (called an *appendectomy*) is the only way to fix this problem.

The exact function of the appendix is unknown. Recently, scientists have found many cells of the immune system in the appendix, which suggests that it may play a role in the immune system. Scientists have also proposed that the appendix may harbor bacteria that are beneficial in the function of the human colon.

Here's the interesting connection between appendectomy and IBD: It appears that appendectomies somehow protect against colitis. However, some researchers have suggested that this is only true if the appendix is removed before the age of 21. Conversely, appendectomies seem to *increase* the chance of developing Crohn's.

Genes Gone Bad: The Role of Genetics

Scientists have discovered that, in a set of twins, if one twin has Crohn's, the other twin is much more likely to also have Crohn's. The risk is even higher if the twins are identical (as opposed to fraternal). The same is true for colitis but to a lesser degree. Because both identical and fraternal twins share the same diet and environment, the higher risk in identical twins shows that genes must play some role in causing Crohn's and colitis. Researchers are looking for those genes. In early 2000, they discovered a gene that increases the risk of having Crohn's. Since then, many other genes have been discovered that increase your risk of having Crohn's or colitis. In this section, I explain the role of genetics in these diseases.

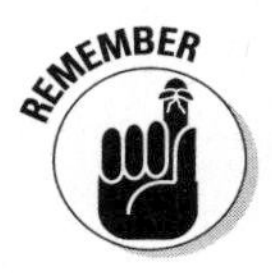

Not everyone who has gene mutation develops IBD. We're still learning about the involvement of genes in the disease.

How genes work

Your body is made up of different organs, like the heart, brain, liver, and intestines. Each organ, in turn, is made up of tissues, which are different cells glued together. Cells act like bricks in your body. The human body is made up of trillions of cells. (Compare that with bacteria, which are made of a single cell.) Each cell is a living organism and has its own command center to carry out its assigned function. This command center is called the *nucleus* of the cell. The machinery inside the nucleus is called *DNA*.

Genes are small portions of the DNA that send signals to your cells to make different products. For example, genes present in the cells of your heart produce proteins to help the heart contract and keep it beating year after year. Similarly, genes of the intestinal cells produce different enzymes and hormones to help the digestion process. They also produce chemicals to help fight against harmful bacteria.

So, DNA contains thousands of genes and in each cell certain genes are turned on to produce specific proteins, and the rest of the genes remain turned off.

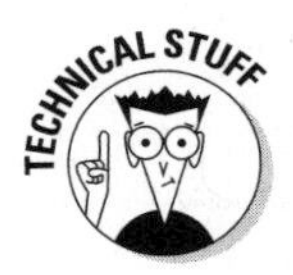

The signal to produce a protein comes from your DNA. This signal is stored in the DNA as a sequence of repeating units, called *nucleotides,* along the DNA chain. There are four types of these units: A, T, G, and C. The sequence of nucleotides storing this information is called *genetic code.* When it's time to produce a protein, the cell copies the genetic code into a similar molecule, called *RNA;* this copying process is called *transcription.* This RNA copy is then used to make amino acids. Proteins are made of a chain of different types of amino acids. This chain folds up into a compact shape. The shape of the protein is determined by the sequence of amino acids, which in turn is determined by the genetic code. This process of copying information from RNA into the amino acids and making proteins is called *translation.* Figure 4-2 illustrates the process of protein synthesis by genes.

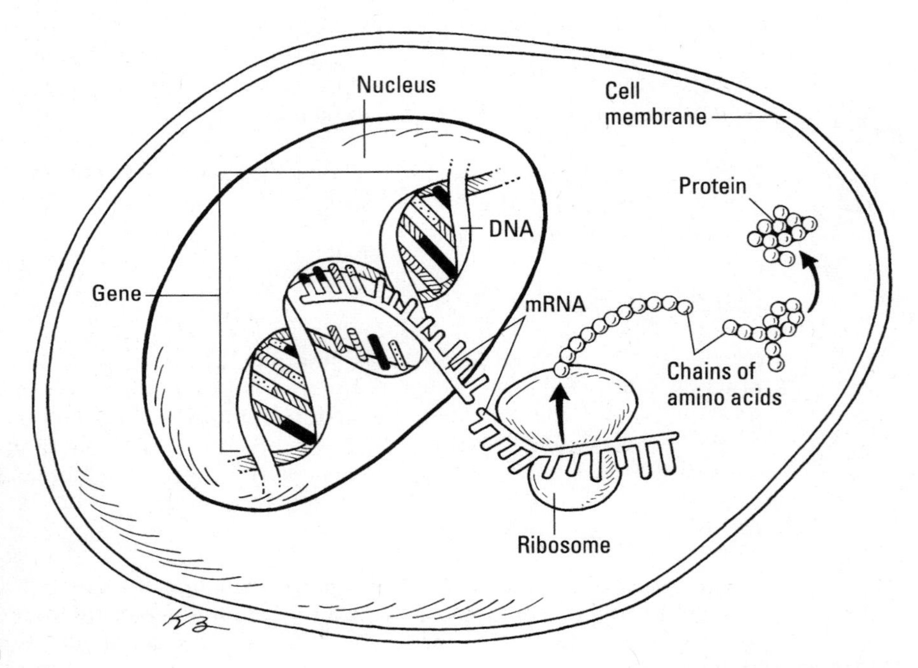

Figure 4-2: The process of protein synthesis by genes.

Illustration by Kathryn Born

If the sequence of nucleotides in a gene is changed, the sequence of amino acids in the protein is also changed. Similarly, if a part of the gene is deleted or mutated, the protein may be shorter. These altered or shorter proteins may not work properly or may not work at all.

The role of family history

If one of your family members has Crohn's or colitis, you may be at risk for developing these illnesses yourself. In fact, one of the greatest risk factors for developing Crohn's or colitis is family history. First-degree relatives (parents, children, or siblings) are at the greatest risk for having this disease.

Here are some numbers to crunch:

- Twenty percent to 25 percent of Crohn's or colitis patients have a first-degree relative with the disease.
- If you have colitis, there is about a 2 percent chance that you'll pass the disease on to your child. If you have Crohn's disease, there is about a 5 percent chance that you'll pass the disease on to your child.
- If both you and your partner have Crohn's or colitis, there is a 45 percent chance that your child will have the disease.

Medical research has shown that first-degree relatives of a Crohn's disease patient are not only at risk for developing Crohn's but also at increased risk for developing colitis, and vice versa. This doesn't hold true for *second-degree relatives* (grandparent, grandchild, uncle, aunt, nephew, niece, or half-sibling) and *third-degree relatives* (first cousins), who are at increased risk for the same disease as their relative has.

Key genes for Crohn's and colitis

Knowing that there is increased risk of Crohn's and colitis in family members, scientists started analyzing different genes to check their association with these illnesses. They have discovered more than 100 genes that are thought to be involved in Crohn's and colitis.

In this section, I tell you about two of them.

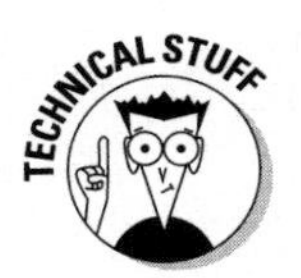

Initially, the process of discovery of these genes was slow because of incomplete understanding of the human genome. Scientists subsequently developed a method to slice DNA in automated machines and were able to study thousands of genes in a very short period of time. This type of study is called the Genome Wide Association Study (GWAS).

NOD 2

The NOD 2 gene serves like a sensor in your immune system. This gene is present in cells in the lining of the *terminal ileum* (the last part of the small intestine). The NOD 2 gene plays an important role in sensing the harmful bacteria that try to break into the cell lining of the terminal ileum to cause inflammation. Besides sending signals to activate other immune cells, the NOD 2 gene also produces a chemical called *defensin* to kill the harmful invader.

Mutation of the NOD 2 gene causes a decrease in production of defensing, which means your body loses an important arsenal to fight against harmful bacteria, and the inflammation process begins. This is also why the terminal ileum is the most common site for Crohn's disease.

Autophagy genes

Autophagy is a self-destructive process inside the cells. If any cell in your body goes wild, the internal process of autophagy kicks in and leads to the death of the cell. This process is very important to keep the inflammation in check.

There are different genes called autophagy genes (ATG) that control this process. ATG16 is one of the genes found mutated in Crohn's disease. This mutation leads to decreased or defective autophagy; inflamed or infected cells stay put and keep on causing more persistent inflammation.

Getting a genetic test

So, if genes play an important role in causing Crohn's and colitis, why not get a genetic test, especially if you have a family member with the disease? Before you jump into genetic testing, keep in mind the following:

- **Genetic testing is very expensive and not readily available everywhere.**
- **Genetic testing is neither sensitive nor specific.** Having a positive gene does not guarantee that you'll develop Crohn's or colitis. In fact, it may just create unnecessary anxiety, and you'll end up rushing to your doctor every time you have an episode of diarrhea or abdominal pain.
- **Mutations of genes are not the only cause of Crohn's and colitis.** Many people have no genetic mutations but still have the disease.
- **Even if we identify Crohn's or colitis before the symptoms appear, it isn't clear that we can give patients anything to prevent the onset of symptoms (or the disease).**

Part II
Getting Medical Help

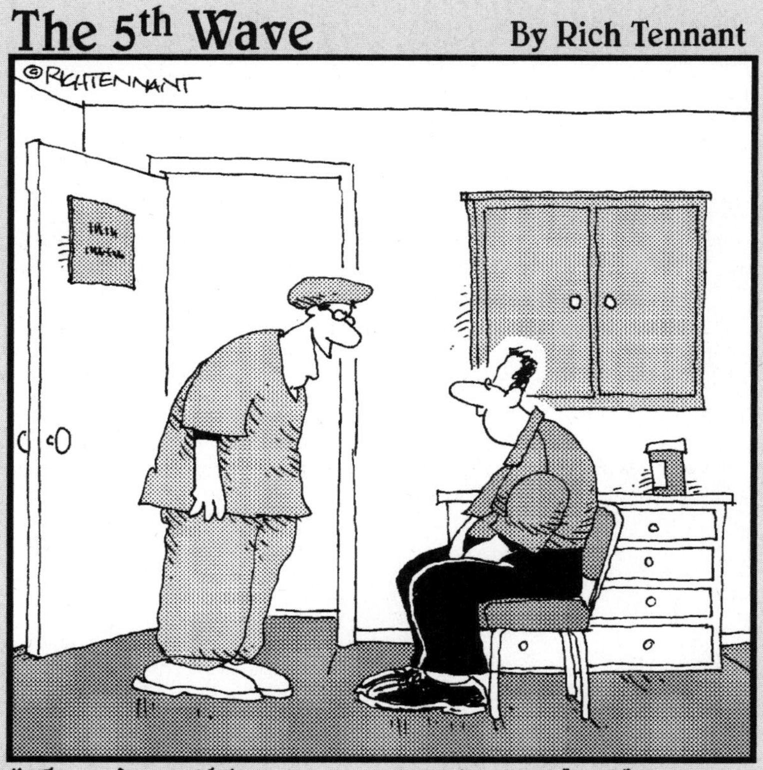

"There's nothing to worry about, Mr. Halloran. I've performed many endoscopies in the past, including an esophagogastroduodenoscopy, which I can also spell."

In this part . . .

Working with your doctor is critical to treating Crohn's and colitis, and in this part I walk you through how to assemble and work with your healthcare team. I also fill you in on what's involved in being diagnosed, including the tests you may have to go through. Finally, I discuss the medications you may have to take and the surgeries you may need to consider if and when the medications are no longer enough.

Chapter 5

Assembling Your Healthcare Team

In This Chapter

- Finding your doctor
- Adding to your healthcare team

Crohn's and colitis are chronic diseases where you have symptom relief at times, but the actual disease may never really disappear completely. Learning more about Crohn's and colitis and understanding your options help you navigate the healthcare decision-making process. A good doctor who can understand you and your disease is as important as managing the disease and keeping it under control.

In this chapter, I present some suggestions to keep in mind when you search for and pull together your healthcare team.

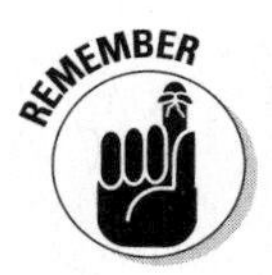

Finding the right doctor is crucial, but you are your own best advocate. Asking questions, expressing your opinion, and sharing your fears and doubts with your friends, colleagues, and doctors will help you make the decisions that work best for you.

Finding the Right Doctor for You

You may have a mild form of Crohn's or colitis and may have spent months or years dealing with annoying symptoms without ever mentioning them to your family members or doctors. Many people live with the troubling symptoms of diarrhea, abdominal pain, and *tenesmus* (a constant sensation of fullness and incomplete relief during a bowel movement) because they're too embarrassed to talk to a doctor. Unfortunately, over time, they may start noticing some alarming symptoms such as bleeding, fever, or worsening pain and diarrhea. You, your primary-care doctor, or an emergency-room doctor (if you let it go that far) may suspect that your symptoms are a result of Crohn's or colitis. If so, it's time to seek help from a specialist to get a diagnosis and discuss a management plan.

Why you need a specialist

Gastroenterologists are trained in diagnosing and managing diseases of the gastrointestinal tract, including Crohn's and colitis. They also master the techniques of performing endoscopy. Primary-care doctors usually don't have such training. Because Crohn's and colitis are very complicated and lifelong diseases, you need a gastroenterologist to manage this disease with you. Not only do you need to get a diagnosis from the specialist, but you need to make sure you aren't having any complications of the disease. You need to be on the right medications to prevent further complications. These drugs may require monitoring of side effects through laboratory tests and careful clinical history and physical examination.

Having a specialist manage these medical issues will not only make your life easier but also keep you safe from many problems and complications that come along with these diseases or the medications used to treat them.

How to choose among the specialists in your area

Choosing a specialist comes down to personal preferences, as well as recommendations from your other doctors, family, and friends. Your primary-care doctor may be the best resource because she's likely to have other patients with Crohn's or colitis and a variety of specialists in your area. But don't hesitate to do your own research, whether online or among your network of family and friends.

As you check out gastroenterologists near you, consider the following questions:

- **Does the gastroenterologist accept your insurance?** This is probably the first question you'll need an answer to. Your health insurance company likely can provide you with a directory of gastroenterologists who accept your insurance.
- **Does the gastroenterologist have a good reputation in your community?** Answering this question can be difficult, but you can check with your primary-care physician, as well as Crohn's and colitis support groups in your area.
- **Is the gastroenterologist an expert in the field?** You can gauge the expertise of a physician in several ways.

  Some gastroenterologists may undergo an extra year or two of training in inflammatory bowel disease (IBD) from well-reputed academic centers. This training provides an opportunity for the gastroenterologists to see and take care of many patients with Crohn's and colitis — from simple cases to those with more complicated disease.

You may also be able to gauge a physician's expertise based on the number of years he has been in practice. Physicians with many years of practice under their belt have probably seen many patients with all kinds of disease severity and complications and may be more comfortable taking care of complex and complicated cases. However, a young physician fresh out of medical school may be more current on the latest information, so don't discount a doctor simply because she's young.

- **Where is the gastroenterologist's office located?** Ideally, you want to find a specialist whose office is convenient for you to get to. If you live in a small town with a larger city nearby, you might sacrifice convenience for expertise and opt for a doctor farther away.
- **What are the gastroenterologist's office hours?** You need a doctor whose hours work with your schedule so you don't end up skipping appointments and sacrificing your healthcare.

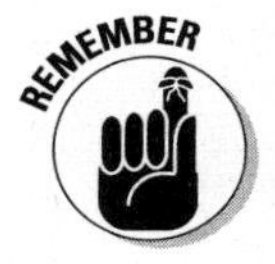

With the fluctuating conditions of Crohn's and colitis, things often go better if you know that your doctor is available when you need her. If you don't have a trusted doctor on your team, even the fear factor can tie your intestines into knots.

Your first visit

When you've landed on a gastroenterologist whom you think may be a good fit, you're ready to make an appointment.

Before your first appointment, write a list of questions that you want to ask. Here are some ideas to get you started, but add to this list with questions that are unique to you and your health:

- What is the difference between Crohn's and colitis, and how do we know I have one and not the other?
- How will you confirm the diagnosis?
- How will we manage and keep track of the disease?
- What are the risks of taking medications?
- What might happen to me in the future?

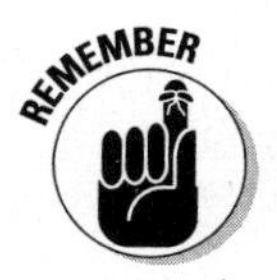

Be sure to be pleasant when asking your questions — you don't want to come off like you're interrogating the doctor. You want her on your team, which means not putting her on the defensive.

Bring a notebook with you to your appointment and take notes on what the doctor says. Better yet, ask a close friend or family member to come with you and be the note-taker. Sometimes when you're dealing with health issues, it's easy to forget or misremember what the doctor said, so having notes can refresh your memory hours or days later.

Considering comprehensive IBD treatment centers

Some people with milder forms of Crohn's or colitis may never need to seek hospital-based care. Other people may go through periods when hospital admission or even surgical treatment becomes necessary. Your doctor may not be able to predict which way your Crohn's or colitis will progress. That's why you should always choose a hospital before the next flare occurs.

Considering the complex nature of the disease, many hospitals are building dedicated Crohn's and colitis clinics or IBD centers to provide comprehensive care under one roof. Usually, these centers are affiliated with academic centers, medical schools, and universities where researchers and clinical doctors collaborate. You can find a center near where you live by searching online or asking your primary-care doctor.

There are several advantages to being cared for at an IBD center:

- The opportunity to enroll in research and clinical trials
- Receiving healthcare from a team of physicians, surgeons, and nurses, all working under one roof
- Access to Crohn's and colitis support groups
- The chance to attend educational seminars
- Direct phone numbers allowing you to communicate with an IBD nurse 24/7

These centers offer the most up-to-date therapies and have experience with complicated cases, but they may not be right for you. For example, you may have to travel a long distance to go to such a center, and that may add to your financial burden or stress. You may also be overwhelmed by a large institution and seeing so many healthcare providers. You may not like being visited by medical students and other trainees. Talk with your doctor before traveling to a specialized center.

Before your appointment, ask the receptionist if you should bring any medical records with you. For example, you might want to bring a list of the medications you take (including the dosages), any surgeries you've had (and when), and endoscopy reports.

After that first office visit, consider the following:

- **Your general impressions of her knowledge and expertise:** Your doctor should take the time to explain your disease to you, and you should feel satisfied with the explanations you get.
- **The doctor's communication skills:** Can the doctor talk to you in plain English, or does he sound like he's quoting from a textbook? If you don't understand what your doctor is saying, you may not understand your disease.

- **How long the doctor spends with you:** Some doctors are in and out of the exam room in five minutes; others spend close to an hour with each patient. Obviously, the more time the doctor spends with you, the better — especially on that first appointment when you may have lots of questions and concerns.
- **How you feel:** You need to feel comfortable with your gastroenterologist. If you can't express your concerns and opinions and ask questions, you may never develop trust, and this may affect your healthcare.

Rounding Up Other Key Players

Your healthcare isn't just in the hands of your gastroenterologist. A whole team of people contributes to your care. In this section, I fill you in on each of these key players.

Your primary-care physician

Your primary-care physician may be the first healthcare provider to suspect you have Crohn's or colitis. If your primary-care doctor thinks you might have Crohn's or colitis, she may order some tests (like an X-ray, CT scan, or blood tests). She may also send you for a colonoscopy or refer you to a gastroenterologist.

Although your gastroenterologist will diagnose and treat your Crohn's or colitis, your primary-care doctor is still the main player on your healthcare team. You may see many doctors, but your primary-care doctor will make sure all the recommendations from all the different doctors are followed.

Your primary-care doctor will also make sure preventive healthcare measures, such as vaccinations, bone tests, and colonoscopies for cancer screening, take place.

At some point, you may have to apply for disability benefits or have some insurance-related issues. Your primary-care doctor's staff can help in these situations. They can write letters to your insurance company and related offices and communicate with them on your behalf.

Nurses

Nurses are very important members of your healthcare team, often acting as a bridge to your doctor. Nurses take care of your day-to-day symptoms and help convey serious problems to your doctor. Here are a few important nursing titles that you may need to be aware of:

- **Ambulatory care nurses:** These nurses usually practice in outpatient clinics. They're assigned different jobs, which can include taking your phone calls and messages and relaying them to your doctor. They work with you and your doctor to manage your disease. If you become acutely sick, they may be able to call in medications ordered by your doctor to the pharmacy. They can also arrange preventive-health measures like scheduling colonoscopies and bone-density tests and administrating vaccinations.
- **Advanced practice nursing:** These nurses have advanced clinical skills and education. They undergo postgraduate training in nursing. They can even work independently when it comes to disease management and decision making. In general, there are two types of advanced practice nurses:
    - Nurse practitioners (NPs): An NP first obtains a bachelor's degree in nursing and then receives a graduate-level education. NPs can provide a wide range of care for patients of all ages. They can complete physical examinations, diagnose and treat short- and long-term illnesses, prescribe and manage medications, and provide training and education for patients. NPs are able to work independently or alongside a physician. Typically, you find them in clinic settings.
    - Clinical nurse specialists (CNSs): A CNS also obtains a bachelor's degree in nursing and receives a graduate-level education. CNSs typically specialize in a certain area — this may be a certain population, a certain type of care, or a certain illness or disease. For instance, you may see a CNS who specializes in IBD. CNSs are able to manage your care much like an NP, but they aren't able to prescribe medications in all states. Typically, you find them either in hospitals or clinics.

  Both receive graduate education, and there are few differences in their scope of practice.
- **Medical case management nurses:** Case management nurses may assess your care and assist in developing, implementing, and coordinating a medical care plan with your doctor. If you're admitted to the hospital, they can work with your insurance company to assist you for prescription approval and enrollment in drug-assistance programs, if available. They may also assist you with completion of disability papers.
- **Home-health nurses:** Home-health nurses provide home care. If you're recently home from the hospital after surgery, these nurses can stop by your home and check on you. They can also administer injections and teach you how to give yourself injections.

- **Ostomy nurses:** More than half of people with Crohn's or colitis end up having surgery within ten years of diagnosis. If you end up needing an ostomy (see Chapter 8), your daily life will need some adjustments. Ostomy nurses can be a great resource during this time. They can work with you and your surgeon to identify the correct spot on the abdomen for ostomy creation and provide you with useful resources to learn to live with an ostomy. They can also help you take care of your ostomy and are available to deal with any complications or problems that arise at your ostomy site.

Physician assistants

Physician assistants (PAs) are healthcare professionals who are trained to practice medicine as part of a team with physicians. There are separate graduate programs for their training. Once licensed, a PA can perform physical exams, diagnose and treat illnesses, order and interpret tests, and prescribe medications. Unlike NPs (see the preceding section), they work directly under physicians and have some autonomy, such as the ability to write prescriptions. Different states have different regulatory laws regarding PAs' scope of practice.

Registered dietitians

One of the important functions of your digestive tract is to provide you with nutrition. Crohn's and colitis jeopardize people's nutritional status by causing inflammation and decreased absorption of nutrients through the intestinal wall. Malnutrition leads to worsening of inflammation, and a vicious cycle starts.

You can see how important a registered dietitian (RD) can be. An RD can help you make sure you're eating the right foods and keeping up with your nutrition. You may have the opportunity to see an RD in private practice (often through a referral from your primary-care doctor or gastroenterologist), or you may see one if you're admitted to the hospital with a flare.

During a hospital stay, RDs work very closely with your doctor to plan the right diet and mode of delivery. During a flare, you may not be able to eat solid foods by mouth, or you may need supplemental nutrition via an IV. An RD will map out nutritional plans for you depending on your caloric requirements and disease activity status. An RD will also check your nutrition status through different laboratory tests and make adjustments to the diet plan accordingly.

Psychiatrists

In the past, people believed that stress was one of the major causes of Crohn's and colitis. Recent studies have not shown that stress actually causes the disease. However, Crohn's and colitis themselves can add stress to your life. Even just getting diagnosed can be stressful. Rushing to the bathroom and having to miss school or work can be stressful and can even cause depression. When you don't feel well or when you're dealing with a chronic illness, you can face physical *and* psychological stress.

Psychological stress may present itself as irritability, anxiety, depression, or even panic attacks. This can aggravate your Crohn's and colitis symptoms. You may require medical therapy for stress, anxiety, or depression. Your primary-care doctor or gastroenterologist may be able to handle a mild form of these stressful conditions, but you may be referred to a psychiatrist for further evaluation. A psychiatrist can provide behavior therapy and other relaxation techniques that can not only help alleviate your mental symptoms but also have a positive effect on your Crohn's and colitis symptoms. Ask your primary-care doctor or gastroenterologist if she knows a psychiatrist who is familiar with Crohn's and colitis.

Surgeons

The goal of medical therapy (see Chapter 7) is to prevent surgery, but more than 50 percent of people with Crohn's or colitis end up needing to have surgery within five to ten years of diagnosis. Choosing a good surgeon is as important as choosing a good gastroenterologist. Surgeons specialize in different kinds of surgery — a brain surgeon won't do a hip replacement. So, as you might expect, you need to find a colorectal surgeon — a person trained to perform surgeries related to Crohn's and colitis (among other diseases). Your gastroenterologist can refer you to a surgeon he trusts.

Friends and family

Your friends and family members are a very important part of your healthcare team. Don't be afraid to ask them for a little support when you need it. They may be able to drive you to the doctor when you're not feeling well, take notes during your doctor visits so you don't have to worry about forgetting something the doctor said, or just help out around the house when you feel lousy.

Chapter 6

Getting a Diagnosis

In This Chapter

- Knowing what to expect on your first appointment
- Having a conversation with your doctor
- Being examined and going through tests
- Differentiating other diseases from Crohn's and colitis

There isn't a magic wand that can tell you or your doctor whether you have Crohn's disease or ulcerative colitis. Plus, many of the signs and symptoms are similar to those of other diseases. To make a diagnosis, your doctor gathers information from multiple sources. You undergo a thorough battery of examinations, lab tests, and imaging studies, not only to confirm the diagnosis but also to rule out other diseases.

A *sign* is something objective that you or your doctor observes or that your doctor finds on a physical exam (for example, being pale, having a rash, or passing blood in the stool). A *symptom* is something you can feel and tell your doctor about (for example, nausea or abdominal pain). Your doctor gathers information through the different signs and symptoms, constructs a diagnosis, and then orders tests to rule in or rule out Crohn's or colitis.

In this chapter, I walk you through your first visit and early conversations with your doctor, fill you in on the tests you may have, and then tell you about some other diseases that look a whole lot like Crohn's and colitis.

Preparing for Your First Visit

In Chapter 2, I describe common signs and symptoms of Crohn's and colitis that may prompt you to seek medical attention. You may start with a visit to your primary-care doctor or arrange a visit with a specialist (a gastroenterologist). You may even have to make a trip to the emergency room if your symptoms are severe.

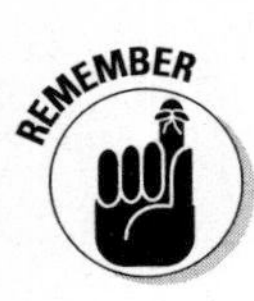

You can help your doctor make a diagnosis if you're able to draw a comprehensive and concise picture of your signs and symptoms. In this section, I show you how.

Charting your signs and symptoms

Before your first doctor's visit, take some time to chart your signs and symptoms. Following is a sample checklist of symptoms — you can use this if you like, or you can use it to jot down a list of your symptoms. Arriving at your first appointment with a list of your symptoms can be a real timesaver — and your doctor will love you for it!

Describe your symptoms. Check all that apply:

❑ Abdominal pain

Duration:	*Frequency:*
❑ Few weeks	❑ Once per month
❑ Few months	❑ Once per week
❑ Less than a year	❑ Every day
❑ Less than 5 years	❑ Several times per day
❑ 5 to 10 years	❑ Constantly

❑ Diarrhea

Duration:	*Frequency:*
❑ Few weeks	❑ Once per month
❑ Few months	❑ Once per week
❑ Less than a year	❑ Every day
❑ Less than 5 years	❑ Several times per day
❑ 5 to 10 years	❑ Constantly

❑ Urgency (the need to go right now)

Duration:	*Frequency:*
❑ Few weeks	❑ Once per month
❑ Few months	❑ Once per week
❑ Less than a year	❑ Every day
❑ Less than 5 years	❑ Several times per day
❑ 5 to 10 years	❑ Constantly

❑ Tenesmus (always feeling like you have to go)

Duration:	*Frequency:*
❑ Few weeks	❑ Once per month
❑ Few months	❑ Once per week
❑ Less than a year	❑ Every day
❑ Less than 5 years	❑ Several times per day
❑ 5 to 10 years	❑ Constantly

❑ Gas and bloating

Duration:	*Frequency:*
❑ Few weeks	❑ Once per month
❑ Few months	❑ Once per week
❑ Less than a year	❑ Every day
❑ Less than 5 years	❑ Several times per day
❑ 5 to 10 years	❑ Constantly

❑ Nausea and vomiting

Duration:	*Frequency:*
❑ Few weeks	❑ Once per month
❑ Few months	❑ Once per week
❑ Less than a year	❑ Every day
❑ Less than 5 years	❑ Several times per day
❑ 5 to 10 years	❑ Constantly

❑ Other: ____

____

____

____

Duration:	*Frequency:*
❑ Few weeks	❑ Once per month
❑ Few months	❑ Once per week
❑ Less than a year	❑ Every day
❑ Less than 5 years	❑ Several times per day
❑ 5 to 10 years	❑ Constantly

Describe your stools. Check all that apply:

❑ Mucus in the stool

❑ Pus in the stool

❑ Blood in the stool

❑ Stool that is black in color

❑ Hard, lumpy stools

❑ Loose, watery stools

❑ Undigested food in the stool

How many times do you go the bathroom during the day? ________________

Do you have to wake up at night to have a bowel movement? ________________

Describe your abdominal pain.

Location: ________________

Intensity of pain (on a scale from 0 to 10): ________________

Anything that makes the pain better: ________________

____

Anything that makes the pain worse: ________________

____

List any red flags. Check all that apply:

❑ Fever

❑ Weight loss

❑ Bloody diarrhea

❑ Nighttime diarrhea

❑ Worsening abdominal pain

Additional questions:

Have you missed school or work because of your symptoms? If so, approximately how much have you missed? ______________________

How are you currently managing your symptoms? Check all that apply:

- ❑ Prescription medications: ______________________
  ____
- ❑ Over-the-counter medications (such as NSAIDs): ______________________
  ____
- ❑ Herbal remedies: ______________________
  ____
- ❑ Other: ______________________
  ____

Are you getting any relief of your symptoms from any of the above? __________

____

____

In addition to charting your symptoms with the preceding questions, you may want to pay attention to your diet (especially alcohol, sugar, dairy, wheat, and processed food). Creating a food journal or diary isn't a bad idea. Your doctor may want to know if certain foods make your symptoms better or worse.

Assembling your medical records

In order for your doctor to develop an accurate picture of your medical condition, she has to review your medical history. You may have undergone tests, procedures, and other investigations in the past that could shed light on your situation today. In this section, I fill you in on what you should try to pull together before that first appointment.

If you're seeing a specialist, your primary-care physician should be able to send him your health records.

Medical history

It may be important for your doctor to know if you have any other health problems, such as thyroid disease, diabetes, heart disease, joint problems, kidney problems, or skin diseases such as eczema. If you have any health problems, write down the date of diagnosis of each illness and any medications you were prescribed.

If a family member has been diagnosed with Crohn's or colitis, definitely make note of that — there is a genetic component to both diseases (see Chapter 4). If you know where the colitis or Crohn's disease occurred (for example, proctitis or Crohn's disease of the colon only), note that as well.

Surgical history

List all your previous surgeries, even if they don't seem remotely related to Crohn's or colitis. Surgery is an important landmark in the natural history of Crohn's and colitis, so your doctor will need to know when, where, and who did your surgery. The type of surgery and exactly what was done during the surgery are also important points to note.

Social history

Make note of whether you've ever smoked, how much, and when you quit (if you have already). Also, make note of how much you drink. Finally, be prepared to talk with your doctor about your dietary habits, as well as your educational background and your job.

Smoking increases a person's risk of developing Crohn's. Alcohol consumption can also worsen the symptoms of Crohn's and colitis.

Drug history

List all the drugs you're currently taking or were recently prescribed. Note their dosages and how long you took them.

Your primary-care doctor can provide a list of medications you've taken.

Talking to Your Doctor

You've assembled your medical records and a summary of your symptoms, and now you're ready to talk to the doctor. In this section, I prepare you for that initial conversation.

Getting over the embarrassment

Many people aren't all that comfortable talking about their poop. When you see a doctor, you need to be specific, detailed, and even graphic. Just telling your doctor, "I go to the bathroom a lot" won't get you very far. If you feel shy talking about your symptoms, imagine you're talking to yourself and just spit it out and get it over with.

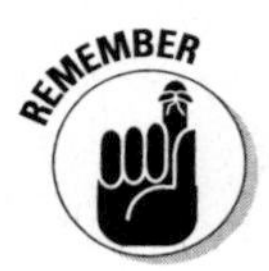

Your doctor has probably heard it all, so you don't need to tiptoe around this topic.

Communicating your symptoms

While your doctor is looking at the written records you've provided, she'll most likely ask you questions about your symptoms. Just tell your story.

Here's an example of the kind of things patients have shared with me:

> I noticed that I was passing loose stools last year. Initially, I would go to the bathroom two or three times a day, and my stools were loose and watery. There was no blood in in the beginning, but as time passed, I noticed that my diarrhea started to get worse with occasional blood. The blood would be mixed with the stool, and usually it was maroon to dark red in color. I also started noticing that I was waking up at night to go to the bathroom to have a bowel movement. I started losing weight, and I didn't have much of an appetite. I've also been experiencing abdominal pain, usually on the lower-right side of my belly. It's crampy and gets worse after I eat certain foods, like salads. Over the past month, the pain has been getting worse. I feel like I can't work comfortably without going to the bathroom three or four times during the day. It's really affecting my job, and sometimes I have to skip important meetings because I'm afraid my stomach will start gurgling and cramping.

When it comes to describing your stools, you can say they're one of the following:

- **Formed:** Like a sausage but with cracks on the surface
- **Semiformed:** Soft blobs with clear-cut edges or fluffy pieces with ragged edges
- **Liquid:** Watery with no solid pieces

Being realistic about your expectations

Your doctor doesn't have a magic wand that he can wave to make the diagnosis and make your symptoms go away in one visit. Think of dealing with Crohn's or colitis like a marathon, not a sprint. It may take time to manage your symptoms. Your doctor will need time to complete his evaluation and confirm a diagnosis. Only then can the treatment begin.

Knowing What to Expect during a Physical Exam

After your doctor has obtained a detailed history of your symptoms, she'll perform a thorough physical examination to look for signs of Crohn's and colitis and their complications. A physical examination can be divided into three parts: a general physical exam, a focused physical exam, and a rectal exam.

General physical exam

In a general physical exam, your doctor assesses your general health. A general physical exam can give lots of clues about your disease status and possible complications.

The doctor (or more likely a nurse) will take your blood pressure, temperature, pulse, and breathing rate; these are called *vital signs.* The doctor then performs a quick head-to-toe examination. She'll be looking for things like hair loss, thin and dry hair, acne, skin rashes, white spots on your nails, spoon-shaped nails, and numbness of the feet. These can indicate a variety of vitamin or mineral deficiencies, steroid use, fungal infections, or drug reactions.

What your doctor can learn from very simple physical signs may surprise you.

Focused physical exam

A focused physical exam includes an examination of your belly. Your doctor will do the following:

- **Feel for any tender spot:** Tenderness indicates inflammation. If your belly is distended, it may be due to entrapment of gas or swelling of your intestines.

  A very distended and tender abdomen may be a sign requiring urgent attention, and your doctor may order an urgent X-ray or even hospital admission.

- **Listen to your bowel sounds with a stethoscope:** Decreased bowel sounds may suggest slowing of your intestines due to inflammation.
- **Look for any signs of abnormal discharge, such as pus or stool:** Abnormal discharge may indicate fistula formation. Fistulas can form on the surface of your abdomen or close to the anus. (See Chapter 2 for more on fistulas.)

Rectal exam

The final part of the physical exam is the rectal exam. Your doctor will ask you to lie on your side, facing away from her, and have you curl your knees up in the fetal position. Alternatively, your doctor may ask you to bend over the exam table, place your elbows on the table, and squat down slightly. Then the doctor will ask you to take a deep breath as he slips his finger into your anus. (Don't worry — he'll wear a glove and use lubrication on his finger.)

During a rectal exam, your doctor is looking for *anal fissures* (cuts on the internal lining of the anal canal), *perianal fistulas* (abnormal openings around the anus), and *masses* (such as rectal cancer) or even an enlarged prostate (in men).

Being Poked and Prodded for Medical Tests

If your doctor suspects that you have Crohn's or colitis, he may order some medical tests. Medical tests are done to help confirm the diagnosis of Crohn's and colitis. They also help assess the degree and severity of inflammation produced by these illnesses. These tests help the doctor select the appropriate therapy for you.

Blood tests

Blood tests provide information about disease severity and may also help your doctor assess your nutritional status. Your doctor may also order a blood test before putting you on immunosuppressive medications. Here are some of the blood tests you may have:

- **Complete blood count (CBC):** A CBC helps your doctor look at the following: your white blood cells, red blood cells, hemoglobin, and platelet count.
    - **White blood cells:** If you have active disease, your white blood cell count may be elevated. This suggests that your body is producing more white blood cells to go to the site of inflammation.

      After getting started on immunosuppressive medications, your white blood cell count may start to go down. Your doctor will monitor your CBC to ensure the white blood cell count isn't going down too much and putting you at risk for more infections.

- **Red blood cells and hemoglobin:** Your red blood cells carry hemoglobin that delivers oxygen to different organs. In case of active disease, your body may not produce enough hemoglobin and you'll be at risk for *anemia* (low hemoglobin). You can also become anemic if you lose blood from your intestines, which can happen during inflammation that may lead to ulcer formation and bleeding from the intestines.
- **Platelets:** When you cut your skin and bleed, you eventually stop bleeding. This happens as a blood clot is formed at the site of bleeding. Platelets play an important role in forming blood clots. In Crohn's and colitis, when the inflammation causes ulcers and those ulcers bleed, your platelets try to form a blood clot and stop the bleeding. So, when you have active inflammation, your body starts producing more platelets and your blood test will show increased platelet count. High platelet count may suggest increased inflammation.

- **C-reactive protein (CRP):** CRP is an indirect marker of inflammation. During active disease, you have higher levels of CRP and when the inflammation is under control, the levels go down.
- **Erythrocyte sedimentation rate (ESR):** ESR is another marker of inflammation. An increase in inflammation will increase your ESR.
- **Liver function tests:** There are several reasons your doctor will check your liver functions:
  - Crohn's and colitis can affect your liver. An abnormal liver function test can alert your doctor to rule out primary sclerosing cholangitis (PSC; see Chapter 2).
  - Prescription medications (including those taken for Crohn's and colitis) can adversely affect the liver. Your doctor may want to check your baseline liver function and then monitor it while you're taking medications.
- **Vitamin B12:** Vitamin B12 is absorbed in the last part of the small intestine called the *terminal ileum*. Inflammation of the terminal ileum, as is seen in Crohn's disease, can compromise the body's ability to absorb vitamin B12. Your doctor may test your B12 levels to see if inflammation is affecting your terminal ileum and compromising your B12 absorption. If your B12 levels are low, you may be put on a vitamin B12 supplement.
- **Vitamin D:** If you have Crohn's or colitis, you may also be at risk for vitamin D deficiency for several reasons. Intestinal inflammation, malnutrition, and steroids put you at risk. Your doctor may want to check your vitamin D levels to make sure you're not deficient. Deficiency of vitamin D puts you at risk for *osteoporosis* (weakening of the bones).

IBD serology

IBD serology is a relatively new blood test — it's still not widely available — but there is a lot of hype about it in the medical community. It detects antibodies against certain bacterial products. The higher the load of these antibodies, the more aggressive disease you may have. So, you can determine the prognosis of the disease based on this test. It can predict with some degree of certainty your risk of having aggressive disease and complications like risk of stricture formation and risk of having surgery in the future. However, it isn't a crystal ball, and it's far from perfect.

Remember: IBD serology can help your doctor understand how aggressive your disease is, but it doesn't help your doctor diagnose and differentiate Crohn's from colitis. The sensitivity and specificity of this test to help diagnose and differentiate the two diseases isn't high. Also, not all people with positive serology will have IBD, and not all people with negative serology won't have IBD.

Stool tests

Stool tests provide useful information about the presence of inflammation in your intestines. They also rule out certain infections that may look like colitis or even coexist with colitis.

When your doctor orders this test, the laboratory personnel can explain to you how to collect the specimen. Usually a specimen container is provided to you, and you can bring back your stool specimen later. Most of the time you have a 24- to 48-hour period in which to return the stool specimen to the lab.

Scans

You can tell your symptoms to a doctor and she can perform a thorough examination, but some unanswered questions may remain. Where exactly is the disease? What is the extent of the disease? And are there any complications, such as fistula formation? To answer these questions, your doctor will need to send you for one or more scans.

Here are some of the scans you may have:

- **Abdominal X-ray:** Abdominal X-ray is one of the simplest radiology tests. You lie down or stand in front of the X-ray machine, it takes a picture, and you're done. Abdominal X-ray is very helpful when you're having acute flare and suffering from abdominal pain, tenderness, and distension. It can rule out any emergency situation, such as severe dilation of the colon (also known as *megacolon*) or obstruction of the intestines.

- **GI series and small bowel follow-through:** For this test, you have to drink a chalky white fluid called *barium,* which makes the gastrointestinal tract visible on X-ray film; you'll have to drink two or three glasses, and X-rays will be taken every 15 to 20 minutes until the barium has passed into the large intestine. In addition, you can't eat or drink dairy products the day before the exam. When an X-ray is done to look at the esophagus and stomach, it's called an *upper GI series;* when it's done to look at the small intestine, it's called *small bowel follow-through.* The test can reveal ulcers and strictures, among other things. It can last anywhere from 30 minutes to many hours depending on how fast the liquid can move through your small intestine.
- **CT scans:** *CT* stands for computed tomography. An abdominal CT scan is an imaging method that uses X-rays to create cross-sectional pictures of the belly. The CT scanner is a large boxlike machine with a short tunnel in the center. You lie on a table that slides into the tunnel. The X- ray tube rotates around you. A computer creates separate images of your abdomen, called *slices.* These images can be viewed on a monitor or printed on film. Three-dimensional models of the belly area can be created by stacking the slices together. The scan usually takes less than 30 minutes to complete.

  CT scans of your abdomen and pelvis can tell your doctor the location of inflammation and any complications such as *abscess* (a collection of pus), fistula, or strictures.

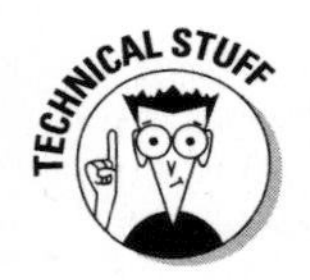

  CT scans expose you to more radiation than regular X-rays. Having many CT scans over time may increase the risk of certain cancers. You and your doctor should weigh this risk against the benefit of getting a correct diagnosis or ruling out complications from Crohn's and colitis.
- **MRIs:** Magnetic resonance imaging (MRI) is a radiology test similar to the CT scan. However, instead of X-rays, MRI uses a magnetic field and pulses of radio waves to make pictures of different organs and structures inside your belly. It may give more detailed information than an X-ray or CT scan. Because no X-rays are involved, there is no increased risk of cancer from repeated MRIs.

  Strong magnetic fields are created during MRIs. Be sure to tell your doctor if you have a pacemaker or other metal implants inside your body — MRIs can be dangerous to people with pacemakers or metal implants.

Endoscopy

Endoscopy is a medical procedure that uses a tubelike instrument called an *endoscope.* The endoscope is put into the body to look inside and perform certain surgical procedures, such as taking a biopsy from the internal lining of the intestines.

Video capsule endoscopy

A capsule endoscopy camera sits inside a vitamin-size capsule that you swallow. As the capsule travels through your digestive tract, the camera takes thousands of pictures. This camera capsule has its own light source, and the pictures are transmitted to a recorder you wear on a belt around your waist. These images can be later seen on a computer screen. Physicians order this test when they suspect Crohn's disease of the small intestine.

This camera capsule comes without any navigating devices and there isn't a driver sitting inside the capsule, so it can get stuck in the small intestine. There is a 5 percent to 7 percent chance of capsule retention in patients with Crohn's disease. If this happens, you may need surgery to retrieve the capsule. Inflammation of the intestines may cause swelling and narrowing of the intestines that pose an additional risk of capsule retention. If your doctor wants to do a video capsule endoscopy, she'll talk to you about the risks and benefits before the procedure.

There are many different kinds of endoscopes. Most have a light source and a small video camera on the end that puts pictures on a computer screen. Endoscopes vary in length. Each type is specially designed for looking at a certain part of the body. In your diagnosis of Crohn's or colitis, you'll likely need to have an endoscopy.

Identifying Other Diseases That Mimic Crohn's and Colitis

Not everyone with abdominal pain, diarrhea, or blood in the stool has Crohn's or colitis. Any disease, including Crohn's and colitis, causing inflammation of the intestines can result in these symptoms.

Similarly, these symptoms can be produced without inflammation. Your doctor may discuss these different situations with you and order some further tests to rule out the other causes.

Here are some of the diseases that mimic Crohn's and colitis:

- **Irritable bowel syndrome (IBS):** IBS and inflammatory bowel *disease* (which Crohn's and colitis are part of) share many symptoms, such as abdominal pain and diarrhea. To complicate things further, about 20 percent to 30 percent of people with IBD also have IBS. The main difference between IBS and IBD is that the symptoms of IBS are produced *without* inflammation.

If you have abdominal pain or discomfort for at least three days in a month associated with two or more of the following, you are most likely to have IBS:

- Improvement in symptoms after having a bowel movement
- Onset of symptoms with a change in bowel habits
- Onset of symptoms with a change in the appearance of stool

- **Celiac disease:** Celiac disease causes damage to the inner lining of the small intestine, called the *mucosa,* and leads to malabsorption of certain foods. The inflammation of the mucosa produces symptoms that can be common to Crohn's and colitis, such as abdominal pain and diarrhea. If you have celiac disease, your intestines are allergic to foods containing *gluten* (a protein found in products made from wheat). A gluten-free diet helps improve celiac disease, but gluten has no bearing on Crohn's or colitis.

- **Microscopic colitis:** As the name implies, this type of colitis is at a microscopic level. You're diagnosed with microscopic colitis only if an endoscopy reveals normal-appearing mucosa, but a biopsy of the mucosal specimens reveals inflammation under the microscope. Microscopic colitis causes watery diarrhea. There is no blood in the stool and no obvious sign of inflammation — except under the microscope.

  Microscopic colitis has not been extensively studied. There may be a genetic or autoimmune phenomenon causing microscopic colitis.

- **Ischemic colitis:** *Ischemia* means restriction of blood supply to an organ. It leads to a shortage of oxygen and glucose, which are vital to the function of the organ and keeps it alive. Ischemia happens when a blood clot causes blockage in the blood vessels. If your heart gets ischemia, you have a heart attack; if your brain gets ischemia, you have a stroke. Similarly when your intestines get decreased blood supply, the inner lining of the intestines get inflamed because of low blood flow, leading to ischemic colitis.

  Usually, ischemic colitis happens in older people when a blood clot or low blood pressure compromises the flow of blood to the colon.

  Ischemic colitis is a medical emergency. If left untreated, it can cause gangrene (death) of the colon cells. The colon can rupture, releasing toxins into the abdominal cavity. Unless treated immediately, it's fatal.

  Symptoms include abdominal pain, nausea, vomiting, and passing blood in the stool. It's treated by correcting the underlying cause of the ischemia. If diagnosed early, you're cured in days or weeks (as opposed to Crohn's and colitis, which are chronic, lifelong diseases).

- **Diverticulitis:** Small pockets or pouches in the inner lining of the colon are called *diverticulosis.* (A single pocket is a *diverticulum;* more than one pocket are *diverticula.*) This condition is very common in people over 50.

You may not even know that you have diverticulosis until you get a colonoscopy for some other reason and your doctor tells you that you have diverticulosis. Diverticula usually don't produce any symptoms. On occasions, they can bleed and you may notice blood in the stool. If they get inflamed, it's called *diverticulitis.*

The exact causes of diverticulosis and diverticulitis aren't known. Some scientists believe that a low-fiber diet puts you at risk for the condition. If you develop diverticulitis, you may experience abdominal pain, blood in the stool, nausea, vomiting, and fever. A CT scan of the abdomen usually confirms the diagnosis.

- **Infectious colitis:** Inflammation of the colon caused by infection is called *infectious colitis.* Just as infection of the skin causes swelling, redness, and even ulcers and bleeding, infection of the colon produces similar findings inside the colon. This infection can look quite similar to Crohn's or colitis. But infection usually happens after you drink water or eat food contaminated with bacteria, viruses, or parasites.

Your doctor may do some tests to rule out these conditions as she's confirming your diagnosis of Crohn's disease or ulcerative colitis.

Chapter 7

Taking Medications for Crohn's and Colitis

In This Chapter

- Recognizing the strong work of steroids
- Acknowledging the work of aminosalicylates
- Identifying medications that suppress your immunity
- Understanding the role of antibiotics
- Looking at other drugs and their uses in Crohn's and colitis

When doctors treat Crohn's and colitis, their primary goal is to bring about remission and keep you there.

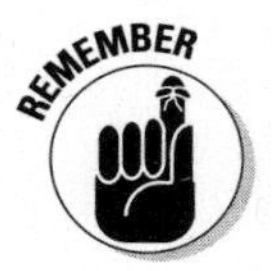

Remission is the state in which the disease is inactive and causing no symptoms. But being in remission doesn't mean you're cured. Though researchers continue to search for a cure, current medications only reduce inflammation or eliminate the symptoms rather than the underlying causes.

When you're in remission, your doctor will use medications for *maintenance* (preventing symptoms from coming back). The majority of patients enjoy long-term remission and relief from symptoms; a small percentage with severe disease may experience unrelenting symptoms that don't respond well to treatment.

Symptom control is not the only goal your doctor will try to achieve with medical therapy. Your doctor also prescribes medications to

- Prevent future flare
- Prevent hospitalization
- Prevent complications such as cancer
- Prevent or delay surgery
- Avoid steroid prescription
- Offer a cost-effective therapy

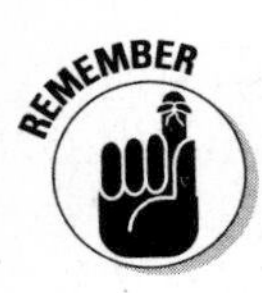

Each individual responds differently to the medications used to treat Crohn's and colitis, so your doctor may try many different treatments to find the drug or combination of drugs that's best for you.

In this chapter, I fill you in on the main medications used to treat Crohn's and colitis, tell you when they're used, and explain some of the side effects you may experience when you take them.

Steroids

You've probably heard of steroids, and you may even have taken them before. *Steroid* is the name commonly used to refer to *glucocorticoids,* a class of drugs related to the natural hormone hydrocortisone, or simply cortisol. This chemical is essential for many bodily processes, including metabolism, bone formation, and regulation of the immune system. The anti-inflammatory properties of steroids can be used to treat many medical conditions, like asthma, certain rashes, arthritis, and many autoimmune diseases. They're commonly prescribed medications in the treatment of Crohn's and colitis, especially in the management of flares.

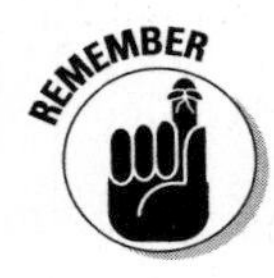

Your doctor may prescribe steroids, but you won't be getting juiced up the way athletes do. Steroid hormones are actually a large class of fatty molecules the human body makes from cholesterol. These include estrogen, progesterone, testosterone, and glucocorticoids. Athletes often abuse anabolic steroids, a kind of synthetic steroid, to gain muscle mass. The effects of the kind of steroids you may be given aren't related to anabolic steroids, so if you were hoping to be able to keep pace with Lance Armstrong, think again.

Types of steroids

Steroids come in oral and intravenous preparations. Most are given orally in pill form. In severe cases that require hospital admission, doctors sometimes administer steroids intravenously. In some patients with colitis, doctors choose to administer steroids with an enema so the steroids can work directly on the walls of the colon. (See the nearby sidebar for more on enemas.)

Steroids can be divided into two groups: systemic and non-systemic.

Systemic steroids

Systemic steroids work on the whole body — their effects are not limited to the gut. Because they work on the whole body, systemic steroids can cause both benefits and side effects for the brain, skin, bones, muscles, and other organs. Commonly used systemic steroids include prednisone, methylprednisolone, and hydrocortisone.

All about enemas

An *enema* is a liquid drug inserted into the rectum for the treatment of colitis. Being liquid in nature, it travels up your colon and treats inflammation in the rectum, as well as the sigmoid, descending, and even transverse colon. For Crohn's and colitis, enemas are often used on their own or, most commonly, in combination with oral pills to treat colitis. Recent studies have suggested that if you take an enema along with oral pills for colitis, you get better and faster results.

Enemas are best taken at bedtime. For best results, empty your bowels before using the enema. Usually the enema comes in a bottle. Make sure you shake the bottle well to thoroughly mix the drug. Then remove the protective sheath from the applicator tip. Hold the bottle at the neck so you don't cause any of the medication to be discharged. For best results, your doctor or pharmacist will instruct you to insert the medication by lying on your left side with your left leg extended and your right knee tucked up toward your stomach. You then gently insert the applicator tip in the rectum, pointing toward the navel. Grasp the bottle firmly and squeeze slowly. With steady hand pressure, most of the medicine is discharged. After using, withdraw the bottle and throw it away. You need to remain in this position for at least 30 minutes to allow complete distribution of the medicine.

Mesalamine enemas can stain fabrics, granite, marble, and vinyl. Keep this in mind before giving yourself a mesalamine enema.

Non-systemic steroids

Budesonide (Entocort) and budesonide MMX (Uceris) are *non-systemic* steroids. Non-systemic steroids' effects are mostly limited to the gut, so they can be great for gut-specific diseases like Crohn's and colitis. Non-systemic steroids provide many of the benefits of systemic steroids with lesser side effects to organs outside the gastrointestinal tract.

Budesonide works best on the last part of the small intestine (the *ileum*) and the first part of the colon (the *ascending colon*), so it's a great drug for Crohn's disease of these locations. Budesonide MMX is a recently approved drug that works on the entire colon and is good for colitis patients.

How steroids work

Steroids have many effects throughout the body, but the most important one for Crohn's and colitis is the anti-inflammatory and immunosuppression effect. Steroids are immunosuppressive drugs that decrease the immune system's ability to fight infection and cause inflammation. This may sound like a bad idea, but if the immune system is attacking things it shouldn't (the way it does in Crohn's and colitis), steroids make sense.

Steroids make it difficult for the white blood cells that cause inflammation to get where they want to go. They keep the cells from sticking to blood vessels, an important way they travel to areas of inflammation. Without this ability, white blood cells are unable to get to the gut to cause problems. Steroids also keep cells from releasing and responding to signals the cells use to recruit more cells to inflamed tissue, thus reducing inflammation.

When steroids are used

Steroids are used to bring about remission when there is active inflammation in the bowel. They shouldn't be used for maintenance of remission because of the side effects they cause and because they aren't good at preventing symptoms from coming back in the long term. For this reason, steroids are a short-term, not a long-term, treatment.

Talk with your doctor about the long-term plan to manage your disease with other anti-inflammatory medications, and not using steroids long term.

A typical steroid regimen may consist of a 6- to 12-week course of the drug with a *taper.* Tapering is when your doctor slowly decreases the dose taken each week to wean you off the medication. This gradual reduction in the dose helps prevent complications that can happen if the drugs are stopped abruptly. Steroids are the only medication you'll be given for Crohn's or colitis that requires tapering. If steroids are used for a short period of time, your doctor may simply have you stop the steroids instead of tapering the dose.

Steroids are especially useful to treat flares. When you have a flare, your doctor may add steroids to another maintenance medication to reduce the inflammation of the flare. But you just can't keep on getting steroids each time you flare. If you're receiving frequent steroid prescriptions (such as more than two or three times a year) or you're becoming steroid dependent, it may be the time to step up your therapy and use more potent drugs such as azathioprine or anti-TNF drugs for remission. Even surgery is sometimes considered a better option than staying on steroids.

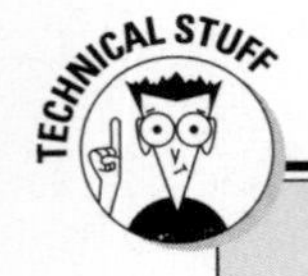

Steroid withdrawal syndrome

Your body makes about 5 mg to 7 mg of prednisone daily in the *adrenal glands* (small glands located on the top of your kidneys). When you take steroids, your body sends a signal to your adrenal glands to shut down the factory of steroid production because there are enough steroids in the body. If you've been taking steroids for a long time, and then you stop it all of a sudden, your body won't have enough time to start making steroids in the adrenal gland. You may suffer from a withdrawal effect. The symptoms include lightheadedness, weakness, and headaches; you may even faint. Be sure to follow your doctor's instructions for tapering off steroids.

For more on steroid withdrawal syndrome, turn to Chapter 8.

Side effects of steroids

The side effects of steroids are numerous and increase with the length of time you take them. When you take steroids less than six weeks, here are the side effects you may experience:

- Weight gain
- Facial swelling
- Mood swings
- Trouble sleeping
- Acne
- Increase in appetite
- High blood glucose
- Headache

If you take steroids more than six weeks, you may experience all the short-term side effects, as well as the following:

- Easy bruising of the skin
- Thinning of the skin
- *Osteoporosis* (weakening bones)
- Diabetes
- High blood pressure
- Cataracts
- Cushing's syndrome
- Infections
- Muscle weakness
- Fatty liver
- Depression
- Growth problems in children

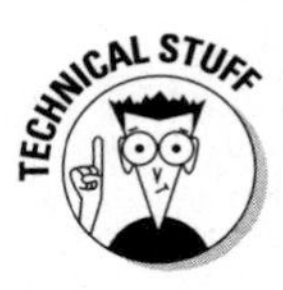

In *Cushing's syndrome,* you develop facial swelling, a fatty hump between your shoulders, a big belly with thin legs, and purple stretch marks on the skin.

Aminosalicylates

Unlike many other treatments for Crohn's and colitis, aminosalicylates do not suppress the immune system. They reduce inflammation without decreasing the body's ability to fight infection. Because they act locally on the bowel wall, aminosalicylates have fewer side effects. They've proven to be much more effective in treating colitis than they are in treating Crohn's, but they still have a role in the treatment of Crohn's colitis. Doctors often use aminosalicylates as a first-line attempt at treatment of mild disease due to their milder side effects.

Types of aminosalicylates

There are two types of aminosalicylates: mesalamine and sulfasalazine.

Mesalamine

Mesalamine (also called mesalazine) is an anti-inflammatory drug that is similar to aspirin. (You may hear it referred to as 5-aminosalicylic acid, or 5-ASA for short.) Mesalamine can be administered orally in a pill, as a suppository, or in an enema. This drug has several brand names and is available in different controlled-release or delayed-release formulas. The different types of mesalamine and their brand names are summarized in Table 7-1.

Table 7-1 Mesalamines

Common Brand Name	*Formulation*	*Use*
Apriso	Capsule	Colitis
Asacol, Asacol HD	Tablet	Colitis
Cannasa	Suppository	Proctitis
Colazal	Capsule	Colitis
Dipentum	Capsule	Colitis
Delzicol	Tablet	Colitis
Lialda	Tablet	Colitis
Pentasa	Capsule	Colitis
Rowasa	Suspension enema	Proctosigmoiditis

All about suppositories

A *suppository* is a drug that is inserted into the rectum where it dissolves or melts. They're usually given for some local action or when you're unable to take anything by mouth. Pain and nausea medications are usually given in the form of suppositories.

For Crohn's and colitis, if the disease is confined to the rectum or rectum and sigmoid colon, you may not need oral pills — just taking a once-a-day suppository may be more than enough. Occasionally, your doctor may prescribe a suppository along with oral pills to control symptoms of urgency and *tenesmus* (always feeling like you have to go). Oral pills or tablets may take longer to relieve these symptoms.

The best time to take a suppository is at bedtime. After emptying your bowels and washing your hands, you remove the foil or plastic wrapping from the suppository. You can moisten the end of the suppository with a little water if you want. Then gently but firmly push the suppository into the rectum with the pointed end first. Push it in far enough so that it doesn't slip out. Sit or lie still for a few minutes. Wash your hands again and try not to empty your bowels for at least one hour.

Sulfasalazine

Sulfasalazine was originally developed for the treatment of another autoimmune disease, rheumatoid arthritis. It's in the class of drugs called sulfonamides and consists of a sulfa molecule connected to 5-ASA. The sulfa molecule was originally added because of its antibacterial properties, but it has little effect in treating bowel inflammation. When the drug is broken down by the bacteria in the gut, the 5-ASA molecule is released and acts with the same mechanism as mesalamine. Doctors prescribe sulfasalazine less often than 5-ASA due to the side effects, such as nausea, vomiting, rash, and even *anaphylaxis* (a severe, whole-body allergic reaction to a chemical) caused by the sulfa portion of the drug.

The common brand name is Azulfidine, and it's given in tablet form for the treatment of colitis.

How aminosalicylates work

5-ASA works by inhibiting inflammatory white blood cells. It removes the free radicals these cells produce. *Free radicals* are volatile molecules used by inflammatory cells to cause destruction and the breakdown of tissue during inflammation. Aminosalicylates also directly inhibit inflammatory cells by blocking their cell-to-cell signaling and their ability to move around the body. Ultimately, they decrease tissue damage in the bowel and relieve symptoms. It may take few weeks before patients see the full benefit of the treatment.

When aminosalicylates are used

Aminosalicylates are more commonly used for colitis than for Crohn's. Doctors use these medications to both induce and maintain remission of mild to moderate colitis.

Your doctor may recommend oral treatment, rectal treatment, or an approach combining both types of treatment. Patients who value convenience may prefer the ease of oral treatment, but rectal treatment can offer added symptom relief.

Rectally administered aminosalicylates are an important treatment for patients with colitis. For patients with symptoms of pain and bleeding limited to the rectum or sigmoid colon, this may be the best option. Your doctor can administer the drugs in a suppository, an enema, or a foam injected into the rectum.

Oral aminosalicylates can be added if rectal treatments alone do not relieve symptoms. Also, if the inflammation involves a large part of the colon, oral drugs will be able to treat the areas of the colon that rectal treatment cannot reach.

Side effects of aminosalicylates

5-ASA has relatively mild side effects, which are related to its local action in the digestive system. Patients commonly report upset stomach and diarrhea. Other side effects such as *pancreatitis* (inflammation of the pancreas) and damage to the kidneys are rare. Your doctor will perform blood tests to check for kidney function at regular intervals.

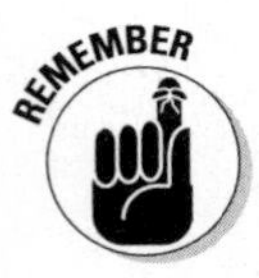

About 3 percent to 5 percent of patients may experience worsening of colitis symptoms on these drugs and are unable to tolerate them.

Patients using sulfasalazine may experience more side effects besides upset stomach and diarrhea. These include a rash, headache, fatigue, and infertility in men (which can be reversed if the medication is stopped). Rarely, it can cause a dangerous drop in white blood cell count. Sulfasalazine can also cause allergic reactions. Patients with a sulfa allergy should avoid sulfasalazine.

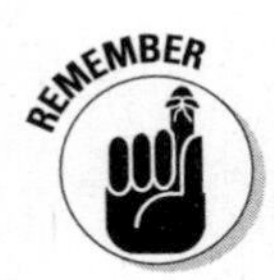

Sulfasalazine inhibits the production of folic acid, and you can develop folic acid deficiency and anemia if you don't take a supplement of folic acid (at least 1 mg daily).

Immunomodulators

Immunomodulators are drugs that decrease the number of inflammatory cells in the body. They're used to treat many autoimmune diseases, to prevent the rejection of transplanted organs, and to treat some types of cancer. Typically, doctors consider immunomodulators for patients who are not achieving remission after treatment with steroids, aminosalicylates, or antibiotics. If your disease is severe or aggressive, you may get started on these drugs as a first line of therapy.

Immunomodulators are often used as steroid-sparing drugs. In other words, they help patients get off steroids when they otherwise would be unable to because of their unrelenting disease symptoms.

Immunomodulators are especially useful for patients with complications such as fistulas caused by the inflammation of Crohn's. Because of their strong inhibition of white blood cells, they come with an increased risk of infection.

Types of immunomodulators

There are three types of immunomodulators: thiopurines, methotrexate, and cyclosporine and tacrolimus.

Thiopurines

Azathioprine and 6-mercaptopurine (6-MP) are classified as thiopurines, a class of drugs that mimics the building blocks of DNA. They look similar to these building blocks, so cells will try to use them, but when they do, the DNA-making process is disrupted and delayed.

6-MP is the active form of the drug that actually works to reduce inflammation, and azathioprine is converted to this active form by the body. Thus, both drugs have essentially the same mechanism of action, with azathioprine requiring an additional step to become active.

Methotrexate

Folic acid, also known as folate, is an essential molecule in the machinery used to create DNA for cells. Methotrexate is a drug that mimics folate, and when it's incorporated into the DNA-producing machinery, cell multiplication is inhibited.

Cyclosporine and tacrolimus

Both of these drugs inhibit special type of white blood cells called T cells or T lymphocytes. They inhibit the production of inflammatory cytokines by T cells.

How immunomodulators work

Immunomodulators work on the DNA of cells to decrease the amount of inflammatory white blood cells circulating in the body. All cells in the body use DNA, and each time a cell divides and multiplies, the DNA is copied. White blood cells multiply very quickly and have to make a lot of DNA to do this. Targeting the DNA slows their ability to proliferate and cause tissue destruction.

You can think of an immunomodulator as a monkey wrench your doctor throws into the machinery of DNA synthesis, disrupting the system and decreasing the speed at which cells can be made. Although inflammatory cells are prominently affected, DNA in other cells is also disrupted, leading to side effects. The overall goal is to decrease the number of inflammatory cells in the body, and decrease the amount of inflammation they can create in the gut.

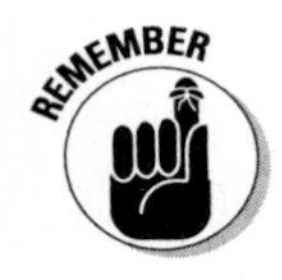

Azathioprine and 6-MP are very effective but slow-acting drugs. It may take two to four months before the full benefit is seen, so your doctor may put you on something else for the short term if your symptoms are severe.

When immunomodulators are used

Doctors use immunomodulators to induce and maintain remission in moderate to severe Crohn's and colitis. Your doctor may use these drugs if you fail to respond to aminosalicylates, steroids, and antibiotics. They aren't routinely used to treat mild disease. For patients who may have trouble weaning off steroids because of recurrent symptoms, immunomodulators can be used to treat the disease so the steroids can be discontinued.

Patients using thiopurines often require months of treatment to see results. Patients may see the greatest benefits within three to six months of use. Thiopurines are typically used as long-term treatment and are taken in pill form by mouth.

Though an oral form of methotrexate exists, the injectable form is more commonly used to treat inflammatory bowel disease (IBD). Your doctor or nurse can administer the shots once a week either under the skin or into a muscle. Some people can even inject themselves with the drug.

Cyclosporine is used in rare cases of severe colitis. It's usually given intravenously to get good levels of the drug in the blood as quickly as possible. When the desired level is achieved, the drug is usually given in the oral form. Cyclosporine is usually given for a few months until other potent but less toxic drugs start working. Tacrolimus is used even more rarely in difficult and tough cases of Crohn's and colitis; more studies are needed before we start using it widely.

Side effects of immunomodulators

These highly effective medications do come with the risk of side effects. You should always discuss risks and benefits of the drug with your doctor.

Common side effects of azathioprine/6-MP include the following:

- Decreased white blood cell count
- Increased risk of infection
- Nausea and vomiting
- Increased liver enzymes
- Muscle ache

Less common side effects of azathioprine/6-MP include the following:

- Hair loss
- Abdominal pain
- Pancreatitis, which causes abdominal pain, nausea, and vomiting
- Lymphoma

Common side effects of methotrexate include the following:

- Nausea
- Fatigue
- Skin rash
- Decrease in sperm count and possible birth defects in babies (people must wait three months after stopping methotrexate before trying to conceive)
- Diarrhea
- Decreased white blood cell count

Less common side effects of methotrexate include the following:

- Dizziness
- Liver toxicity
- Joint pain
- Kidney and lung toxicity

Women who are pregnant or may become pregnant cannot use methotrexate. Methotrexate can cause miscarriage or severe birth defects. For this reason, women of child-bearing age who are taking this drug should use two forms of birth control.

Biologics

Biologics are drugs manufactured through a biological process using human, animal, or microorganism sources. (This is in contrast to pharmaceutical drugs, which are manufactured from chemical processes.) Vaccines, insulin, and different blood products used from transfusions are examples of biologics. Biologics can also act as antibodies to certain inflammatory signals in the body. This is useful in Crohn's and colitis because, by binding up these signals, they inhibit the immune system's ability to attack the bowel.

Types of biologics

Different types of biologics are used in the treatment of Crohn's and colitis. They're often used when other drugs (such as 5-ASA or immunomodulators) fail to work.

Choosing a biologic

Because the cost, effectiveness, and potential side effects are all comparable, the choice of biologics depends on personal preference (both yours and your doctor's). Insurance coverage and availability of the drug may be the limiting factors in your decision.

Some of my patients like Remicade because it gives them an opportunity to visit their health-care team members. They want to have the drug given to them where doctors and nurses are available in case there is an infusion or other drug reaction. The infusion process last for a few hours. They get a chance to catch up on book reading or watch a movie during the infusion process. However, infusion involves missing work or school, which may not be desirable. Travel plans can be affected because you have to go to an infusion center on a regular schedule (for example, every six to eight weeks).

Other people like the convenience of giving themselves shots of Humira or Cimzia at home. Self-administered injections are also helpful for patients who travel a lot. However, some of my patients are scared of needles — even though it's a short, fine needle like the kind found in insulin syringes or the EpiPen. These patients usually come to my office or go to a clinic to have a nurse administer the injection. You may be able to arrange for a home-health nurse to visit your home or office and give you the injection.

Losing response to anti-TNF therapy

Anti-TNF drugs are highly effective and potent, but they aren't very long lasting. After one year, approximately one-third or even more people may lose response to these medications.

There are many reasons people lose response to the drugs. The most common cause is developing antibodies against the drugs. Your body considers the drugs foreign proteins and can make antibodies to counteract their effect.

When you lose response to the drug, your symptoms come back and you no longer feel better after an injection of the anti-TNF drug. Your doctor may check for drug levels and presence of antibodies by doing a simple blood test. Commercial blood tests to check drug levels or antibodies aren't available for all anti-TNF drugs. In the absence of these blood tests, your doctor may try to increase the dose or shorten the interval in an effort to increase the drug levels and overcome the antibodies. If this approach is unsuccessful, she may switch you to another anti-TNF drug or to a drug with a different mechanism of action.

Remember: Taking anti-TNF drugs on a regular basis makes them more durable. If you take these drugs irregularly or have unnecessary breaks in between doses, your body has a chance to develop antibodies, and you have greater chance of losing response early.

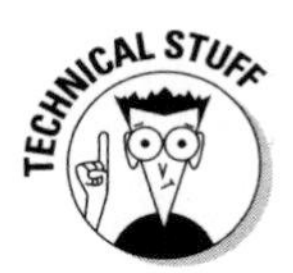

Scientists have recently discovered that early use of biologics in certain high-risk patients who have aggressive disease may be more helpful. When used early in those patients, it may change the natural course of the disease and prevent complications such as strictures or fistulas, which will eventually lead to lesser surgeries. However, considering the cost and side effects of biologics, they may not be suitable as first-line drugs for everyone at this point.

Anti-TNF drugs

Tumor necrosis factor–alpha (TNF-α) is a powerful component in the inflammatory process and has a large role in the disease process of Crohn's and colitis. Anti-TNF drugs attach to TNF-α to prevent it from working to cause inflammation.

There are three anti-TNF drugs currently available to treat Crohn's or colitis: infliximab (Remicade), adalimumab (Humira), and certolizumab pegol (Cimzia). These drugs are highly effective at controlling inflammation and lead to the healing of the mucosa.

Infliximab is the first biologic used in the treatment of Crohn's and colitis. It has been on the market for more than ten years. It's engineered to be 75 percent human and 25 percent mouse protein. Adalimumab and certolizumab pegol are made from human proteins.

Anti-TNF drugs derived from animal proteins may be associated with increased risk of infusion reactions, but even human proteins can cause reaction.

Before putting you on anti-TNF drugs, your doctor may order a hepatitis panel to check for hepatitis infection, especially hepatitis B. Crohn's and colitis themselves don't increase your risk of hepatitis B infection, but certain immunosuppressive medications such as anti-TNF drugs put you at a higher risk of hepatitis B reactivation. If reactivated, hepatitis B can be fatal.

Other biologics

Natalizumab (Tysabri) is another biologic. It binds to another protein that is important for the creation of inflammation. Sites of inflammation leave a type of protein sign post that white blood cells use to find where they should go. The cells travel through the bloodstream, latch onto these proteins, and leave the blood vessel to go into the tissue and cause inflammation. Natalizumab blocks these sign-post proteins to prevent the white blood cells from getting to the site and causing problems.

How biologics work

Biologics are protein antibodies designed to target specific molecules of the immune system. These specific molecules, such as TNF-α, are involved in inflammation and play important roles in inflammatory diseases such as rheumatoid arthritis, Crohn's, and colitis. The anti-TNF drugs bind these molecules and prevent them from promoting the process of inflammation.

When biologics are used

Biologics are used similarly to immunomodulators. They're considered steroid-sparing drugs, allowing patients to reduce or eliminate their use of steroids. And they're typically reserved for moderate to severe disease and are especially useful for Crohn's patients with fistulas and those who have failed to respond to more conventional treatments.

Biologics are fragile proteins that are destroyed in the body's digestive system. So, they don't come in tablet or pill forms. Adalimumab and certolizumab are administered in an injection under the skin, avoiding digestion. Infliximab has to be administered by *infusion* (the process by which a medication is injected slowly into a vein); this process takes a few hours to complete and requires a short visit to a clinic while the infusion takes place.

If you have an infection (such as a respiratory tract infection) or if you have a history of cancer or are currently being evaluated for cancer, you may not be a suitable candidate for biologics, and your doctor may defer the treatment until the infection is clear or your oncologist is okay with using these drugs.

Similarly, biologics have to be used very carefully in patients suffering from heart failure. If you have cardiac problems, your doctor may want to consult and work with your cardiologist before prescribing biologics.

Side effects of biologics

Biologics are protein antibodies that are administered into the body. Your body can sense these proteins as foreign bodies and develop its own antibodies to attack them. This can lead to a more serious infusion reaction or allergic reaction causing shortness of breath, fever, and rash. Luckily, this happens very rarely. Sometimes, your doctor may pre-medicate you with antihistamine (such as Benadryl), Tylenol, and a shot of steroids to prevent this hypersensitivity reaction from happening. If the reaction is severe enough, you may be switched to a different drug.

Another common side effect with self-administered biologics is simple injection-site reaction. Swelling and redness at the injection site pose no risk to the patient, but they can be very uncomfortable.

Biologics suppress the immune system. In doing so, they increase the risk of serious and *opportunistic infections* (infections that are usually rare in people with healthy immune systems). Examples of opportunistic infections are fungal lung disease, certain types of pneumonia, and severe viral infections.

Patients using biologics are also at increased risk of getting *tuberculosis* (TB), a serious bacterial lung infection. All patients who plan to start biologics should have a TB test before they start the drug. If patients already have TB in their lungs when they start an immune-suppressing drug, the disease can spread and get worse. (See the nearby sidebar for more on testing for TB.)

Testing for tuberculosis

Although Crohn's and colitis themselves do not increase your risk of TB, taking medications that suppress your immunity can certainly increase your risk for TB. You may have been exposed to TB bacteria in the past, and your body has successfully contained the bacteria without it causing any illness. For example, you may have inhaled TB and your lungs have TB, but your immune system successfully walled off the bacteria. If you take immunosuppressive medications, this wall can be weakened and TB bacteria can spread and cause illness. This is especially true in the case of anti-TNF therapy (biologics).

Your doctor can check if you've been exposed to TB in the past by doing a TB skin test. If the test is positive, he may want to do a chest X-ray and send you to an infectious disease doctor or TB expert for complete evaluation before putting you on immunosuppressive medications.

Counting the benefits of biologics

Some patients consider biologics scary drugs because they're associated with risks of infections and lymphoma. The risks with these drugs can't be denied, but they should always be weighed against the benefits you achieve with these drugs.

Risk of infection and cancer can be minimized by proper screening and monitoring. Without using these drugs, your options may be very limited, and surgery may be the next step. Some patients don't want to have an ostomy or scars on their abdominal skin, as well as suffer the risks and complications of surgery. In those situations, biologics come in handy.

Also, the latest research is showing that if we use biologics early in the disease, we may be able to change the disease course and prevent complications and risk of surgery altogether.

Remember: Every action or decision has risks and benefits. Would you stop driving a car because of the risk of getting in an accident, or stop swimming because of the risk of being attacked by a shark? Studies show that using biologics is associated with a decreased in risk of hospitalization, an increase in quality of life, and an overall ease in the burden of living with Crohn's and colitis by reducing disease activity and prolonging the time between flares.

Biologics also slightly increase the risk of developing a type of cancer called *lymphoma.* Scientists are still researching the association of biologics with the risk of lymphoma. Even though there is some risk of lymphoma with biologics, the risk is very small. In a normal population, the risk of lymphoma is 2 per 10,000. With biologics, the risk is 4 to 6 per 10,000. This risk increases especially in patients who take other immunosuppressive medications, such as azathioprine or who have taken anti-TNF drugs for a long time. Talk with your doctor and assess the risks and benefits of the drug before choosing any therapy.

Natalizumab activates a virus called JC virus, which causes a fatal brain infection called progressive multifocal encephalopathy (PML). PML is incurable and leads to permanent disability and even death. Therefore, patients and their doctors have to take special precautions when using this drug.

Antibiotics

Antibiotics are drugs that kill bacteria. Because bacteria are thought to play a role in the inflammation of Crohn's and colitis, reducing the number of bad bacteria in the gut with antibiotics makes sense.

Antibiotics are used in Crohn's and colitis in different scenarios. Your doctor will prescribe antibiotics if you develop a fistula, an abscess, pouchitis, or any other infection. The scientific evidence to treat Crohn's and colitis with antibiotics as primary medications isn't very strong — antibiotics are usually used as adjunct therapy, along with mainstay anti-inflammatory drugs.

Types of antibiotics

Metronidazole (Flagyl) and ciprofloxacin (Cipro, Proquin) are the antibiotics doctors most commonly use to treat Crohn's and colitis. Not all antibiotics are created equal, and some work better than others to kill different types of bacteria. Your doctor will choose the antibiotic that will work best to treat the type of infection you have.

There are many antibiotics doctors can choose from besides metronidazole and ciprofloxacin. Vancomycin (Vancocin) and rifaximin (Xifaxan) are two examples of other antibiotics your doctor may use.

How antibiotics work

The word *antibiotic* means "opposed to life." Fortunately, antibiotics are typically opposed to the life of bacteria. They do this by targeting specific parts of bacterial cells that are either absent in humans or are so different that the antibiotics affect the bacteria and don't affect you.

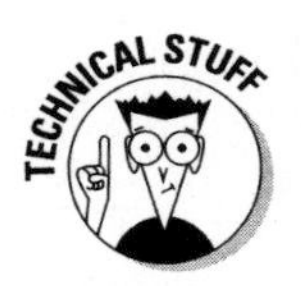

Ciprofloxacin blocks an enzyme in bacteria that unwinds their DNA, so it can be copied. This blocked enzyme prevents the bacteria from dividing and causes the DNA to split apart. Without functional DNA, the bacteria are unable to make proteins, and they die.

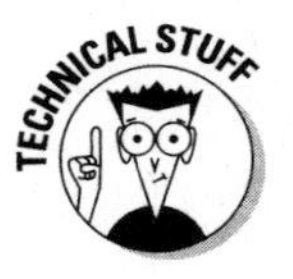

Metronidazole works by destabilizing bacteria DNA as well. The drug is absorbed by the bacteria, where it reacts with the organisms' DNA, causing breaks. The bacteria are then unable to make new proteins or multiply, and eventually they die.

When antibiotics are used

Doctors don't treat Crohn's and colitis with antibiotics alone. They're added to one or a combination of the drugs discussed in this chapter. But antibiotics are very important in the treatment of infection when bacteria get outside the bowels.

Common conditions treated with antibiotics in Crohn's and colitis include the following:

- Active Crohn's fistula
- Abdominal abscess
- Intestinal infections such as *Clostridium difficile*
- Pouchitis

Side effects of antibiotics

Antibiotics are generally considered to be safe, but some patients find it difficult to take metronidazole because of its side effects. It can cause a metallic taste in the mouth. Other common side effects include nausea, vomiting, indigestion, and diarrhea.

Long-term use of metronidazole, especially with high doses, may cause damage to the nerves in the feet and legs. This leads to numbness or tingling in the feet. Fortunately, these effects are usually reversible.

If you drink alcohol while taking metronidazole, you can become quite ill. You can experience flushing of the face, shortness of breath, severe headache, and rapid heartbeat. You may also develop nausea and vomiting and may even collapse. Many people prefer simply to avoid alcohol rather than risk being very ill from a reaction.

The other commonly used drug, ciprofloxacin, is also generally very safe. However, it does increase caffeine's stimulant effect. You don't need to avoid caffeine while on ciprofloxacin — you just need to be aware of this interaction and cut down on the amount of caffeine you consume if the side effects bother you.

Ciprofloxacin can cause ruptured tendons, particularly the Achilles tendon. This is especially true in young kids.

Other Medications

Besides the medications used to treat the specific symptoms of Crohn's and colitis, many others aim to treat the downstream effects of these diseases. Diarrhea is a serious problem common to both Crohn's and colitis, and it's often a target of treatment. Nutritional deficiencies are also common, especially in Crohn's disease. This can be due to an inflamed bowel that does not digest and absorb nutrients well. Some patients may have a large portion of their intestines removed due to severe disease, and what remains may not be adequate to absorb all the nutrients the body requires; this is called *short bowel syndrome.* In these cases, nutritional supplementation is used to replace deficiencies that develop.

In this section, I fill you in on other medications you may take as part of your treatment of Crohn's or colitis symptoms.

Top-down and bottom-up therapies

The goals of therapy are changing with increased knowledge about Crohn's and colitis. New research has also provided scientists with a better understanding of how the diseases behave. In the past, the main goal of therapy was symptom control. If you were feeling better, your doctor continued the same medications. If you had a flare, your doctor would prescribe steroids. But today we're learning that if we don't control the inflammation, we may not be able to change the natural course of the disease, and you may end up needing surgery. We've also learned the harmful consequences of steroid therapy if it's given for a longer period of time.

So, the current goals of therapy are to control inflammation, prevent steroid use, prevent surgery, and delay surgery as much as possible. This sometimes requires your doctor to use immunosuppressive medications early in the disease process. Even combination therapy with biologics is chosen earlier to prevent damage and keep you in good shape. This is called *top-down therapy* (as opposed to the traditional approach, or *bottom-up therapy,* where biologics are introduced after failure of immunosuppressive medications, which themselves are introduced after failure of mesalamine).

Scientists are working hard to identify which patients would benefit the most from the top-down therapy. This will soon help individualize medical therapy depending on your personal risk factors.

Antidiarrheals

A common symptom of Crohn's and colitis is diarrhea. There are many causes for diarrhea related to these diseases, and treating the underlying cause with the medications discussed earlier in this chapter often treats the diarrhea. However, sometimes this isn't enough, and your doctor may want to add another medication to treat symptoms of diarrhea.

Loperamide is a common first-line drug used for this purpose. It's also the safest of all the antidiarrheal drugs. It goes by a variety of brand names you may recognize, including Imodium. Other antidiarrheal medications include diphenoxylate, codeine, and other narcotics.

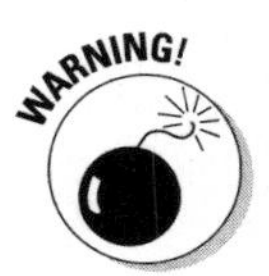

If you're having active flare and severe inflammation is causing you to have diarrhea, don't take an antidiarrheal. It will only mask the symptoms, and you may not get the medications you need. There is also a danger that slowing your intestines with an antidiarrheal will build up more inflammation and increase the risk of severe inflammation, colon dilation, and perforation.

Bile salt binders

Bile salts are absorbed in the ileum, which is the most common site of inflammation in Crohn's disease. Chronic inflammation in the ileum or a surgery in which the ileum is removed can cause bile salts to go unabsorbed until they're taken up by the colon. Bile salts are irritants to the colon lining and cause it to secrete water, producing diarrhea. Bile salt binders trap these molecules in the feces and prevent them from irritating the colon. Three common bile salt binders are cholestyramine (Questran), colestipol (Colestid), and cholesevem (Welchol). These drugs are effective in treating diarrhea because of ileal disease or previous ileal resection.

Bile salt binders can also bind and inhibit the absorption of certain vitamins. They can trap vitamins that otherwise would be absorbed by the body, preventing the body from using them. Vitamins A, D, E, and K can all be affected in this way. Your doctor may recommend that you supplement your diet by taking a multivitamin containing A, D, E, and K if you're taking a bile salt binder.

Bile salt binders also trap other medications and prevent them from being absorbed. If you take bile salt binders, do so one or two hours before or after you've taken your other medications.

Analgesics

When you have abdominal pain or fever, analgesics can help. But sometimes, the side effects of analgesics can be very dangerous, especially in Crohn's and colitis. The main analgesics that you may be familiar with are acetaminophen (Tylenol); non-steroidal anti-inflammatory drugs (NSAIDs), such as ibuprofen (Advil, Motrin), naproxen (Aleve), and aspirin; and narcotic pain killers such as codeine and morphine.

Acetaminophen (Tylenol) is safe and preferred for fever and pain. But taking large doses of acetaminophen or taking it for a long period of time may cause injury to your liver and kidneys.

NSAIDs, on the other hand, can cause ulcers in the stomach and intestines. When you have Crohn's or colitis and your intestines have inflammation, NSAIDs can sometimes cause worsening of the inflammation.

Narcotics are strong analgesics and are usually given after surgery to control pain. During acute flare of Crohn's and colitis, they can be used to control the severe pain. However, narcotics also have undesirable side effects. They slow your intestinal movement, which could be dangerous during acute flare, because it causes toxic material to build up, causing more dilation of the intestines and putting you at risk for perforation of the intestines. Narcotics are also associated with dependence, addiction, and increased risk of infections. Studies have even shown that these drugs may be associated with increased risk of death.

Talk to your doctor before taking any medication to treat fever or pain.

Iron

Iron is an important nutrient. It's used to make red blood cells that carry the oxygen your body needs. Crohn's patients may become iron deficient due to inflammation in the bowel, limiting its ability to absorb iron. Another common problem that affects both Crohn's and colitis is bleeding from the intestines. Chronic bleeding causes loss of blood cells that are packed with iron. Eventually, this can deplete the body's stores.

Supplemental iron is usually given in an oral pill, but in the most severe cases, its elemental form can be given intravenously in the hospital. Supplementation can prevent or treat iron-deficiency anemia.

Some patients with Crohn's and colitis may not tolerate oral iron pills — it may upset their stomachs. Talk with your doctor if you develop intolerance to oral pills. There are different preparations of oral iron that your doctor may want to try, or he may even consider prescribing you iron infusions as an alternative.

A diet rich in iron may help improve your iron stores. Iron is found in two different forms in food: heme iron, which is found in meat, and non-heme iron, which comes from plants. The body readily absorbs heme iron. Doctors and dietitians usually recommend taking vitamin C along with non-heme iron to increase the iron's absorption. Beef, chicken, and turkey are good sources of heme iron. Lentils, soybeans, spinach, and tofu contain non-heme iron.

Calcium and vitamin D

Patients with Crohn's and colitis often have problems with low levels of calcium and vitamin D. These nutrients are very important because of their role in maintaining strong, healthy bones. Their deficiency can cause bones to become weak and increase the risk of bone fractures. In children, the risk of calcium and vitamin D deficiency is even more dangerous; it can stunt their growth.

Several factors in Crohn's and colitis increase your risk of developing low levels of these nutrients. Inflammation in the intestines decreases their ability to absorb vitamin D and calcium. The poor absorption of fats by your intestines can also become a problem because these fats can bind to calcium, preventing its absorption and use by the body. Because the body doesn't make calcium and must get it from food, it will start breaking down its own bone when the levels become low.

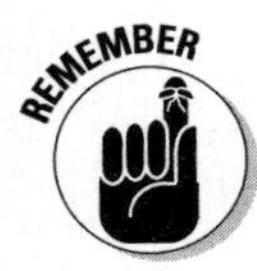

Your body also uses calcium for regulation of muscle contractions, forming blood clots when you bleed, and transmitting impulses through your nervous system.

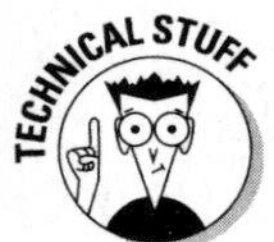

Along with low calcium and vitamin D, frequent use of steroids can also lead to thinning of the bones, a problem called *osteoporosis.* They do so by interfering with the absorption of calcium, causing bone breaks, and preventing new bone formation.

Your doctor can check the levels of calcium and vitamin D in your blood. Your doctor may also order a bone scan to check the thickness of your bones. If your levels of calcium and vitamin D are low or your bones look too thin, your doctor will have you take supplements. You may even be prescribed special medicines called *bisphosphonates* if you've already developed osteoporosis. Some doctors may also prefer to have their patients with Crohn's and colitis take calcium and vitamin supplements without these tests, as a preventive treatment.

You need at least 800 IU of vitamin D and 1,200 mg to 1500 mg of calcium every day to keep your bones healthy. This is especially true if you're taking steroids.

Vitamin B12

Vitamin B12 is an important nutrient used to build red blood cells and maintain healthy nerve cells. If you have low levels of B12, you may develop anemia because your body is unable to make enough blood cells without the vitamin. You may also experience confusion and loss of sensation related to dysfunction of the nervous system cause by low B12 levels.

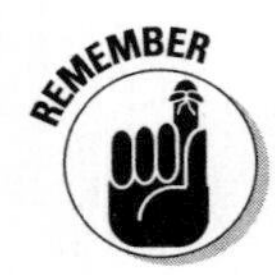

If you develop numbness or tingling in your hands or feet, you may be suffering from vitamin B12 deficiency.

Vitamin B12 is absorbed in the terminal ileum of the small intestine. If you have chronic inflammation in this area or have had surgery to remove the terminal ileum, you may develop a deficiency of B12. This typically happens with Crohn's disease and not colitis (colitis spares the terminal ileum).

Animal products such as meat are the best source for vitamin B12. Strict vegans are at risk for B12 deficiency. Excessive alcohol consumption also increases your risk for deficiency of this vitamin. If you're at risk for deficiency, you doctor may suggest you take extra vitamins, either in your diet or as a supplement.

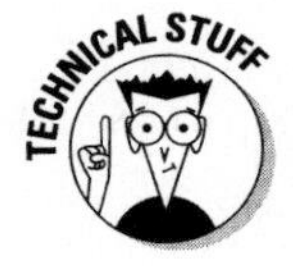

The body stores B12 that can last for years, so typically only those who have had disease for many years have a B12 deficiency.

Your doctor may check vitamin B12 levels with a blood test. If the levels are low, the vitamin can be administered with an injection under the skin using a small needle. A nasal spray for B12 is also available.

Chapter 8

Considering Surgery

In This Chapter

- Understanding when you need surgery for Crohn's or colitis
- Identifying the different types of surgery
- Considering the complications of surgery
- Dealing with an ostomy

If medications fail to control your symptoms and you have persistent inflammation, your doctor may recommend surgery as the next step. Because there is no cure for Crohn's and colitis, patients with these diseases will have to live with them for years. As time goes on, complications may arise that eventually necessitate surgery. One of the goals of therapy is to prevent and delay surgery, but unfortunately many patients with Crohn's and colitis will need surgery after several years of medical therapy.

In this chapter, I walk you through the types of surgery you may need and when you may need them.

When You May Need Surgery

There are different reasons to undergo surgery for Crohn's disease and ulcerative colitis. In this section, I fill you in on when surgery may be required for each disease.

For Crohn's disease

Most Crohn's patients will ultimately have surgery — 25 percent within 3 years of diagnosis and 75 percent within 20 years of diagnosis. Unfortunately, the management of Crohn's often requires multiple surgeries. One-fourth of people who undergo surgery will require another surgery within five years, and one-third of those people will eventually require a third surgery.

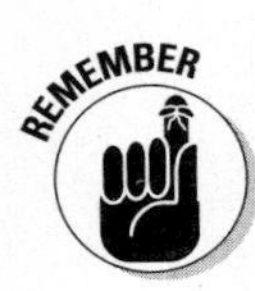

Having surgery for Crohn's disease gives you a fresh start. It gives you a chance to control the disease — possibly in a better way — before it gets a grip on you again.

As someone with Crohn's disease, you may need surgery if any of the following occurs:

- Medical intervention fails to control inflammation and symptoms persist.
- Complications (such as an abscess) develop.
- One or more fistulas develop that aren't successfully treated by medical therapy.
- A stricture with symptoms of obstruction develops.
- You become severely ill and your colon dilates to a dangerous level (called *toxic megacolon*).
- You experience severe bleeding.
- You develop cancer in your intestines

Some people also choose surgery over the complications caused by drugs that suppress the immune system. Additionally, children may need surgery if they aren't growing normally.

Because surgery does not cure Crohn's disease, one of the goals of postoperative care is the prevention of recurrence. Other than the obvious goal of avoiding repeat surgery because it's unpleasant, removing too much of your intestines can cause *short-bowel syndrome* — a condition in which you can't digest and absorb nutrients sufficiently because you don't have enough bowel.

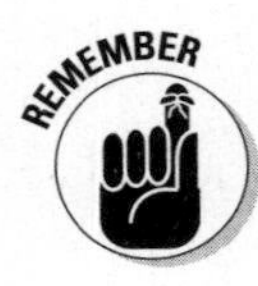

For people with Crohn's disease, surgery is not a last resort. It's simply another treatment option. Your doctor will help you decide if surgery is the best option for you.

For ulcerative colitis

You can't live without your brain, heart, or lungs, but you can survive without your colon. Your colon processes waste matter to be expelled as solid stool. This process is important, but thanks to modern medical advances, you can live just fine without it. And the news gets better: Removing the colon and rectum *cures* ulcerative colitis. After surgery, many patients return to my clinic saying, "I wish I'd had the surgery earlier!"

Your doctor will suggest surgery for you if any of the following situations applies:

- You fail to respond to medical therapy and continue having troubling symptoms.
- You can't tolerate medical therapy due to side effects or complications.
- You develop uncontrollable bleeding.
- You develop toxic megacolon.
- Your colon perforates.
- You develop *dysplasia* (a precancerous lesion) or cancer.

If a child with colitis is not growing normally, surgery may be necessary.

Your doctor will help you determine if surgery is the right course.

Types of Surgery

There are different types of surgeries for Crohn's and colitis. In this section, I cover the most important ones.

Resectioning the small intestine

Resection is the most common type of surgery for Crohn's disease. It involves cutting out the diseased part of the small intestine. Usually, the remaining two parts are joined together in what is called an *anastomosis* (see Figure 8-1). The most common site of Crohn's disease is the last part of the small intestine, the *terminal ileum,* which is connected to the colon. When the inflammation of this area becomes resistant to medical therapy, when you become dependent on steroids to control inflammation, or when you develop complications, your doctor may want to have this part of your intestine taken out. Besides persistent inflammation, the other reasons for resections include strictures, fistulas, perforation, and cancer.

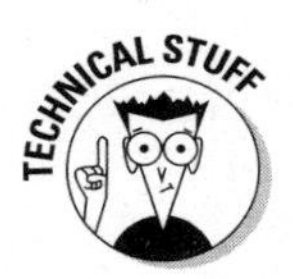

Sometimes the surgeon creates a temporary ostomy, bringing the end of the upper intestine out of the skin and closing the end of the lower intestine instead of joining them together. This usually happens when there is severe inflammation, presence of infection, or technical difficulties making it difficult to perform anastomosis during the first surgery. After few months of healing, the surgeon will go back and join the two ends together. This is called *temporary ileostomy,* and the surgical process of joining the intestines later is called *takedown.*

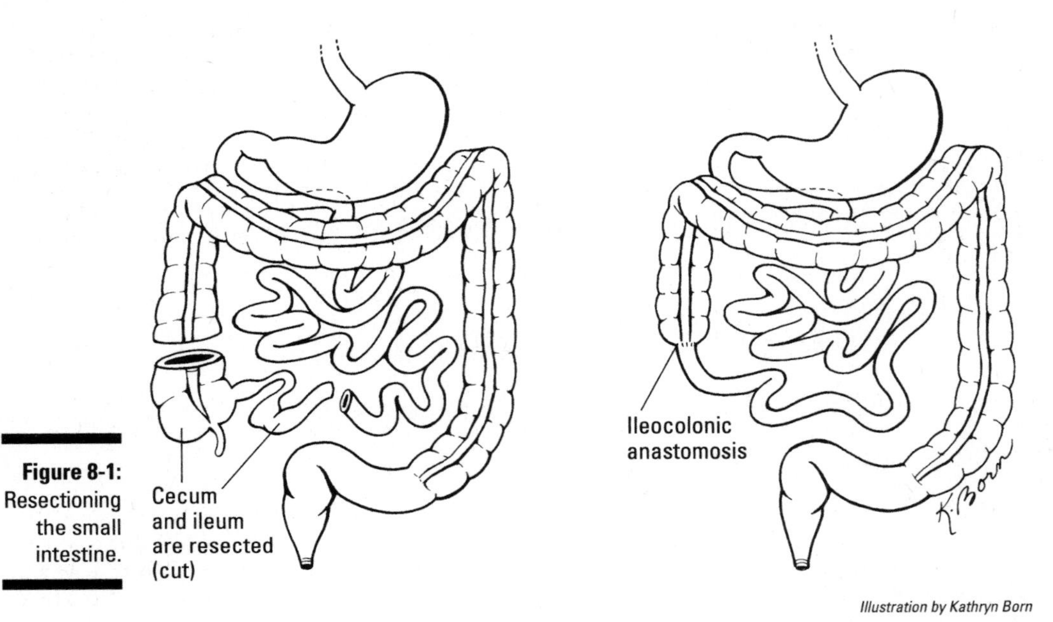

Figure 8-1: Resectioning the small intestine.

Illustration by Kathryn Born

Removing the end of the ileum can cause the following problems:

- **Diarrhea:** The ileocecal valve acts like a gate between your small and large intestines and allows a controlled flow of waste matter into the large intestine. With resection, you lose this gate and can experience frequent bowel movements due to lots of waste matter being dumped into the colon that your colon will try to squeeze out. This is one of the most common reasons for having diarrhea after resection.
- **Bile-salt-induced diarrhea:** Bile salts play an important role in the digestion and absorption of fats. Bile is secreted into the upper part of your small intestine, and 90 percent or more is absorbed by the terminal ileum and recycled back to the liver. By removing the terminal ileum, the recycling process is disturbed. Bile salts have a laxative effect and cause diarrhea when excreted into the colon in large amounts. As more bile salts are lost, the total bile salt pool decreases, affecting the absorption of fat and causing more fat to be excreted into the colon. Unabsorbed fat is broken down by bacteria in the colon, producing chemicals that have a laxative effect. Luckily this happens only if more than 100 cm or more of your ileum are removed.

- **Vitamin B12 deficiency:** An important function of the terminal ileum is to absorb vitamin B12 from the diet. With resection of the terminal ileum, you may develop vitamin B12 deficiency. When you become deficient in vitamin B12, you can't simply replenish it by taking extra B12 capsules — you don't have the part of intestine that absorbs it. For this reason, your doctor will recommend vitamin B12 injections instead.

There is now a nasal spray for vitamin B12. The nasal spray may be easier and more convenient than injections, but it's also more expensive.

Removing a stricture

When the inflammation in the intestines becomes severe, it can cause narrowing of the *lumen* (hollow space) of the intestines due to swelling. This narrowing is called *stricture.*

Initially, the stricture consists of swollen and inflamed intestine. But as time progresses, the inflammation turns into scar tissue, and more collagen and fiber forms inside the stricture. This is called *fibrotic stricture* (as opposed to *inflammatory stricture*). Inflammatory strictures can be treated using anti-inflammatory drugs, including immunosuppressive therapy. But fibrotic strictures are permanent, and medical therapy can't reverse the obstruction. Fibrotic stricture can eventually cause severe obstruction, making you unable to process food and causing symptoms such as abdominal pain and abdominal swelling. When this happens, it's time to surgically open the area.

One option is to cut out the area of the small intestine with the stricture and reattach the remaining intestine (resection and anastomosis; see the preceding section). If you've had multiple surgeries already, or if you have more than one area of stricture, you could end up with short-bowel syndrome.

The good news is, surgeons have developed a technique to cut open a stricture without causing further resection of the small intestine, to preserve the length of the small intestine and allow the process of digestion and absorption to continue. This technique is called *stricturoplasty* (see Figure 8-2). It generally involves opening the stricture by cutting through the bowel wall parallel with the intestine over the affected area. The slit is pinched open in the opposite direction and sewn closed, leaving a slightly shortened but widened opening without losing intestines.

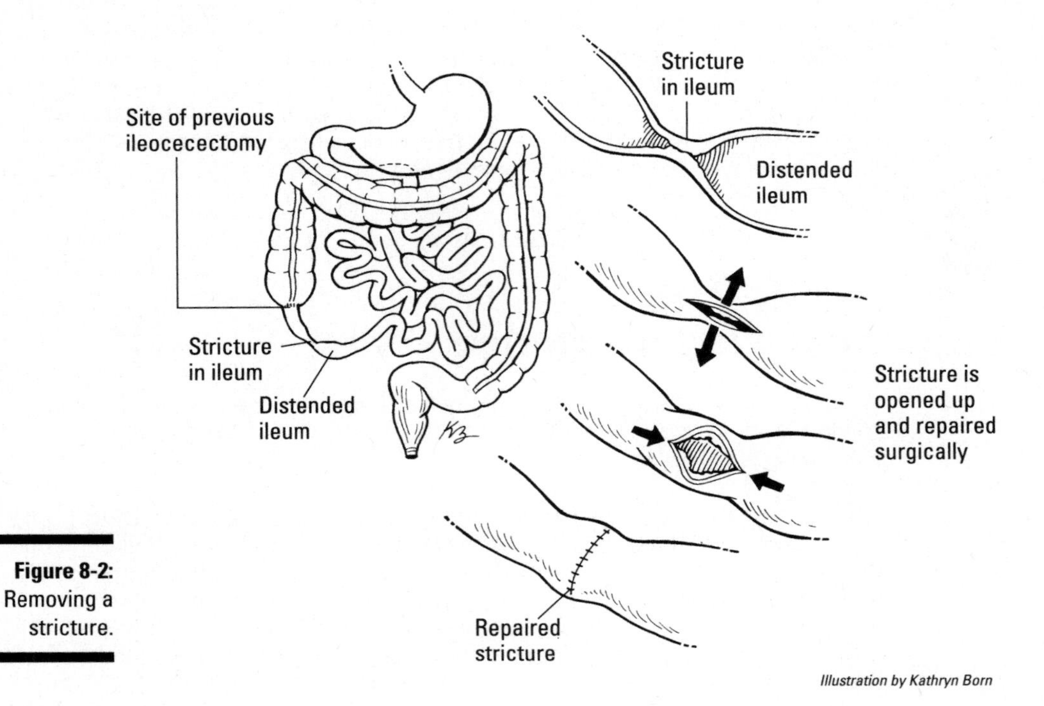

Figure 8-2: Removing a stricture.

Illustration by Kathryn Born

Treating fistulas

A *fistula* is an abnormal connection between two parts of the intestine or between the intestine and another organ. When medical therapy fails to close a fistula, you may need surgery to have the fistula removed; this procedure is called *fistulectomy*.

Another type of fistula in Crohn's disease is the *perianal fistula*. Here, the abnormal connection develops between the rectum and the skin surrounding the anal opening. This could cause stool, mucus, and pus discharge from these abnormal openings. Sometimes perianal fistulas can get complex and have more tortuous and long connecting tunnels between the rectum and perianal skin. Occasionally, these tunnels can get clogged and develop into abscesses. This requires drainage by the surgeon.

One way to drain these fistulous tracts is to place a *seton* (see Figure 8-3). Setons are simply rubber bands that are sewn into place as a temporary measure across the fistula tract while medical therapy helps to heal the inflammation around the area. Setons can stay in place for months to years. After healing occurs, the seton can be pulled out easily, just like stitches after surgery.

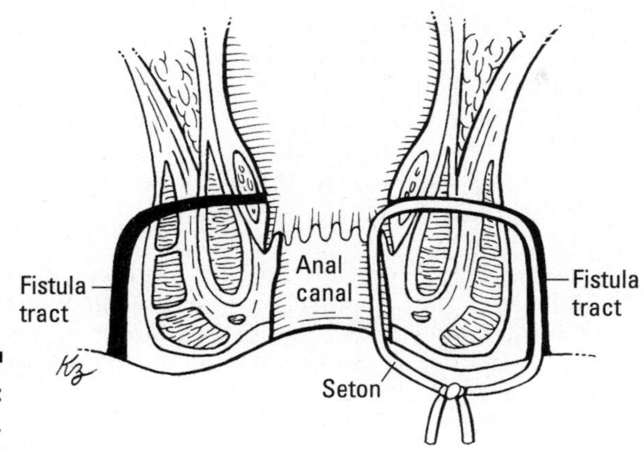

Figure 8-3: A seton.

Illustration by Kathryn Born

Draining abscesses

An abscess is a collection of *pus* (dead white blood cells). When you get an infection, your immune system reacts and tries to contain it to prevent it from spreading to other parts of the body. Skin boils and pimples are types of abscesses. Patients with Crohn's and colitis are at an increased risk of developing abscesses inside their bellies. The inflamed intestines become leaky and can easily let bugs enter the abdominal cavity, causing infection. Certain immunosuppressive medications, especially steroids, also increase the risk of abscess formation.

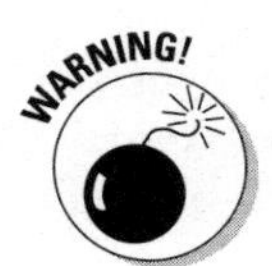

Fever, chills, or worsening abdominal pain may be the signs of an abdominal abscess. If you experience these symptoms, contact your doctor immediately. Untreated abscesses can cause widespread infection, which can lead to sepsis and even death.

Abdominal abscesses are usually diagnosed through CT scans. After they're diagnosed, your doctor may send you to a surgeon. If the abscess is small, the surgeon can make a small hole in your belly and drain the abscess. If the abscess is big, the surgeon will operate by making an incision in the belly and cutting it open to remove the abscess and wash the abdominal cavity with sterile water.

After draining the abscess, the surgeon may also remove the inflamed intestine, which could have been the source of the abscess.

A small abdominal abscess can also be drained by radiologists by placing a needle or catheter. They usually perform this procedure under CT guidance, which helps them locate the precise site of the abscess. This minimally invasive procedure can avoid having to cut your belly open.

Resecting the colon

If the inflammation is not being controlled with medications, or if you're unable to tolerate the side effects of medications, a surgeon will need to remove part of your colon or your entire colon (in a procedure called *colectomy*). Your colon will also need to be resected if you develop *dysplasia* (precancerous lesions) or cancer.

How much of the colon needs to be resected depends on the type of disease and site of inflammation. In Crohn's disease, only the inflamed part needs to be removed, and the remainder can be joined together. In colitis, disease progresses from the rectum upward and may eventually involve the entire colon. The persistent inflammation puts you at risk for colon cancer, so once the decision for surgery is made, the whole colon is resected along with the rectum. The remaining small intestine is either brought out to the skin surface as ostomy — bypassing the anus — or joined with the anal canal creating a pouch; this is called *ileoanal pouch anastomosis* (IPAA).

Here are the various types of colectomy:

- **Partial colectomy:** During a partial colectomy, your surgeon removes the diseased portion of the colon and a small portion of the surrounding healthy tissue (see Figure 8-4, top). The cut ends of the colon are then joined together. This procedure is more common for people with Crohn's disease. If the disease involves your terminal ileum, ascending colon, and part of the transverse colon, the right side of the colon along with part of the ileum is removed; this is called *right hemicolectomy.* The end of the remaining ileum is joined to the healthy transverse colon. Similarly, if the left colon is involved, as in Crohn's disease of the left transverse colon, descending colon, and sigmoid colon, *left hemicolectomy* is performed, and the healthy end of the transverse colon is joined to the rectum. Sometimes the rectum is also inflamed and the transverse colon can't be joined to the inflamed rectum. (The surgeon won't be able to stitch the inflamed intestine.) In this case, the remaining end of the transverse colon is brought out to the abdominal wall; this is called a *colostomy.*
- **Total colectomy:** If the entire colon is inflamed or if you develop multiple areas of precancerous lesions, your surgeon will advise you to have a total colectomy. In this procedure, the entire colon is removed and the healthy small intestine is either joined to the rectum (see Figure 8-4, middle) or an ostomy is created.
- **Proctocolectomy:** Proctocolectomy involves cutting out the entire colon and rectum (see Figure 8-4, bottom). This is a typical surgery for colitis and is considered a cure.

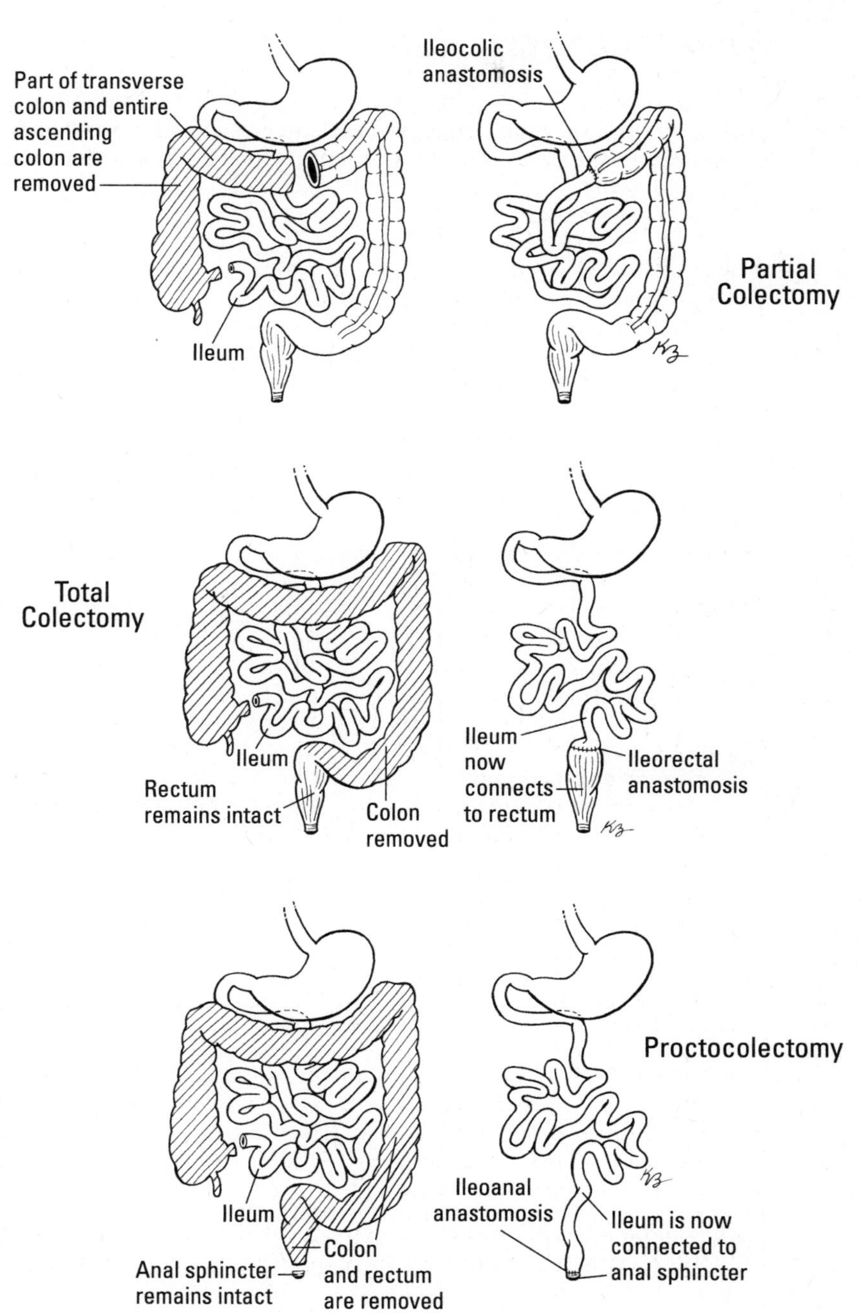

Figure 8-4: Partial colectomy (top), total colectomy (middle), and procto-colectomy (bottom).

Illustration by Kathryn Born

Pouch surgery

Pouch surgery is the most important surgery for people with colitis. In this procedure, the surgeon connects your small bowel to your anus by creating a pouch that acts as a rectum (see Figure 8-5). This surgery eliminates the need for ostomy.

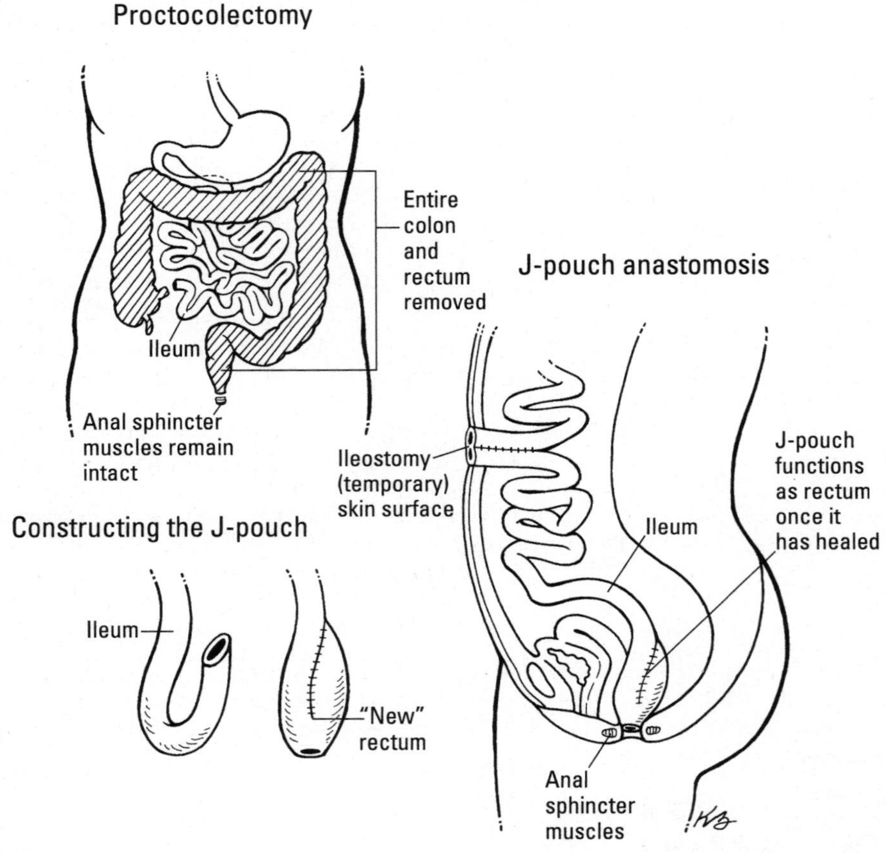

Figure 8-5: Pouch surgery.

In one of the techniques for pouch surgery, the terminal ileum is sewn back onto itself to form the shape of the letter *J*. That's why it's often referred to J-pouch surgery. In some cases, the ileum is sewn into a different shape such as *S* or *W*. These are less common than the usual *J* shape.

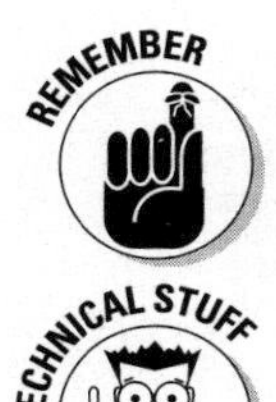

Pouch surgery is not for everyone. Your doctor may suggest ileostomy rather than pouch if you have anal-sphincter problems, especially in old age, where pouch surgery is associated with more complications. Pouch surgery may also decrease fertility in women, so you should discuss this type of surgery with your doctor if you're planning to become pregnant.

Pouch surgery is usually performed in different stages:

- **Stage 1:** In the first stage, the entire colon and rectum are removed. A reservoir or pouch is made out of the small intestine and then connected to the anus. Next, a temporary ileostomy, bringing one end of the small intestine to the skin of your abdominal wall, is created. This diverts the stool and protects the reservoir (the pouch) while it heals. You wear an ileostomy bag to collect waste. Learning to care for the ileostomy can be a little tricky, but with practice it becomes very manageable. You may occasionally pass a small amount of mucus or blood through the anal opening. About six weeks after the surgery (pouch creation and diverting ileostomy), an X-ray of the pouch is performed. If it shows healing of the pouch, the second surgery (Stage 2) can be scheduled.
- **Stage 2:** The second surgery (takedown surgery) is usually performed after two or three months. At this stage, the ileostomy is removed and the small intestine is reconnected to the rest of the bowel, restoring its original functionality. The pouch now becomes functional, and waste matter passes through the pouch. Your new pouch starts learning to accommodate the stool so that it can perform the same storage function as your rectum did. So, when you feel an urge to go, the stool can be squeezed through the anus. In the beginning, you'll be passing frequent and loose stools. This improves over time as the pouch adapts to its new function. Your small intestine will absorb more water, so the stool also becomes thicker. Your doctor may prescribe medications to control diarrhea and advise you to stay away from foods that may cause gas and diarrhea.

  For the first six months after takedown surgery, you can expect about six to eight semi-formed stools during the day and one at night. Sometimes it may take up to one year to fully adapt. In most patients, functioning of the pouch continues to improve over time.

Pouch surgery can be modified to a three-stage procedure. Stage 1 is removal of the colon and creation of the ostomy, Stage 2 is creation of the pouch, and Stage 3 is takedown. Sometimes, the procedure is performed in only one stage. How many stages are needed depends on how severe the colitis is, as well as on the expertise of your surgeon and the surgeon's protocol for performing surgery.

Although pouch surgery cures colitis, it may be associated with some side effects:

- **Sexual dysfunction and infertility:** Sexual function usually remains unchanged or actually improves following pouch surgery. This is because your general health improves. However, 1 percent to 2 percent of men become impotent or unable to achieve orgasm after pouch surgery. Four percent may also experience *retrograde ejaculation* (where the semen goes into the bladder instead of coming out the penis) after the pouch surgery. The fertility rate in women is reduced after pouch surgery; the exact cause is not known, but scientists believe that it may have to do with dense scar formation involving the ovaries or Fallopian tubes.
- **Frequent bowel movements:** You may continue to have four to six semi-formed bowel movements a day and one bowel movement per night. This varies from person to person. You may even have more frequent bowel movements. Your doctor may prescribe you antidiarrheal drugs to control these symptoms.
- **Incontinence:** Some people may experience frequent, unpredictable bowel movements called *incontinence.* This can happen while you're sleeping. Everyone passes gas from the rectum, even while sleeping. But if there is no rectum, such as after pouch surgery, there is less-than-normal sensitivity in the anal canal. This becomes even more of a problem when you have loose stools. While trying to pass some gas, you may also accidentally pass some amount of liquid stool. In this case, your doctor may advise that you wear a pad at night.
- **Stricture:** About 5 percent of people who undergo pouch surgery may develop narrowing at the site where the pouch and anal canal are surgically connected. This is called formation of stricture at the anastomosis site. It can usually be treated by *dilation* (stretching), which is a simple procedure performed with local anesthetic or sedatives and does not require general anesthesia.

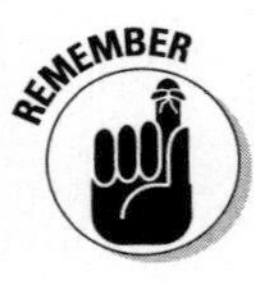

Your pouch will get larger with time and learn to store more stool. This usually solves the problems of frequent bowel movements and incontinence.

Complications from Surgery

Surgery isn't without its complications. When you're considering surgery, it's important to weigh the pros and cons with your doctor so that you go into it confident you've made the right choice. In this section, I walk you through the short-term and long-term complications.

Short-term complications

Short-term complications happen right after surgery and usually last for only days to weeks. You doctor and surgeon will keep a good eye on these possible complications and try to prevent them.

Ileus: Sleeping intestines

During the surgery, you're given drugs that put your body to sleep. This is called *general anesthesia.* After the surgery is complete, you wake up from the state of being unconscious. After few days, your surgeon will let you start a clear liquid diet. Most of the time, you start tolerating food and your doctor will slowly advance your diet to regular food. Normally, your intestines wake up within three to five days after surgery. However, sometimes your intestines go into a deep sleep and don't wake up for quite some time. This condition is called *ileus.*

Doctors don't know why some people get ileus. A few things may increase your risk:

- If your surgery was complicated and required a lot of manipulation
- If you were taking a lot of narcotics (pain medications) before the surgery
- If you take a lot of narcotics after the surgery for pain control

Your doctor may suggest few things to wake up your intestines. Walking, deep breathing, and even chewing gum sometimes help jump-start your intestines. In difficult cases, a tube may be passed through your nose into your stomach to suck all the fluids and secretions that are pooling and not moving forward. This will reduce the risk of aspiration of fluids into the lungs.

Thrombosis: Blood clots

After surgery, you're at risk of developing blood clots in your veins. This condition is called *deep venous thrombosis* (DVT). The clots can develop in the veins of your legs, abdomen, and, rarely, your lungs. Clots in the leg veins can travel upward and lodge in the veins of the lungs, causing difficulty breathing, which can be life threatening.

People develop clots for different reasons. Scientists believe that during active inflammation, certain chemicals are released that lead to formation of clots in the veins. Remaining immobile after surgery and having catheters in your veins cause decreased blood flow in the veins, which can then lead to clot formation.

Compared to surgeries in other people, the risk of forming blood clots is nearly double in Crohn's and colitis patients after surgery.

To avoid blood clot formation, your doctor will encourage you to get up and get moving as quickly as possible after the surgery. Even sitting up on the bedside or in a chair is an important step to prevent clot formation. Your doctor may also put you on blood thinner such as heparin to prevent clot formation. Heparin is usually given as an injection under the skin two to three times a day while you're in the hospital.

Wound infections

You may be at increased risk of developing infection at the wound site after surgery. If you were on steroids prior to surgery or you've been diagnosed with malnutrition, you're particularly at risk for developing wound infection. Pay special attention to any wounds on the skin, and notify your doctor or surgeon of any abnormal discharge or swelling. Usually, a simple course of antibiotics will take care of the infection.

Abscesses

If your wound becomes infected, and you aren't paying attention to it, it can turn into an abscess. An *abscess* is a collection of fluid and dead cells (commonly known as *pus*) that has a thick wall around it. Wound infections can be easily treated with antibiotics, but treating abscesses is difficult. The thick wall of the abscess makes it hard for the antibiotics to penetrate. Abscesses can develop on the skin at the site of the wound or inside your belly at the site of surgery. If an abscess doesn't improve with antibiotics, a radiologist has to drain the abscess with a needle or catheter or a surgeon will have to operate to drain the pus.

Leaking intestines

When a plumber replaces an old pipe with a new one, he creates a new joint connecting the new piece with the existing pipe. Sometimes, there could be leakage around the new joint for a variety of reasons — the old pipe wasn't completely taken out, the pipes weren't glued properly, or debris inside the pipe is causing blockage and back pressure.

The same concept applies to surgery in Crohn's and colitis. The new *anastomosis* (joint) can leak, causing fluid and stool inside the intestines to leak out into the abdominal cavity. This situation can be very dangerous — not only can it cause infection or abscess, but it can cause sepsis, a life-threatening event. Your surgeon will make every effort to ensure that all the inflamed and diseased part is out and the new connection between the intestines is made between two healthy parts. Even so, there could be leakage at the anastomosis. This is especially likely to happen if you're taking steroids (because steroids interfere with healing) or if there is residual active disease. Malnutrition can also cause poor wound healing and leakage.

Narcotic withdrawal

If you were taking large doses of narcotics (pain medications) before the surgery, you may not receive the same amount after the surgery. This may make you experience more pain, nausea, vomiting, or even hallucinations. This is called *acute narcotic withdrawal syndrome.* Working with your doctor to minimize the narcotics before the surgery and making sure that your surgeon knows the exact doses of the narcotics before the surgery can help you avoid such complications.

Steroid withdrawal

If you're taking high doses of steroids before surgery, you may suffer from *acute steroid withdrawal syndrome.* This condition happens when you don't receive the same amount of steroids after the surgery as you were getting before. Withdrawal may cause sleep problems, lethargy, and restlessness. Sometimes, steroid withdrawal can be severe and life threatening.

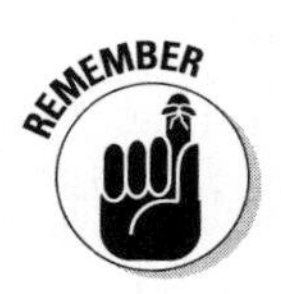

Don't worry about steroid withdrawal — your surgeon and other doctors are trained to follow protocols for steroid dosing during and after surgery.

Long-term complications

Some complications of surgery can persist long term (for months and even years). You need to be aware of these problems so you can identify them and notify your doctor if they occur.

Pouchitis

After pouch surgery, about half of all patients experience at least one bout of *pouchitis* (inflammation of the pouch). The exact cause of this inflammation is still unknown. Symptoms of pouchitis usually include diarrhea, urgency, cramps, or even bleeding in severe cases. Endoscopy of the pouch will show inflammation, and your doctor typically will prescribe antibiotics. In some people, pouchitis becomes difficult to treat, and long-term antibiotics are required to keep the inflammation suppressed. If inflammation is severe enough, it can also lead to excision of the pouch and creation of ostomy.

One study found that certain probiotics (especially a formulation called VSL#3) right after surgery can prevent pouchitis.

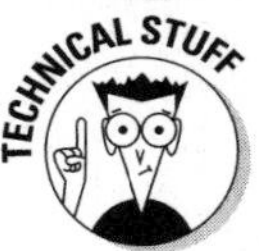

Sometimes a tiny piece of rectal lining is left while taking out your colon and rectum during the pouch surgery. The pouch is joined to this rectal lining instead of actually getting hooked up to the anal canal. In about 10 percent of people, this part of the rectum gets inflamed and produces symptoms of urgency or bleeding. The inflammation of this cuff of rectal lining is called *cuffitis.*

Short-bowel syndrome

Crohn's disease tends to come back even after surgery. So, you may have more than one resection surgery for Crohn's disease. Usually, after one or two resections, the rest of the intestine catches up in terms of nutrient absorption. When the surgeon takes multiple pieces of your intestine, you may end up with too little small intestine to absorb adequate nutrients, minerals, and water. The remaining short segment of small intestine won't be able to catch up. This is called *short-bowel syndrome.*

When you have only 100 cm or less of small intestine left, your ability to absorb nutrients and water significantly decreases and you may need nutrition support through other means.

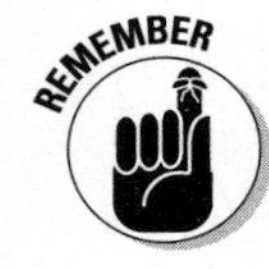

Short-bowel syndrome is associated with other complications such as gallstones, kidney stones, weight loss, and weak bones.

If you start having signs and symptoms of short-bowel syndrome — such as diarrhea and nutrient deficiencies (such as low vitamin and mineral levels) — your doctor will consider adding supplements and putting you on a special diet that's easy to absorb, known as an *elemental diet.* If this doesn't solve the problem, she may start intravenous nutritional support, also known as total parenteral nutrition (TPN). For more on TPN and elemental diets, turn to Chapter 9.

Nutritional deficiencies

Because your intestines are the only channel to absorb nutrients from food, if they're taken out, you can become deficient in nutrients. After an intestinal surgery, you're at risk for the following:

- Vitamin B12 deficiency
- Iron deficiency
- Fat and bile acid malabsorption
- Deficiency of trace elements, fluids, and electrolytes
- Food intolerance

When you have an ileostomy for Crohn's or colitis, you're at risk for dehydration. You can easily lose electrolytes through ostomy. Your doctor usually will advise you to add more fiber to your diet, take antidiarrheal medications, and drink plenty of water, especially drinks containing electrolytes (such as Gatorade).

A recurrence of Crohn's disease

Crohn's disease never leaves you. Even after surgery, it usually comes back within a few years. Most of the time, it comes back at the site where the inflamed intestine was removed and the healthy ends were reconnected.

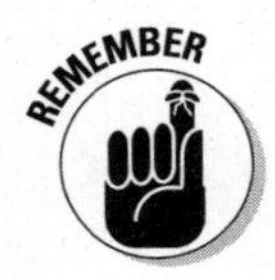

Within three years of surgery to remove the inflamed or narrowed intestine, 70 percent of patients will have a recurrence of Crohn's disease.

If you've had multiple surgeries in the past, if your small intestine and colon are involved, or if you've had a long segment of intestine removed during the first surgery, you may be at higher risk of Crohn's coming back. Being young, having fistulas, and smoking are additional risk factors for early recurrence of Crohn's. Your doctor may start some medications right after the first surgery to reduce your chances of needing further surgery.

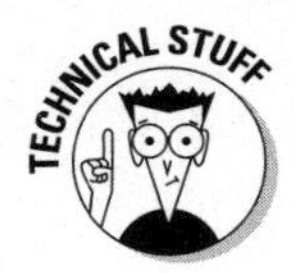

There are different definitions of Crohn's disease recurrence referred to in the medical literature:

- **Endoscopic recurrence:** In endoscopic recurrence, Crohn's disease is said to be back when a doctor performs an endoscopy and sees ulcers in the mucosa. This type of recurrence doesn't produce any symptoms, and you have to perform endoscopy at regular intervals to watch for Crohn's coming back. Seventy percent of Crohn's disease patients can have endoscopic recurrence within one year of their surgery.
- **Clinical recurrence:** In clinical recurrence, signs and symptoms of Crohn's disease come back. About 50 percent to 70 percent of Crohn's disease patients have clinical recurrence within five years of their surgery.

To make things more confusing, some scientists define recurrence as *surgical recurrence,* when you need another surgery for Crohn's disease.

Rarely, a patient diagnosed with colitis who has undergone colectomy and pouch surgery develops inflammation in the pouch along with deep ulcers and fistulas that is difficult to treat with medical therapy. This is actually Crohn's disease of the pouch — the patient had Crohn's all along but was misdiagnosed. This condition happens in only 5 percent to 10 percent of colitis patients. In this case, the doctor did nothing wrong — sometimes it's just hard to tell the difference between Crohn's and colitis.

Ostomy: What It Is and How to Deal with It

If you have Crohn's or colitis, you may need to have surgery and possible ostomy someday. Better awareness and understanding can eliminate lots of fears associated with ostomy.

The terms *ostomy* and *stoma* are often used interchangeably, but they have different meanings. An *ostomy* is an opening on the skin of your belly that the surgeon creates for the discharge of waste matter. A *stoma* is the actual end of the small or large intestine you see protruding through the abdominal wall.

Types of ostomy

There are different types of ostomies. The two main categories are *colostomy* (large intestine ostomy) and *ileostomy* (small intestine ostomy), shown in Figure 8-6.

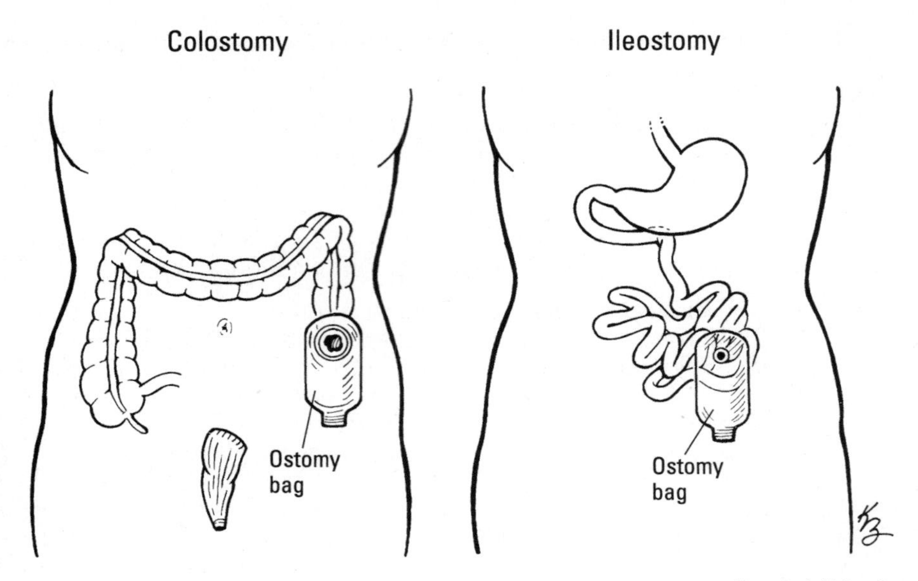

Figure 8-6: Types of ostomies.

Illustration by Kathryn Born

Based on the permanence of the colostomy there are two different types:

- **Temporary:** This type of colostomy allows the lower portion of the colon to rest and heal. The end of the upper portion of the colon is brought to the surface of the abdomen. After the lower portion is healed, the two portions are reconnected.
- **Permanent:** This usually involves the loss of the colon (because of issues such as persistent inflammation that can't be treated with medical therapy). The diseased colon is taken out, and the rest of the colon is brought to the surface in the form of permanent colostomy.

Similarly, there are temporary and permanent ileostomies.

When you may need ostomy

Your doctor will make every attempt to preserve the integrity of the intestines with medical therapy, but sometimes surgery is the only or best choice. Your surgeon will try to connect your intestines together, but sometimes this isn't possible and you may end up with ostomy. The reasons for having ostomy surgery include the following:

- **To treat severe and fulminant colitis and toxic megacolon:** These are emergency conditions with a great risk of perforation and sepsis. Your surgeon may have to perform urgent surgery and create a temporary ileostomy.

- **As an alternate to pouch surgery for ulcerative colitis or when you develop pouchitis.**
- **For healing of rectal fistulas:** Sometimes your surgeon may create a temporary colostomy to divert the stool and let the rectum and fistulas around it heal.

How to care for your stoma

After ostomy creation, your *stoma* (the end of your small or large intestine) looks like a shiny, wet, red, round opening. Usually the stoma shrinks in size during the first few months. Knowing how to care for your stoma is important so that you can prevent things from going wrong.

You may be wondering how stools are handled when they come out of the stoma. A plastic bag is attached around the stoma to collect the stool, which is liquid (in the case of ileostomy) or semi-solid to solid (in the case of colostomy). Stool takes the form of a solid shape only when it reaches the colon, so stool that comes out of an ostomy isn't solid.

The skin surrounding the stoma (called *peristomal skin*) must be protected from the irritating waste matter. The stools coming out of the ileostomy are particularly rich in digestive enzymes that can be very irritating to the skin. The best way to prevent skin irritation is to carefully clean the skin with residue-free soap and dry it every time the pouch system is changed. Moisturizing soap can leave residue that can interfere with the adhesion of the pouch to the skin, and it can easily fall off, which may cause embarrassment.

Usually, bacteria and fungi are on the skin all the time. You can get a yeast infection if the fungi grow in number, especially if the skin is kept moist most of the time.

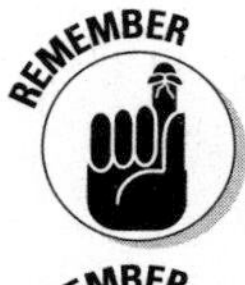

Your stoma has no nerve endings. That means it can't feel anything, including pain. It's rich in blood vessels, though, and may bleed if rubbed or irritated. If you develop any persistent irritation, rash, swelling, and skin breakdown on the stoma, talk to your doctor.

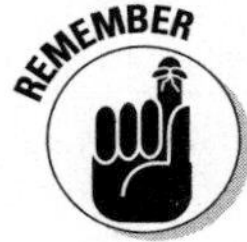

Water cannot enter the stoma, so you have to cover it while bathing and showering.

Your ostomy pouch

The ostomy pouch is made of lightweight, odor-proof material. It's available in one- or two-piece systems. The two-piece system includes an adhesive skin barrier and a pouch. The pouch can be transparent or opaque. Most of the time, the pouch fits nicely under your clothes, and no one can even guess that you have an ostomy or are wearing an ostomy bag.

There are two types of pouches: drainable and disposable pouches. Drainable pouches have an opening on the bottom and close with a clip. You can release the clip to allow the stool to drain. Disposable pouches can be discarded completely after they're filled with waste matter.

When you're in the hospital getting your ostomy, you'll have a visit by an ostomy nurse, also known as *enterostomal therapist.* The nurse will instruct you on how to choose, change, and take care of the ostomy bag. The type and location may influence your choice of pouch. The pouch should be the correct size, and you should measure your stoma size every time you purchase supplies, because the stoma size and shape may change with your body weight.

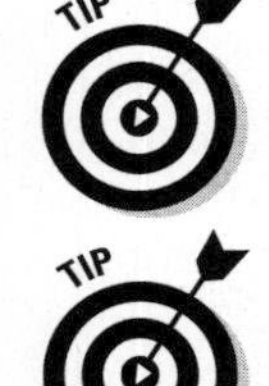

You may want to experiment with different types of pouches to determine which one is best for you and suits your daily needs.

Empty your pouch several times a day. Consider emptying it after each meal or when it's one-third full. Here's how to change your ostomy pouch:

1. **Gather all the necessary supplies.**

   You'll need adhesive remover, skin protector, a plastic bag, a washcloth, scissors, and a new pouch.

2. **Wash your hands before touching and handling your pouch.**

3. **Empty your pouch as instructed by your ostomy nurse or by the written instructions given to you when you're discharged from the hospital.**

4. **Wipe the tape surrounding the old *wafer* (the baseplate, plasticlike substance that surrounds the actual stoma and protects the skin from waste) with the adhesive remover.**

5. **Put the old pouch, wafer, and the other waste into a plastic bag for disposal.**

   Resealable sandwich bags from the grocery store can work great.

6. **Clean your skin and stoma with a washcloth and warm water.**

   If you can, take a shower. Any stool coming out of your stoma can easily get washed down the drain. If you aren't in the shower, stand over an old towel or some paper towels when changing bags to catch any waste from the stoma.

7. **Pat your skin dry and measure the stoma with the measuring guide.**

   Leave only 1/8 inch to 1/16 inch between the measuring guide and the stoma.

8. **Trace the correct size onto the back of the wafer, and cut out the hole with the scissors.**
9. **Apply skin protector to the surrounding skin where you'll put the wafer.**
10. **Peel the paper from the wafer and apply adhesive paste, if needed; then place it over the stoma, making sure that stoma is in center of the hole.**

    Press it firmly.
11. **Snap the new pouch onto the wafer, and close the bottom of the bag with the clip, if needed.**

    Consider adding a few drops of peppermint oil, a teaspoon of baking soda, or a little mouthwash to the pouch each time you change or empty it to help reduce the odor.

    You're good to go!

Note: These instructions can vary slightly depending on the exact type of pouch and the manufacturer's instructions. Always consult your ostomy nurse or read the manufacturer's package insert for guidance.

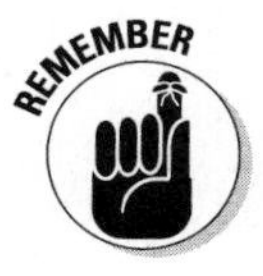

In the beginning, you may feel uncomfortable emptying and changing your pouch. With time and experience, though, you'll learn to take care of your pouch with ease and confidence.

Ostomy-pouch accessories

The ostomy pouch comes with some accessories. During your stay in the hospital, the ostomy nurse will help you get familiar with the different appliances. Here is a list of some common items:

- **Ostomy belts:** These are belts that you wrap around the abdomen and attach to the loops found on certain pouches. They can be very helpful to support the pouch and keep it in place.
- **Pouch covers:** These are made with a cotton or cotton-blend backing and easily fit over the pouch. They protect your belly skin. They come in handy during intimate occasions.
- **Skin barrier liquid/powder:** These help protect the skin under the wafer and around the stoma from irritation caused by waste matter.
- **Tapes:** Tapes are used for waterproofing. A wide range of different tapes is available to meet the needs of different skin sensitivities.
- **Adhesive remover:** This is helpful in cleaning the adhesive that may stick to your skin after removing the wafer or tape.

Ostomy fashion

You may be concerned about covering the stoma and ostomy pouch and wondering how they'll affect the clothing you can wear. Luckily, pouch systems are designed to be as thin as possible and fit under most clothes, so they're virtually invisible. Emptying the bag and not letting it get too full will help keep it discreet and comfortable under your clothes. ***Remember:*** You see people in public with ostomies all the time without knowing it.

The proper placement of the stoma will ensure the greatest possible comfort and privacy. An ostomy nurse can help you decide the best location to place the stoma to avoid irritation from clothes, especially from belts and pants waistbands.

Here's some advice on clothing choices when wearing an ostomy pouch:

- **Stick with looser clothes, and pay attention to fabric choice.** Stiff or thick fabrics will do a better job of hiding any bulges the bag may cause, while thin or clingy fabrics like silk and linen may accentuate the bag and allow it to show through.
- **Women can wear skirts, trousers, and even pantyhose as long as they're comfortable and the waistband doesn't cut into the stoma.**
- **For men, suspenders may be a better option if belts are uncomfortable.**
- **Pants and skirts with pleats can help hide the location of the ostomy bag.** They can also have some "give" when the bag starts to fill up.

Commercially available ostomy belts are great for use in saunas and during intimate moments.

You can even go swimming with a pouch, though women may want to stick to a one-piece and use boy shorts for better coverage. The right choice of fabric, cut, and style will hide the pouch. For example, dark-colored fabric with a busy pattern can camouflage the appliance better than light colors, which can become transparent when wet. For men, boxer-style swimming trunks work better than Speedo-type suits.

You can find more information about clothing and ostomy from ostomysecrets (`www.ostomysecrets.com`).

Ostomy complications

The ostomy is a special structure that requires lots of attention and care. With good care and maintenance, you can avoid many problems, but even with the best care, complications can arise.

Certain patients are more at risk for complications than others. Older patients, those who are malnourished, and those who have difficulty properly caring for the stoma are at an increased risk. Patients with Crohn's disease may run into trouble if they have inflammation at the stoma site.

Many of the complications that occur with ostomies need to be cared for by a doctor or an ostomy nurse. Let your provider know if you notice any changes in the stoma, bowel function, or anything else that concerns you.

Skin irritation

Irritation is likely to occur in many patients with stomas. It can be caused by the frequent changing and removal of adhesive parts related to an ostomy bag. This also causes tearing and stretching at the skin that can be irritating. If you're gentle when changing bags on the stoma, you'll reduce the amount of irritation.

When stool comes in contact with bare skin, it can also cause irritation. This type of irritation is most common in patients with ileostomy (because their stool contains more digestive enzymes that can break down skin on contact) and patients who have stomas that are retracted below the skin. Make sure your ostomy pouch is the correct size for your stoma, and use barrier powders to reduce this type of irritation.

Allergic reactions against products used on the ostomy can cause irritation as well. The barrier, powders, adhesives, and materials in the pouch can contain products that some people are allergic to. This can cause redness, itching, and blistering on contact. If you notice any of these complications after starting a new product, discontinue its use, and let your doctor know about the problem.

Infection

Bacteria and some types of fungi love warm, moist environments. Unfortunately, an ostomy is just such a place, so you have to be on the lookout for signs of infections. Rashes, redness, skin breakdown, and pain can all be signs of infection. Let your doctor know if you're having any of these problems. They most common infection at a stoma site is with a fungus called *candida.* This fungus causes the common yeast infection, and it can be treated with an antifungal power you can get from your doctor.

Parastomal hernia and prolapse

The word *parastomal* means "next to the stoma." A *parastomal hernia* occurs when intestines or other organs present inside the abdomen bulge through a weakness in the muscle that surrounds the stoma. Conditions that increase the pressure on the stoma — like obesity, lifting heavy objects, and persistent cough — are risk factors for developing a parastomal hernia.

Minor hernias can be treated with special compression belts that keep the skin from protruding. Hernias that persist and those that cause symptoms such as pain or vomiting should be evaluated by a doctor.

The same factors that increase pressure and can cause a hernia near a stoma can also cause a prolapse. A *prolapse* occurs when the bowel protrudes through the stoma itself. When the intestine is sticking out away from the skin, it's more prone to injury. Initial treatment of a prolapse consists of gently pushing the bowel back through the stoma and using a compression belt. Similar to hernias, prolapses that persist or cause pain require the attention of a doctor.

Retraction

Normal stomas usually stick out of the skin a little bit. If the stoma sits below the skin surface, this is called *retraction.* This complication can make it difficult to attach an ostomy pouch. It also puts the skin around the stoma at risk of irritation from constant contact with stool. Mild retraction can be treated with special compression belts and ostomy pouches. If the problem persists, the surgeon may have to revise the ostomy with another surgery.

Obstruction

Any surgery on the bowel creates a risk for the formation of strictures. This complication causes a narrowing of the intestine and may lead to obstruction. Mild blockages can be treated by eating a low-residue diet (see Chapter 9), using laxatives, and using enemas. Severe blockages must be treated surgically.

If you experience severe abdominal pain with vomiting or notice a complete stoppage of stool and gas passing from the stoma, contact your doctor for treatment right away.

Part III
Healing and Dealing with the Disease

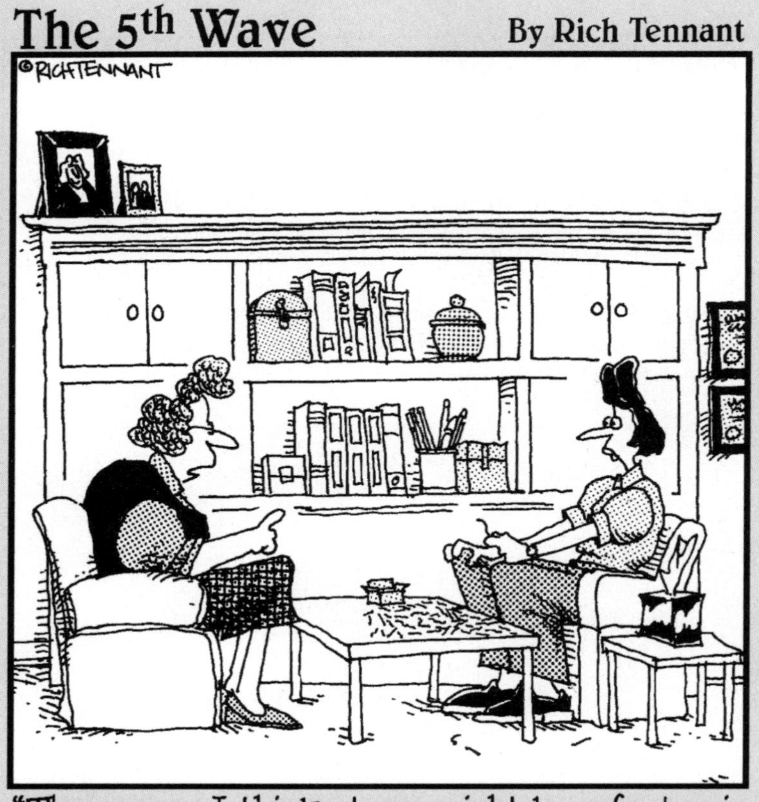

"The reason I think stress might be a factor in your colitis is because of research, statistics, and the fact that you've straightened out an entire box of paper clips during our conversation."

In this part . . .

Nutrition is important for everyone, but when you have Crohn's or colitis, it's especially important. In this part, I explain why it matters and tell you how to ensure you're getting the nutrients you need. I also offer guidelines for preventing health problems when you have Crohn's or colitis. I end the part with complementary and alternative therapies you may want to consider for treating the disease.

Chapter 9

Paying Attention to What You Eat

In This Chapter

- Recognizing the effects of nutrition
- Exploring the nutrients your body needs
- Looking at special diets for Crohn's and colitis
- Considering other ways of getting the nutrients you need

Nutrition is involved with two important tasks: First, food provides energy. The amount of energy a food provides is measured in calories. Without enough food, you won't have enough energy. Second, nutrition provides your body with chemical substances, called *nutrients,* to help build, maintain, and repair your body organs.

In this chapter, I walk you through the important role nutrition plays for the immune system, wound healing, and growth. Then I fill you in on the different nutrients you need. I cover special diets used for people with Crohn's and colitis. And I end the chapter with information on how to boost your nutrition if you're not getting what you need from food alone.

Considering the Impact of Nutrition

Crohn's and colitis can impact your nutritional status. For example, if you've had a large part of your intestines removed, you may have decreased absorption of nutrients. The medications prescribed for Crohn's and colitis can have the same effect — for example, steroids cause decreased absorption of calcium and phosphorus, and cholestyramine (used to control diarrhea) decreases the absorption of vitamins A, D, E, and K.

Just as Crohn's and colitis can impact your nutritional status, your nutrition can affect the illness. For example, nutrition can have important effects on the process of inflammation. Similarly, if your nutritional status is not optimal, it may take longer for your *mucosa* (the inner layer of the intestines) to heal, which may contribute to more complications such as frequent disease flares or affect other organ systems, such as skin, hair, bones, and liver.

In this section, I cover two major ways in which nutrition impacts your health.

The impact on your immune system

Nutrition's effect on the immune system is a two-way process: Nutrition can influence the function of your immune system, and the immune system can affect your nutrition.

How the immune system affects your nutrition

Your immune system protects you against bacteria, viruses, and other disease-causing organisms. It's an efficient, complex defense system. When you get an infection, your immune system is activated and the process of inflammation begins. During the process of inflammation, your immune system actively recruits inflammatory cells and releases protein chemicals to fight infection and invading organisms. Fuel is needed to process, handle, and recruit those inflammatory cells.

If the process of inflammation continues (as happens in Crohn's or colitis), lots of energy will be used, sometimes at the expense of your body muscles and fats. If you don't give your body the fuel it needs, you can easily become malnourished.

How nutrition affects your immune system

Malnutrition can affect your immune system in a number of ways:

- **It can reduce the numbers and functions of immune cells, such as T and B cells.** T and B cells are special types of white blood cells that help defend your body against intruders such as bacteria, viruses, parasites, and other toxins in the environment. They're found in abundance in the intestinal wall where they come in contact with these intruders every day and kill them before they gain entry into your body. If these cells are low in number or unable to function properly, you'll easily get sick with infections. Bacteria will also damage the *mucosa* (the protective inner layer of the intestines) and trigger inflammation, which is the hallmark of Crohn's and colitis.
- **It can cause shrinkage or impaired development of organs (such as the spleen) and lymph nodes.** These are an integral part of your immune system and are involved in clearing infection-causing microorganisms and other toxins from your system.
- **It leads to a decrease in the levels of complements.** *Complements* are important proteins that fight the invading microorganisms and toxins.

- **Copper and zinc deficiency can impair the functions of T cells.**
- **Deficiency of vitamins A and D have been found to impair the immune system.** These vitamins play an important role in suppressing inflammation by decreasing the production of certain chemicals from the T cells.

The impact on wound healing

During the later stages of inflammation, the mucosa begins to heal. And healing requires extra calories, proteins, vitamins (such as vitamins A and C), and minerals (such as zinc). Making sure you're getting enough nutrients will help your mucosa heal better and faster.

I cover the key nutrients you need later in this chapter, but protein, carbohydrates, fat, vitamins, and minerals are all important to wound healing.

Identifying the Nutrients You Need

The food you eat provides you with two different groups of nutrients: macronutrients and micronutrients. In this section, I cover both.

Macronutrients

Macronutrients constitute the majority of your diet. They're important because they provide fuel for the body. Without the energy that comes from macronutrients, your body wouldn't be able to perform even the most basic of tasks, such as breathing and walking.

There are three macronutrients: carbohydrates, protein, and fat.

Carbohydrates

Carbohydrates are sugar compounds that are great sources of energy. They come in two varieties:

- **Simple carbohydrates:** Simple carbohydrates contain only one or two sugar units. A carbohydrate with one unit of sugar is called a *simple sugar* or a *monosaccharide.* A carbohydrate with two units of sugar is called a *double sugar* or a *disaccharide.*

  Fructose and glucose are examples of simple sugars. Table sugar (made of one unit of fructose and one unit of glucose) is a double sugar.

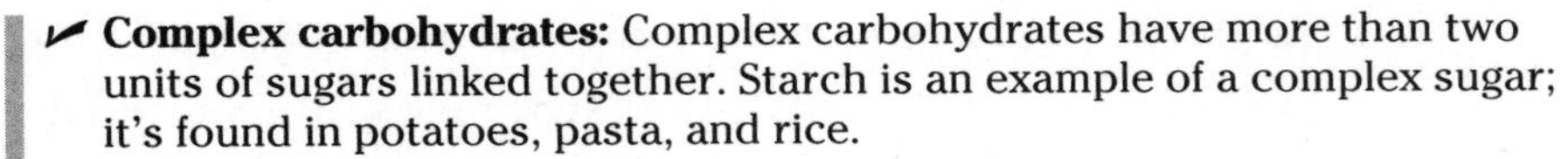

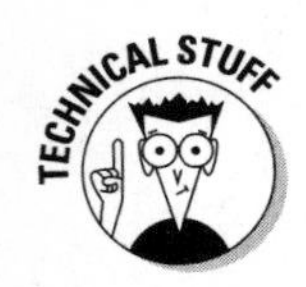

- **Complex carbohydrates:** Complex carbohydrates have more than two units of sugars linked together. Starch is an example of a complex sugar; it's found in potatoes, pasta, and rice.

  Complex carbohydrates may have anywhere from three to several thousand units of sugars. So, your body needs more time to digest them than it does simple sugars.

Your body runs on glucose. When carbohydrates are digested and broken down to release glucose, the glucose enters your cells and is burned to produce heat and a molecule called adenosine triphosphate (ATP). ATP stores and releases energy as required by the cells. Your cells budget energy very carefully — they don't store more than they need. Any glucose the cells don't need for their daily work is converted to glycogen and tucked away as stored energy in your liver and muscles.

Providing energy isn't the only thing carbohydrates do for you. When your body needs energy, such as during the inflammation process, your body first uses glucose to make energy. If you run out of glucose, you begin to pull energy out of fatty tissue and then move on to burning protein tissue (muscles). A diet that provides enough carbohydrates keeps your body from eating its own muscles. That's why a carbohydrate-rich diet is sometimes described as a *protein-sparing diet.* Carbohydrates also provide nutrients for the friendly bacteria in your intestinal tract that help digest the food.

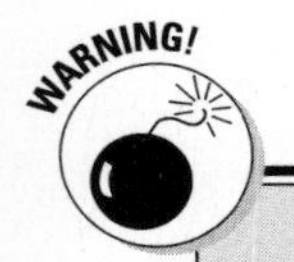

Avoiding the Specific Carbohydrate Diet

In the Specific Carbohydrate Diet, you avoid complex carbohydrates. You can eat nuts, aged cheeses, fish, beef, and unsweetened juices, but sugars, oats, pasta, potatoes, rice, and wheat are off limits. The theory behind the Specific Carbohydrate Diet is that complex carbohydrates can be the food for the bad bacteria residing inside your intestines. If these bacteria are starved, they won't be able to multiply and will eventually die.

Some people find the Specific Carbohydrate Diet very helpful for their Crohn's and colitis. On the downside, if you exclude starchy vegetables and grains, you eliminate a dietary source of short-chain fatty acids, which are an important source of fuel for your colon cells.

The bottom line: This diet is not endorsed by any professional medical societies, and in the absence of good scientific data to prove its effectiveness in the treatment of Crohn's and colitis, I don't recommend the Specific Carbohydrate Diet to my patients.

The most important sources of carbohydrates are plant foods, such as fruits, vegetables, and grains. Milk and milk products also contain carbohydrates in the form of lactose. Meat, fish, and poultry don't have any carbohydrates.

Proteins

Protein is made of small units called *amino acids,* which are linked together in a chain. Your body uses proteins to build new cells and maintain the health of existing tissues and organs.

Your muscles have proteins that make it possible for them to contract and function. Your red blood cells contain *hemoglobin,* another type of protein, which helps carry the oxygen throughout the body. Similarly, proteins are required to make neurotransmitters, which send signals from your brain to different parts of the body. Finally, each cell of your body has a central headquarters that makes proteins; this headquarters, known as DNA, is made of amino acids, which are the subunits of protein molecules.

To make all the proteins your body needs, you require 22 different kinds of amino acids. Ten of these amino acids are labeled *essential;* you can't synthesize these amino acids in the body and must get them from your diet.

Proteins from animal sources such as meat, fish, and poultry are called *high-quality proteins.* Your body absorbs these proteins more efficiently. The proteins from plants (such as fruits, legumes, and nuts) often have a limited amount of some essential amino acids. The prime exception is soybeans, a legume that contains abundant amounts of all the essential amino acids.

When you have Crohn's or colitis, you're at very high risk for protein deficiency. There are several reasons why protein deficiency may occur:

- **You may consume less protein.** During periods of sickness, your appetite may be suppressed and you simply may not want to eat. You may even not be *able* to eat, if you develop ulcers in your mouth (a result of deficiencies of various vitamins or of Crohn's disease itself), making it painful to swallow food.
- **You may not be able to absorb protein.** If your intestines are inflamed, you may not be able to digest and absorb nutrients, including proteins, from the diet.
- **You may not be taking in as much protein as your body is using.** During the process of inflammation, your body is constantly burning calories and using energy to fuel the inflammatory cells. Your immune system produces lots of chemicals called *cytokines* that stimulate, recruit, and maintain the health of immune cells such as T cells and B cells. So, you need more proteins to ensure proper functioning of the immune system.

- **You could be losing protein.** During the process of inflammation, your intestinal layers become leaky, and you can easily lose proteins from your intestines. This is called *protein-losing diarrhea* or, in medical terms, *protein-losing enteropathy.*

One of the first signs of protein deficiency is muscle weakness. You may also have thin hair or sores on the skin. Your blood tests may also show that you're *anemic* (a condition in which you don't have enough red blood cells) or that you have low blood levels of a protein called *albumin,* which helps maintain your body's fluid balance. A low level of albumin allows your body to retain more water, and you can develop leg swelling; in severe cases, your whole body may swell like a balloon.

Fats

Fats are high-energy nutrients. In fact, fats have *twice* the energy (calories) as proteins and carbohydrates do. Your body needs fat to build tissues and make chemicals such as hormones. Fat provides a source of stored energy, gives shape to your body, and cushions your skin — imagine sitting on a chair without your buttocks to pillow your bones. Fat also acts as an insulation blanket to reduce heat loss from the body.

Although dietary fat has more energy per gram than protein and carbohydrates do, our bodies can't extract energy from fats as easily. Bile, a liquid chemical released by the gallbladder, comes in handy here — it acts as an emulsifier and enables fat to mix with water so that enzymes can start breaking down the fat into fatty acids. From there, fatty acids easily get absorbed through the intestinal cells.

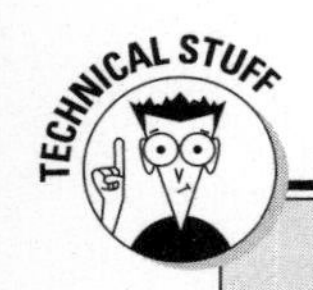

Why whey?

Whey is one of the two proteins found in milk. During the cheese-making process, the protein called *casein* is separated out to make cheese, and the remaining liquid is filtered, dried, and processed into whey protein powder, a very digestible protein that provides all the essential amino acids. Researchers have found a beneficial effect of whey protein for Crohn's and colitis because of the two amino acids — threonine and cysteine — that are present in a very high concentration in whey protein. These two amino acids have been found to be necessary for the production of *mucin,* which forms the protective layer around your intestinal inner wall, allowing it to be protected against harmful bacteria and viruses.

For this reason, taking whey proteins when you have Crohn's or colitis makes sense, but these findings and observations are based on studies performed on animals, and we still need larger human studies before accepting whey proteins as essential supplements in the diet.

The fats in food are combinations of fatty acids. They're divided into three categories:

- **Saturated:** Saturated fats are solid at room temperature; an example is butter.
- **Monounsaturated:** Monounsaturated fats are liquid at room temperature and become thicker when chilled; examples include olive oil and canola oil.
- **Polyunsaturated:** Polyunsaturated fats are liquid at room temperature and stay liquid when chilled; examples include corn oil and soybean oil.

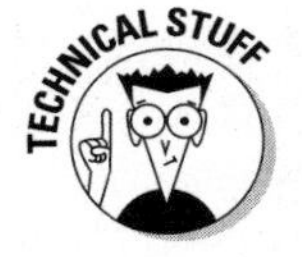

How fatty acids are categorized is based on how many hydrogen atoms are attached to the carbon atoms in the chain. The more hydrogen atoms, the more saturated the fatty acid.

All fats were once thought to be unhealthy and the cause of many illnesses, including heart disease. Today we know that all fats are not created equal and that there are good fats, bad fats, and very bad fats:

- Unsaturated fats — both monounsaturated and polyunsaturated — are the good kind. They actually help lower cholesterol and are a good source of omega-3 fatty acids, which help reduce inflammation. You find unsaturated fats in nuts, oils, and seeds, as well as in dark, leafy vegetables.
- Saturated fats, on the other hand, are the artery-clogging ones. Butter and red meat contain saturated fats.
- The worst kind of fat of all is trans fat, which is made by the hydrogenation process, in which liquid vegetable oils are converted into solid fats. Trans fats not only increase the bad cholesterol in your blood (LDL) but also decrease your level of good cholesterol (HDL). Often, French fries and cookies contain trans fats. Some nutrition labels today list the amount of trans fats, or you may see "Zero trans fats!" on the package.

So, how does fat affect you if you have Crohn's or colitis? A high-fat diet can create two problems in Crohn's and colitis:

- It can speed up the movement of food through the intestines, causing diarrhea — the last thing you want, especially during active disease.
- If you have Crohn's disease involving the ileum or you've had your ileum removed by surgery, you may become deficient in bile, a necessary chemical for fat absorption, which means your body may not get the fat it needs.

Omega-3s versus omega-6s

Omega- 6 fatty acids are unsaturated fatty acids that are found in red meat, cooking oils, and margarine. When omega-6 fatty acids are metabolized in the intestines, they produce chemicals that can cause inflammation. So, many studies have linked high consumption of omega-6 fatty acids to increased risk of developing colitis.

Omega-3 fatty acids, on the other hand, are found in foods such as fish, flaxseed, and kiwifruit. Unlike omega-6 fatty acids, omega-3s have *anti*-inflammatory properties and are considered to be beneficial in many inflammatory diseases, including Crohn's and colitis.

The clinical studies looking at the effects of omega-3 have not shown consistent results. Some studies have proved its effectiveness in the treatment of Crohn's and colitis, but other studies have failed to show any benefit. So, it remains unclear if omega-3s actually improve the symptoms and the process of inflammation.

Considering the overall health benefits of omega-3s, I find no harm in supplementing your diet with it. One well-respected brand is Nordic Naturals (`www.nordicnaturals.com`), but the key is to find one that's labeled as being free of mercury and other heavy metals.

Experts usually recommend a daily supplement of 500 mg to 1,000 mg of omega-3. The most common side effect from fish oil is indigestion and gas. Getting a supplement with an enteric coating can help with this problem.

You may want to talk with your doctor about supplementing with omega-3s to make sure you're getting the benefits you need.

Micronutrients

You need micronutrients in smaller quantities than macronutrients (see the preceding section), but they're just as important for healthy living as macronutrients are.

There are two kinds of micronutrients: vitamins and minerals.

Vitamins

Vitamins are organic chemicals required by the body to regulate a variety of functions; they're also essential for growth of tissues, such as bones, skin, glands, nerves, and blood. Nutritionists classify vitamins into two main groups: fat soluble and water soluble.

Fat-soluble vitamins

Fat-soluble vitamins dissolve in — you guessed it — fat, and they're stored in fatty tissue. They require fat in order to be absorbed through the intestines. Here are the fat-soluble vitamins:

- **Vitamin A:** Vitamin A is the moisturizing nutrient that keeps your skin and the *mucous membranes* (the internal lining of the nose, mouth, throat, intestines, and vagina) smooth and supple. Vitamin A also helps makes a protein that enables you to see even when the lights are low. You can find vitamin A in apricots, cantaloupe, carrots, liver (from chicken and turkey), mango, and peas. If you're deficient in vitamin A, you may experience poor night vision; dry skin; slow wound healing; nerve damage; a reduced ability to taste, hear, and smell; and decreased resistance to infections.
- **Vitamin D:** Vitamin D helps in the absorption of calcium, an important mineral for bones and teeth. Vitamin D has recently been shown to help prevent cancers and suppress inflammation in the intestines. You can find vitamin D in eggs, milk, salmon, and tuna. If you're deficient in vitamin D, you may experience muscle and bone pain, osteopenia or osteoporosis, and fatigue.
- **Vitamin E:** Vitamin E helps maintain your nerves, muscles, heart, and reproductive system. You can find vitamin E in almonds, apricots, green vegetables, peaches, and sunflower seeds. If you're deficient in vitamin E, you may experience muscle and nerve weakness, as well as decreased resistance to infections.
- **Vitamin K:** Vitamin K helps in the making of proteins that help in blood clotting. You also need vitamin K for bones and kidneys. You can find vitamin K in egg yolks; green, leafy vegetables; and liver (from beef, chicken, and turkey). If you're deficient in vitamin K, you may tend to bleed easily.

Many medical conditions, including Crohn's, can lead to difficulty absorbing fat. Fat malabsorption causes you to pass greasy, sticky, foul-smelling stools. If your body isn't absorbing fat properly, your doctor will advise you to take extra supplements of the fat-soluble vitamins to ensure you're getting enough.

Water-soluble vitamins

Water-soluble vitamins don't require fat for their absorption. Here are the water-soluble vitamins:

- **Vitamin B1 (thiamine):** Vitamin B1 helps in extracting energy from carbohydrates. It's also important for the health of your heart, liver, and kidneys. You can find vitamin B1 in bagels, carrots, corn, English muffins, ham, honeydew melons, liver (from beef), and sunflower seeds. If you're deficient in vitamin B1, you may experience poor appetite, weight loss, upset stomach, depression, an inability to concentrate, and fatigue.
- **Vitamin B2 (riboflavin):** Vitamin B2 helps in the digestion of proteins and carbohydrates. Like vitamin A, it protects the health of the mucous membranes. You can find vitamin B2 in bagels, English muffins, liver

(from beef, chicken, and turkey), milk, and yogurt. If you're deficient in vitamin B2, you may experience cracked lips, a sore tongue, burning eyes, and skin rashes.

- **Vitamin B3 (niacin):** Vitamin B3 is essential for proper growth; it also helps moves the oxygen in the body. You can find vitamin B3 in bagels, chicken, lamb, peanuts, pork, salmon, and veal. If you're deficient in vitamin B3, you may experience diarrhea, skin rashes, mental confusion, and fatigue.
- **Vitamin B5 (pantothenic acid):** Vitamin B5 helps extract energy from food. It also helps in forming hormones and defending the body against infections. You can find vitamin B5 in avocados and broccoli. If you're deficient in vitamin B5, you may experience fatigue, numbness, tingling, and muscle cramps.
- **Vitamin B6 (pyridoxine):**Vitamin B6 plays an important role in extracting energy from food. It's good for the health of your heart and brain. You can find vitamin B6 in bananas, chicken, lamb, liver (from beef), plantains, and prunes. If you're deficient in vitamin B6, you may experience anemia, seizures, skin rashes, upset stomach, nerve damage, and fatigue.
- **Vitamin B7 (biotin):** Vitamin B7 plays a role in the growth of the body. It's also thought to strengthen hair and nails. You can find vitamin B7 in berries; eggs; liver; leafy, green vegetables; and peanuts. If you're deficient in vitamin B7, you may experience loss of appetite; pale, dry, and scaly skin; hair loss; and depression.
- **Vitamin B9 (folic acid):** Vitamin B9 is very important to make new proteins in cells. It's vital for normal growth and wound healing. It also plays an important role during pregnancy for the growth of the baby. We also require vitamin B9 to produce healthy red blood cells and healthy sperm in males. You can find vitamin B9 in beans; green, leafy vegetables; beef liver; and pita bread. If you're deficient in vitamin B9, you may experience anemia and fatigue.
- **Vitamin B12 (cobalamine):** Vitamin B12 is important for the health of red blood cells and nerves. You can find vitamin B12 in beef, eggs, lamb, milk, pork, veal, and yogurt. If you're deficient in vitamin B12, you may experience anemia, fatigue, and numbness and tingling in your hands and feet.
- **Vitamin C:** Vitamin C is important for your muscles and bones. It also plays an important role in wound healing and protecting your immune system. You can find vitamin C in broccoli, Brussels sprouts, oranges, grapes, sweet peppers (also known as bell peppers), and tomatoes. If you're deficient in vitamin C, you may experience bleeding gums, loose teeth, easy bruising, painful joints, muscle pain, and skin rashes.

Inflammation and surgery of the intestines lead to decreased absorption of water-soluble vitamins and can cause deficiencies. Vitamin B12, in particular, is absorbed in the terminal ileum, which is the most common site for Crohn's disease. Inflammation or surgical removal of the terminal ileum may leads to vitamin B12 deficiency. In addition, certain medications (such as sulfasalazine) can cause decreased absorption of vitamin B9, and you may need to take a supplement to get what your body needs.

Minerals

When you hear about minerals, the first things that may come into your mind might be gold and silver. Those are minerals, but some types of minerals are also found in your food. Like vitamins, minerals help your body grow, develop, and stay healthy. They're divided into two categories: major minerals and trace elements.

Major minerals

Major minerals are minerals your body needs in larger quantities. The major minerals are

- **Calcium:** Calcium is important for your bones and teeth. You can find calcium in broccoli, dairy products, fish (such as sardines and salmon), spinach, and tofu.
- **Chloride:** Chloride helps maintain the right amount of water in your body. You can find chloride in celery, lettuce, olives, rye, and tomatoes.
- **Magnesium:** The body uses magnesium to move nutrients in and out of the cells and to send messages between cells. You can find magnesium in artichokes, nuts, peas, seeds, and whole wheat bread.
- **Phosphorus:** Like calcium, phosphorus is essential for strong bones and teeth. It also helps in building the protective sheath around your nerves. You can find phosphorus in broccoli, dairy products, spinach, and tofu.
- **Potassium:** Potassium, like chloride, helps maintain the right amount of water in your body. You can find potassium in bananas, broccoli, citrus fruits, and tomatoes.
- **Sodium:** Sodium, like potassium and chloride, helps maintain the right amount of water in your body. It also helps with nerve and muscle function. You can find sodium in beets, celery, cheese, green olives, milk, and salt.
- **Sulfur:** Sulfur is important for the health of your liver and heart. It also promotes healthy hair, skin, and nails. It's found in broccoli, cabbage, egg yolks, garlic, and onions.

Trace elements

These are naturally occurring chemical substances necessary for the optimal development and metabolic functioning of all living things. They're called *trace elements* because we require only minute amounts of their consumption for proper body functioning.

The important trace elements are as follows:

- **Chromium:** Chromium keeps your blood sugar under control. You can find it in American cheese, broccoli, and beef liver.
- **Copper:** Copper is an anti-aging mineral. You can find it in almonds, barley, cashews, crabmeat, lobster, peas, prunes, and shrimp.
- **Fluoride:** Fluoride prevents cavities and strengthens bones. It's usually added to your water system; food prepared in fluoridated water contains fluoride. Seafood and tea are other sources of fluoride.
- **Iodine:** Iodine is important for protein synthesis, regulation of body temperature, and many other body functions. You can find iodine in iodized salt and in seafood.
- **Iron:** Iron is an essential part of the protein hemoglobin, which stores and transports oxygen to different parts of the body. You can find iron in apricots, clams, lentils, nuts, oysters, peas, seeds, and soybeans.
- **Manganese:** Manganese keeps your bones, kidneys, intestines, and liver healthy. You can find it in cereal, tea, and whole grains.
- **Molybdenum:** Molybdenum helps extract energy from proteins and is also involved in waste processing in the kidneys. You can find it in beans; green, leafy vegetables; lentils; and peas.
- **Selenium:** Selenium is important for your heart. You can find selenium in dairy products, eggs, organ meat (such as liver and kidney), and seafood.
- **Zinc:** Zinc protects your nerves and brain tissues and boosts your immune system. You can find zinc in beef, chicken, oysters, and veal.

Fiber or No Fiber? That Is the Question

Fiber is a class of complex carbohydrates. The human body can't extract nutrients from certain fibers — we don't have the digestive enzymes in our intestinal tracts the way, say, cows do. But not being able to digest and absorb fiber doesn't make them less valuable. Consuming fiber has a variety of benefits.

In this section, I walk you through the types of fiber, tell you why fiber matters in general (for all people), and what role fiber plays when you have Crohn's or colitis.

Types of fiber

There are two types of fiber: insoluble and soluble.

Insoluble fiber

Insoluble fiber doesn't dissolve in water. It gives bulk and softness to the stool and stimulates your colon. Insoluble fiber is great for preventing constipation. This type of fiber is present in

- Whole-grain foods
- Legumes (such as beans and peas)
- Potato skins
- Tomato skins
- Vegetables such as celery and zucchini

Soluble fiber

Soluble fiber dissolves in water. It's also fermented by the bacteria present in your colon. You find this type of fiber in

- Oats
- Barley
- Fruits and fruit juices
- Psyllium seed husk
- Flaxseed

Why fiber matters

There are many benefits of consuming fiber. Medical research has shown that fiber can help

- Decrease the risk of colon cancer
- Control blood sugar and decrease the risk of diabetes
- Reduce blood cholesterol and decrease the risk of heart disease
- Prevent constipation

Although fiber is not digested and absorbed by the intestines, it does get broken down into smaller pieces in the stomach and intestines and performs important functions:

- **It slows the emptying of the stomach and lengthens the time it takes for sugar to be absorbed.** This helps improve your blood sugar level and is beneficial in preventing and controlling diabetes.
- **Insoluble fiber stimulates the intestine and moves solid material through the intestinal tract.** Not only does this help if you're constipated, but it also helps remove the old intestinal cells from the intestinal lining so that they can be replaced by new, healthy cells.
- **When fiber reaches the colon, the good bacteria residing there convert soluble fiber into short-chain fatty acids.** The colon cells use short-chain fatty acids for energy and to stay healthy.

The American Dietetic Association recommends that adults consume a minimum of 25 g to 35 g of fiber per day. If you want to get really specific, you need at least 14 g of fiber per 1,000 calories you consume.

Fiber's role in Crohn's and colitis

When your disease is under control and your intestines aren't inflamed, you should be able to tolerate the recommended amount of fiber (see the preceding section). Some people may still feel abdominal discomfort and bloating when they consume fiber.

During active disease, you may want to avoid fiber. Fiber makes the stool bulkier, and when the intestines contract to push the stools down, the rough surface of the fiber and bulkier stool can cause mild scraping of the tissue. When your intestines are inflamed, this can cause pain and further damage to the mucosa.

If you have narrowing of the intestines, such as a stricture, fiber can get stuck and cause abdominal swelling and pain. Most of the time, this gets better if you rest the intestines and take a break from eating. However, it can also cause severe obstruction, and you may need to be admitted to the hospital and even require surgery.

When you achieve remission and your intestines are no longer inflamed, you may want to add fiber back to your diet. But be sure to do so very slowly — add a few more grams to your diet every week until you're at the recommended level.

Be sure to chew your food very well to break down the fiber into smaller pieces to avoid obstruction at narrowed areas of the intestine. Also, drink plenty of water —fiber absorbs water, which keeps it soft and easy to pass. If you don't get enough water, constipation can occur.

Considering Specialized Diets for Crohn's and Colitis

As I mention earlier, there is no single magic diet for Crohn's and colitis. What works for one person may not work for others. I usually tell my patients to simply watch their diet; keep track of any foods that are causing bothersome symptoms; and eliminate those foods from the diet.

However, sometimes you need to follow a specific diet. For example, before going for a procedure such as a colonoscopy or surgery, you may be asked to consume a liquid diet. Similarly, if you have disease with active inflammation or stricture formation, you have to be on a low-residue diet. Finally, some people can't tolerate lactose and need to follow a lactose-free diet. In this section, I explain all these different types of diets.

Liquid diets

When you have Crohn's or colitis, you can get sick for a variety of reasons. You may develop severe inflammation, leading to increased abdominal pain, diarrhea, or blood in the stool. You may develop a narrowing of the intestines. You may develop complications from the drugs you take, including ulcers in the stomach or infections in the gut. When you're sick, you may not be able to tolerate solid food, and your doctor may advise you to be on a liquid diet because it's easily digestible. You may also be on liquid diet immediately before and after surgery and before a colonoscopy.

Liquid diets can be divided into two categories:

- **Clear:** A clear liquid diet consists of transparent liquids, such as water, clear fruit juices (apple juice, but not orange juice, for example), vegetable broth, popsicles, and clear gelatin (such as Jell-O).
- **Full:** A full liquid diet consists of both clear and opaque liquids with a smooth consistency. It includes milk; milkshakes; ice cream; smooth, cooked cereals (porridge, but not oatmeal, for example); butter; and honey.

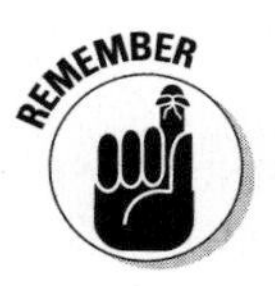

You can't stay on a liquid diet for more than a few days. A liquid diet is the kind of thing your doctor may put you on, but it's not something you should do on your own without consulting your doctor. (Of course, odds are, you won't want to anyway!)

Low-residue diets

Crohn's and colitis may cause a narrowing of the intestine. This can happen because of two main reasons:

- You get swelling of your mucosa during active inflammation, leading to narrowing of the *lumen* (the inside space of your intestines).
- When inflammation subsides, you can develop a scar in your intestines, which leads to a narrowing of the lumen.

In either case, you may have difficulty moving the food inside your intestines, and it can get stuck, causing obstruction. This especially happens when you have a lot of fiber in the diet.

During periods of active inflammation or after intestinal surgery, your doctor may put you on a low-residue diet. Low-residue diets also help with diarrhea. Low-residue diets typically allow no more than 10 g to 15 g of fiber per day.

Foods you may be able to eat on a low-residue diet include the following:

- White bread
- Cereals
- Crackers
- White rice
- Tender, ground, well-cooked meat
- Fish
- Eggs
- Poultry
- Butter
- Mayonnaise
- Vegetable oils
- Margarine
- Plain gravies
- Pulp free, strained, or clear juices

You typically can't have more than 2 cups of dairy products per day on a low-residue diet. Dairy products that you can have on a low-residue diet are milk, yogurt, cottage cheese, pudding or 1½ ounces of hard cheese.

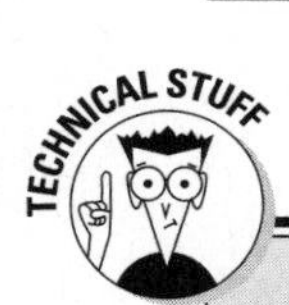

Low fiber versus low residue: Solving the mystery

The terms *low-fiber diet* and *low-residue diet* are often used interchangeably, but there is actually a difference between the two diets. Fiber is the part of plant food that can't be digested, and residue is the undigested part of plants that contributes to the stool. A low-fiber diet, as the name says, is low in fiber. A low-residue diet is more restrictive than a low-fiber diet and limits more foods, including fiber. For example, a low-fiber diet allows some fruits and vegetables, but a low-residue diet allows only fruit and vegetable juices without seeds or pulp. Some foods (like dairy products and coffee) are low in fiber but can increase residue; other foods (like seedless peaches and ripened bananas) are low in residue but high in fiber. A low-fiber diet helps to decrease the number of bowel movements you have, and a low-residue diet also reduces the size of your stool.

Foods to avoid when you're on a low-residue diet include the following:

- Whole-grain breads and pastas
- Cornbread or muffins
- Raw vegetables
- Tough meat and meat with gristle
- Peanut butter
- Millet
- Flax
- Oatmeal
- Dried fruits
- Berries
- Fruits with skins or seeds
- Highly spiced foods and dressings
- Pepper
- Hot sauces
- Popcorn
- Nuts
- Seeds

One size doesn't fit all. You may not be able to tolerate some of the foods in the first list, or you may be able to tolerate some of the foods on the second list. Work closely with your doctor and dietitian to come up with an individual plan that works best for you.

Lactose-free diets

Many people are deficient in *lactase,* the enzyme that splits *lactose* (milk sugar) into glucose and galactose, the simple sugars. If lactose-intolerant people drink milk or consume milk products, they end up with lots of undigested lactose in their intestines. The result: gas, cramps, and diarrhea.

About 15 percent to 20 percent of people with Crohn's and colitis have lactase deficiency.

Lactose intolerance is most often controlled through adjusting your diet. For young children, all lactose-containing foods should be avoided. For adults and older kids, the amount of lactose that can be tolerated varies. Some people may be able to eat butter and aged cheeses (which have low levels of lactose). Others can tolerate one glass of milk, but drinking two will give them trouble. For most people, figuring out how much dairy they can consume is a matter of trial and error.

Watch out for hidden lactose. Lactose is used in some prescription medicines (such as birth control pills) and over-the-counter medicines (like drugs to treat stomach acid and gas). Checking the ingredients on food labels is helpful in finding possible sources of lactose in food products.

Common foods that may contain lactose include the following:

- Bread
- Candies
- Commercial pie crusts
- Pancakes
- Pudding and custards
- Salad dressings
- Soups

Because milk and other dairy products are rich sources of calcium, avoiding these foods can put you at risk for calcium deficiency. Your doctor or dietitian may recommend other sources (such as a daily calcium supplement or nondairy sources of calcium, such as broccoli, salmon, shrimp, and turnips).

Elemental diets

An elemental diet is a predigested liquid diet that contains all the nutrients your body needs. The nutrients in this diet require very little digestion and are easily and quickly absorbed. An elemental diet meets all your nutritional requirements while giving rest to your digestive system. (For this reason, it's also called a *bowel-rest diet.*)

Instead of having protein, carbohydrates, and fat, this diet has amino acids, glucose, and fatty acids that are easily absorbed. Your intestines don't have to work hard to break down the nutrients. The stool that results from consuming an elemental diet is small in volume and usually liquid, allowing your colon to heal faster.

Vitamins, minerals, and electrolytes are usually added to the formula. Usually flavor is added as well, to make it more palatable.

An elemental diet is given either through the mouth or through a *nasogastric tube* (a tube passed directly through the nose into your stomach). Obviously, this isn't a diet you follow on your own — it's one your doctor may prescribe if you're having bothersome symptoms such diarrhea and abdominal pain and/or if the regular diet is worsening your symptoms of Crohn's and colitis. Some clinical studies have shown the benefit of an elemental diet in healing the inflamed intestines, especially in Crohn's disease.

Nutritional Support: When You Can't Go It Alone

When you have Crohn's or colitis, you may have periods when you can't get the nutrients you need by mouth. This situation can arise when you have mouth sores and swallowing is painful. It can also occur when you just don't have an appetite, and you aren't eating enough to stay nourished.

In order to prevent or correct malnutrition, your doctor may suggest tube feeding or nutrition through the veins to provide you enough calories and nutrients so that you stay healthy. You may also take nutrition supplements. In this section, I cover all three.

Enteral feeding: Feeding through a tube

Enteral feeding, also known as *tube feeding,* is a way to deliver nutrients through a tube if you can't take food or drink through your mouth. In most cases, you only need tube feeding for a short period of time (such as during a hospital stay or shortly after surgery). In some cases, you may need to go home from the hospital with a tube.

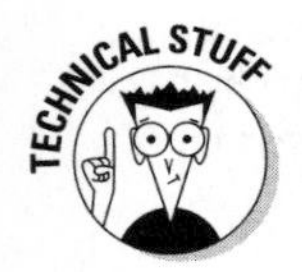

Depending on the situation, you may get a tube that leads from the nose to the stomach (a *nasogastric tube*), a tube that leads directly from the skin to the stomach (a *gastrostomy tube*), or a tube that leads from the skin to the intestines (a *jejunostomy*).

Unfortunately, you can't feed yourself a hamburger through a tube. The food you use for enteral feeding is specialized. Although you can use blenderized food, most of the time you get commercially made liquid formulas.

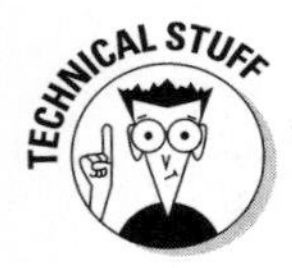

The foods you consume through a tube could be *polymer feeds* (containing whole proteins, fats, minerals, and fiber) or *elemental feeds* (containing predigested proteins, fats, carbohydrates, and other supplements).

Total parenteral nutrition: Feeding directly into your veins

Parenteral nutrition is a method of feeding a person through the veins. When this is the only way of getting nutrition, it's called *total parenteral nutrition* (TPN). TPN is a liquid formula that contains all the important nutrients your body needs (such as glucose, amino acids, fats, vitamins, and minerals). The formula is connected through a pump and infused to one of your larger veins through a catheter.

You can get TPN even at home with the help of a family member who can help you prepare and attach the formula to the pump and connect it to your veins. Also, you don't have to get nutrition through this method around the clock — formulas are calculated and concentrated, so you can give yourself nutrition lasting for 12 to 16 hours, especially through the nighttime, and freely move around during the day to perform most of your daily chores.

Typically, you get TPN if you have severe Crohn's or colitis and are unable to tolerate an oral diet, leading to a compromised nutritional status. TPN helps you get all the calories and nutrients you need to function and remain healthy and alive. It gives rest to your intestines during time of active inflammation and provides adequate nutrients to help with the process of healing.

However, because TPN is an unnatural way of feeding, it does come with side effects and complications, such as infection at the site where the tube is inserted into your veins, blood clots, *fatty liver* (deposits of fat in your liver that can affect its functioning), and gallstones. Your doctor will carefully review your medical condition and discuss with you the risks and benefits before recommending and starting this form of therapy.

Nutrition supplements: Boosting your diet

If you've recently recovered from an acute flare or had Crohn's or colitis surgery, you may be malnourished, and simply getting extra food may not provide you with enough nutrients. In this case, you may need to take extra supplements. Similarly, your doctor may suggest supplements to help with inflammation and aid the process of healing.

Supplements come in variety of forms:

- Protein and energy shakes (such as Ensure Immune Health)
- Organ tissues, such as liver
- Hormones, such as melatonin
- Vitamins and minerals
- Probiotics and prebiotics (see the nearby sidebar)

The supplements may come as a single-ingredient product (such as vitamin E capsules), or they may be combination of products (such as multivitamins or energy drinks).

Many nutritional supplements are not regulated by food and drug authorities and may even contain harmful ingredients that could interfere or interact with your medications. Always talk with your doctor before taking any supplement, no matter how safe it seems.

When choosing a supplement, pick a well-known brand. Follow the storage requirements on the label (for example, keeping the bottle out of extreme heat or cold), and pay attention to the expiration date. Follow the dosage on the bottle (as long as your doctor says it's okay).

The story of probiotics and prebiotics

The bad bacteria inside your intestines play an important role in causing inflammation and may lead to Crohn's or colitis (see Chapter 4). This theory sparked interest among many physicians and scientists, and led them to explore the option of using *good* bacteria as a therapy for Crohn's or colitis.

Probiotics are live bacteria that provide you with different health benefits. They replace the bad bacteria by directly killing them and also taking away their food and starving them to death. Probiotics also do the following:

- Decrease inflammation of the intestines
- Boost the immune system

(continued)

(continued)

- Treat and prevent intestinal infections such as *Clostridium difficile*
- Manage symptoms of irritable bowel syndrome
- Prevent antibiotics-associated diarrhea
- Improve symptoms of lactose intolerance

Many different types of probiotics have been used to manage Crohn's and colitis. However, there are trillions of bacteria inside the intestines, and scientists have yet to find the right bacteria that can treat and cure the inflammation. In the meantime, they've combined some important kinds of bacteria and developed different formulations. These different combinations are found to have stronger anti-inflammatory properties. One such probiotic, called VSL#3, is readily available in the United States, Canada, and Europe. It contains billions of live bacteria belonging to three different classes — *Bifidobacterium, Lactobacillus,* and *Streptococcus.* This combination of bacteria has been found useful in preventing *pouchitis* (inflammation of the pouch) after colitis surgery. Many doctors recommend VSL#3 to their patients if they're at a higher risk for developing pouchitis.

Remember: Research on probiotics controlling active symptoms and inflammation of Crohn's and colitis has produced mixed results. Some studies have shown a benefit, while others show no significant difference. Talk to your doctor to see if this form of therapy is right for you.

The good bacteria and bad bacteria in the intestines are constantly battling for food to survive and reproduce. How about creating a special food for these good bacteria to increase their numbers and keep them healthy and alive? Scientists are a step ahead and have discovered *prebiotics* — the food for *probiotics.* Besides keeping the good bacteria alive and well in the intestines, prebiotics can

- Increase the health of healthy bacteria
- Increase the absorption of calcium and magnesium
- Lower blood cholesterol levels
- Enhance immune function
- Normalize bowel function
- Reduce the risk of intestinal infections

Most types of grains contain prebiotics. Many vegetables and fruits also contain prebiotics, including bananas, beans, kiwifruit, and onions. Most of the commercially available prebiotics are mixed with probiotics and sold as a supplemental food. They're also added as additives to foods like breads, cereals, yogurts, and spreads.

Chapter 10

Preventing Health Problems

In This Chapter

- Knowing which vaccinations you need and why
- Uncovering skin problems
- Dealing with bone issues
- Identifying your cancer risk

No one can argue with Benjamin Franklin's famous saying that an ounce of prevention is worth a pound of cure. If you have Crohn's or colitis, old Ben's adage should become your mantra. These chronic lifelong illnesses, along with the drug therapies you receive to manage the troubling symptoms associated with them, put you at various risks.

Crohn's and colitis can affect many body systems — even ones you may not expect. For example, they can cause skin problems and increase your risk of various cancers. The drugs for Crohn's and colitis can put you at risk for infections, as well as cause weakening of your bones. The good news is, you can prevent or at least minimize these risks by adopting different preventive strategies. In this chapter, I give you a closer look at these risk factors and different measures that you can take to prevent them.

Getting Vaccinated

Just as wearing a seat belt protects you from injury in a car accident, vaccines protect you from serious infections that could even be fatal. A vaccine is a drug used to enhance or induce immunity to a particular disease. It usually contains an agent that resembles the disease-causing microorganism. Vaccines are usually made from weakened or killed forms of the microorganism or its toxins. Your body's immune system recognizes the vaccine as a foreign object and destroys it. In doing so, it also preserves a memory of that invader so that if your body is exposed to the bug or toxin again, your body can easily recognize and destroy it.

Why vaccination matters

When your immune system is trained to resist an infection, you are said to be *immune* to it. Before vaccines, the only way to become immune to an infection was to actually *get* the infection. This is called *naturally acquired immunity,* but it comes with its own price tag — you suffer the symptoms of the disease and also take the risk of complications, including serious and deadly ones. You may also become contagious and pass the disease on to others. Vaccines provide *artificially acquired immunity.* They're a much less risky way to acquire immunity — they prevent the disease from happening in the first place.

Immunity is especially important when your immune system is already weak, as it is when you're taking drugs that suppress your immunity. Not only do these drugs put you at risk for infections, but you may not be able to tolerate the infections without becoming seriously sick. Some of these infections can even be fatal if your immune system fails to control them properly. Vaccines are essential in these situations.

Which vaccines you need

You need to make sure you get all the recommended vaccines indicated for your age. You can review your vaccination status with your doctor to make sure you're up to date. If you have any incomplete vaccination series, your doctor may suggest getting a catch-up vaccination.

Demystifying the measles vaccines story

The virus that causes measles infects your respiratory system and then spreads to the lymph nodes. During the acute infection, lymph cells in your intestines also are infected and may cause inflammation. This observation by scientists led to a speculation that the measles virus vaccine, which contains live attenuated virus, may cause inflammatory bowel disease (IBD). However, this has not been proven by medical research.

Some studies in the early 1990s showed a *possible* association between the vaccine and Crohn's and colitis, but these studies were methodologically weak. Subsequently, many larger studies failed to show *any* increased risk from measles vaccines. Scientists also failed to find any active measles virus in the inflamed intestines.

Currently, all experts recommend continuing measles vaccines as indicated.

You may not be able to receive live vaccines if you're taking certain medications that suppress your immunity, such as anti-TNF drugs. If you have any concerns about receiving a vaccine, talk with your doctor.

In the following sections, I cover the vaccines you may need.

Note: For information on vaccines required for international travel, check out Chapter 14. And for more information on vaccinations for children, see Chapter 15.

The influenza vaccine

Influenza, also known as the *flu,* is a contagious illness that affects your respiratory system. It's caused by flu viruses. The flu is different from a cold. It usually comes on suddenly and causes fever, cough, sore throat, muscle or body aches, and fatigue. Most people who get the flu will recover in a few days to a few weeks. But if you have suppressed immunity, you're at a higher risk of developing complications, including ear or sinus infections and pneumonia. Other people at risk for developing complications include older people, pregnant women, and people suffering from certain chronic medical conditions such as heart disease, diabetes, or asthma.

There are two types of flu vaccines:

- **Flu shot:** The flu shot is an inactivated vaccine — it contains killed virus. It's given with a needle into a muscle, usually in the arm.
- **Nasal-spray flu vaccine:** The nasal spray is vaccine made with live but weakened flu viruses. It's given to healthy people who are not pregnant or immunosuppressed. You should avoid this vaccine if you're taking steroids, other immunosuppressive drugs, or biologic therapy for Crohn's or colitis. (Talk with your doctor if you're not sure whether it's safe to have the nasal spray — or, if you prefer, just opt for the flu shot instead.)

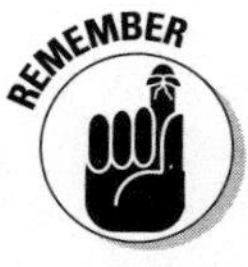

It takes about two weeks after vaccination for antibodies to develop in the body and provide protection against the flu. In the meantime, you're still at risk of getting the flu. That's why it's better to get vaccinated early in the fall, before the flu season really gets under way.

Some people should *not* get flu vaccines without first consulting a doctor. These include people with severe allergy to chicken eggs, children under the age of 6 months, and people who have moderate to severe illness with a fever.

The pneumococcal vaccine

Pneumococcal disease is an infection caused by bacteria named *Streptococcus pneumoniae* (pneumococcus). There are different types of pneumococcal diseases, including

- **Pneumonia:** Pneumonia is an infection of the lungs. The common symptoms include fever, cough, and shortness of breath.
- **Meningitis:** Meningitis is an infection of the brain. It can cause a stiff neck, fever, mental confusion, and sensitivity to light (called *photophobia*).
- **Otitis media:** Otitis media is an infection of the ear. It typically causes a painful earache.

Pneumococcal diseases can be fatal. In some cases, they can cause long-term complications such as brain damage or hearing loss. The vaccine can prevent these complications. There are two types of vaccines:

- **Pneumococcal conjugate vaccine (PCV 13):** This is also called Prevnar 13. A four-dose series is recommended for all children under 5 years of age. A singe dose is recommended for children between 6 and 17 years of age and for adults 50 years or older.
- **Pneumococcal polysaccharide vaccine (PPSV):** This is also called Pneumovax. It's currently recommended for
    - All adults 65 years of age and older
    - Any person 2 years of age or older who is at high risk for the disease (such as someone receiving immunosuppressive medications)
    - Adults ages 19 through 64 years of age who smoke or who have asthma

The hepatitis B vaccine

Hepatitis B is a contagious liver disease that results from infection with the hepatitis B virus. It can range in severity from a mild disease lasting a few weeks to a serious and lifelong illness. Hepatitis B is usually spread when blood, semen, or another body fluid from a person infected with the hepatitis virus enters the body of someone who is not infected. This can happen through sexual contact with an infected person or through the sharing of needles. Hepatitis B also can be passed from an infected mother to her baby at birth.

The best way to prevent Hepatitis B is by getting vaccinated. Experts recommend that all children get their first dose of hepatitis B vaccine at birth and complete the vaccine series between 6 and 18 month of age.

Hepatitis B can cause chronic hepatitis without producing any symptoms — you may not even know that you're infected with the virus. If you get immunosuppressive medications, such as anti-TNF therapy for Crohn's or colitis, you can get fatal hepatitis B virus reactivation. So, doctors usually perform blood tests to ensure that you have good immunity against the virus and to rule out any unknown hepatitis B infection before starting these medications.

The HPV vaccine

Human papillomavirus (HPV) is the most common sexually transmitted infection. In the majority of cases, the immune system clears the virus within two years. But sometimes HPV infection is not cleared and can cause *genital warts* (small bumps in the genital area), cervical cancer, and even vaginal cancer. Taking immunosuppressive medication may increase your risk of getting HPV infection and not being able to clear it. Women who take drugs like azathioprine or 6-MP have been shown to have increased risk of abnormal Pap smears.

There are two HPV vaccines licensed in the United States to prevent genital warts and cervical cancer:

- **Cervarix:** Recommended only for females ages 19 to 26
- **Gardasil:** Recommended for both males and females ages 19 to 26

Varicella

If you can't provide a clear history of chicken pox, you should have a blood test for *varicella* (the virus that causes chicken pox). If you're not naturally immune to it, you should get a varicella vaccine.

Shingles

The varicella virus can also cause shingles, a very painful skin rash. Taking immunosuppressive medications increases your risk of shingles. Unlike chicken pox, shingles does not produce natural immunity.

The shingles vaccine has been approved for people over 50 years of age as a one-time dose regardless of previous varicella infection. Your doctor may suggest this vaccine if you're receiving or about to receive immunosuppressive drugs.

Meningococcal vaccine

Meningococcal disease is a serious bacterial infection that can cause meningitis, pneumonia, and infection in the blood. People between 16 and 21 years of age are at particularly increased risk. College freshmen living in dorms are also at increased risk. The risk of getting the disease and the complications from the disease increase if you're on immunosuppressive drugs. Experts recommend vaccinating kids at 11 or 12 years of age and then giving another booster shot at age 16.

Caring for Your Skin: It's Not Just Cosmetic

The skin is the largest organ in the body — and it's a very important one at that. Skin covers and protects everything inside your body. Without skin, your muscles, bones, and other organs would be hanging out all over the place — skin holds it all together. It helps regulate body temperature and acts as a filter. When you have a fever or you're working hard physically, you tend to sweat, which is the body's way of lowering its temperature. Your skin also makes vitamin D, which is important for your bone health. Skin problems aren't just cosmetic — they can affect some of the important functions your skin performs.

Identifying the skin complications you may face

Skin problems are very common in people with Crohn's and colitis. About one-quarter of patients may suffer from skin problems. These include problems related to the disease itself, as well as drug reactions.

Skin conditions associated with Crohn's or colitis are as follows:

- **Acrodermatitis enteropathica:** In acrodermatitis enteropathica, red patches appear around the mouth and also on the hands, feet, and scalp. It's caused by zinc deficiency.
- **Apthous stomatitis:** Apthous stomatitis is marked by small painful ulcers in the *mucosa* (inner lining) of the mouth, also known as canker sores. The ulcers frequently appear on the inside of the lower lip or cheeks.
- **Crohn's disease:** Yes, Crohn's disease can occur on your skin, too! It especially can appear as ulcers or plaques around an ostomy site and in the female genitals.
- **Erythema nodosum:** Erythema nodosum are skin lesions appearing as painful, red nodules that develop most commonly on the lower legs. (See Chapter 2 for more information.)

- **Pyoderma gangrenosum:** Pyoderma gangrenosum develops as deep ulcers filled with pus. It's also commonly found on the lower legs. (See Chapter 2 for more information.)
- **Sweet's syndrome:** Sweet's syndrome is characterized by small, red bumps that appear suddenly on the arms, neck, face, or back, accompanied by a fever. You can also get pinkeye and joint pains with Sweet's syndrome.

You can also get skin rashes as a reaction to the drugs you're prescribed for Crohn's or colitis, such as aminosalicylates (such as mesalamine) and azathioprine.

The most fearful complication in Crohn's and colitis patients is skin cancer (see the next section).

Recognizing and reducing your risk of skin cancer

Skin cancer is the most common form of cancer in the United States. More than 3.5 million skin cancers in more than 2 million people are diagnosed annually. There are two main categories of skin cancer:

- **Melanoma:** Melanoma is the skin cancer that arises from pigment-making cells of the skin called *melanocytes.*
- **Non-melanoma:** Non-melanoma cancers arise from the outermost layer of the skin. Basal cell carcinoma and squamous cell carcinoma are the main types of non-melanoma skin cancers. About eight out of ten skin cancers are basal cell carcinomas. They most often start on skin that has been exposed to the sun, like the face, ears, neck, lips, and backs of the hands.

So, why is skin cancer a problem among those with Crohn's and colitis? The sunlight contains ultraviolet (UV) rays. These UV rays can damage the genes in your skin cells, which puts you at risk for skin cancer — and this is true for everyone (whether they have Crohn's or colitis or not). The immune system helps the body fight cancers of the skin and other organs. Therefore, weakening of the immune system — as happens with immunosuppressive drugs — increases your cancer risk. This risk of skin cancer in Crohn's and colitis is especially increased in patients taking azathioprine and 6-MP, because these medications get metabolized in the body and some of the drugs enter the skin cells, making these cells more sensitive to the UV rays and thereby increasing the risk of skin cancer.

Besides UV radiation and immunosuppressive medications, your risk of skin cancer increases even more if you have fair skin, are older, are male, or smoke.

The most important thing you can do to lower your risk of skin cancer is to limit your exposure to UV radiation. You may have heard the catch phrase “slip, slop, slap, and wrap” from your dermatologist — this phrase helps remind you of four important steps in preventing skin cancer:

- ***Slip* on a shirt.** Long-sleeved shirts, long pants, or long skirts protect you from UV radiation. Dry fabric is more protective than wet fabric.
- ***Slop* on sunscreen.** Many groups, including the American Academy of Dermatology, recommend using products with a sun protection factor (SPF) of 30 or more. Generously apply sunscreen over your entire body 30 minutes before going outside. Reapply every two hours or immediately after swimming or excessive sweating.
- ***Slap* on a hat.** A hat with at least a 2- to 3-inch brim all around is ideal because it protects areas that are often exposed to intense sun, such as your ears, eyes, nose, and scalp. Wearing a baseball cap can protect the front and top of your head but not the neck or the ears.
- ***Wrap* on sunglasses.** Sunglasses provide protection for the eyes and the skin area around the eyes. Look for sunglasses labeled as blocking UVA and UVB light.

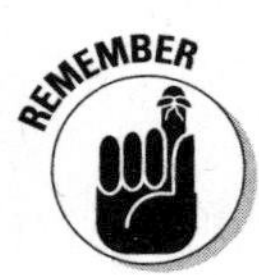

Don’t forget to examine your skin head to toe every month and see your doctor for a yearly skin exam if you’re on immunosuppressive medications such as azathioprine and anti-TNF drugs.

Caring for your skin “down there”: Perianal skin care

Just as infants gets diaper rash because of frequent contact with feces and sweat, going to the restroom and wiping your bottom frequently during the active phase of Crohn’s and colitis can lead to skin problems around the anus and surrounding area. Medically speaking, this skin inflammation is called *perineal dermatitis.* The resulting skin injury can range from redness and itching to ulcer formation and bleeding from the ulcerated skin. These skin problems can extend to the buttocks, groin, and even your upper thighs.

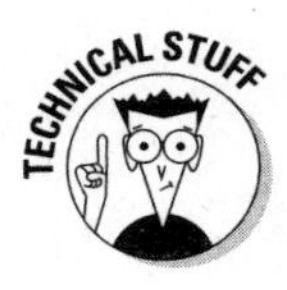

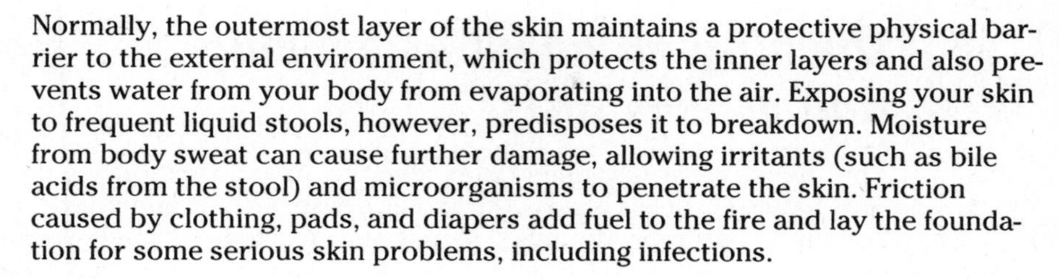
Normally, the outermost layer of the skin maintains a protective physical barrier to the external environment, which protects the inner layers and also prevents water from your body from evaporating into the air. Exposing your skin to frequent liquid stools, however, predisposes it to breakdown. Moisture from body sweat can cause further damage, allowing irritants (such as bile acids from the stool) and microorganisms to penetrate the skin. Friction caused by clothing, pads, and diapers add fuel to the fire and lay the foundation for some serious skin problems, including infections.

Here are a few important tips for keeping your perianal skin clean and healthy:

- **Manage moisture.** Cleanse and pat dry your skin, especially after having a bowel movement. You can even use a hairdryer on a cool setting for this purpose. Also, wear cotton underwear, instead of nylon or other fabrics. If you use pads or briefs, try to avoid plastic-backed products.
- **Use a good cleanser and moisturizer.** Cleaning your skin as soon as possible after going to the bathroom is critical to prevent skin damage. Moisturizers help maintain the barrier function of the skin. Select a product that's easy to apply and that stays on the skin. Pastes and ointments are better than creams and lotions for this purpose. Avoid products with irritants, such as fragrance and alcohol.
- **Rule out infections.** Consider talking to your doctor or consulting a dermatologist if a rash doesn't respond to cleansers and moisturizers. Bacterial infections and yeast rash are common problems and can be easily treated with local antibiotic or antifungal medications.

Boning Up on Bone Health

Healthy bones are very important. Whether you're lifting your baby, enjoying a day in the park, or going grocery shopping, your bones make it possible. Without bones, your body would be nothing more than a shapeless blob of tissue. Bones protect your nervous system (in the form of your skull and backbone). Most of the bones are filled with a jellylike material called *bone marrow.* Your red blood cells (which take oxygen throughout the body) are made here. Bone marrow also produces white blood cells (which are needed for the immune system) and fat cells.

Bones live on calcium and vitamin D. If you're deficient in these important nutrients, your bones will be weak and fragile and can easily break. Many diseases, including Crohn's and colitis, can affect your bones by affecting the balance of calcium and vitamin D in your body.

Opening up about osteopenia and osteoporosis

Your bones are programmed to regenerate. New bones replace the old ones. This natural process keeps your bones dense, strong, and sturdy. If there is a fault in this process, though, you may start losing bone mass too fast or may not be able make new bones fast enough. As a result, your bones become weak over time, and if the situation isn't addressed and treated, something as ordinary as lifting a stuffed grocery bag can cause a fracture. Medically speaking, this condition is called *osteoporosis.*

Osteopenia is when your bone mineral density (BMD) is lower than normal peak BMD but not low enough to be called osteoporosis. BMD is a measurement of minerals in the bones, telling how strong they are. Osteopenia, if untreated, can lead to osteoporosis.

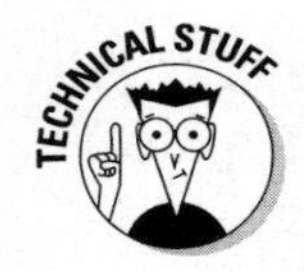

Osteoporosis means "porous bone." When you look under the microscope at a bone, it looks like a honeycomb. If you have osteoporosis, the holes and spaces in the honeycomb become much bigger than they are in a healthy bone. The bone has become less dense. As the bones become less dense, they become weaker and can break easily.

The risk factors for osteopenia and osteoporosis include the following:

- Being white (Caucasian)
- Having a family member with osteoporosis
- Being thin and slim (with a body mass index of 19 or lower; you can find yours at `www.nhlbisupport.com/bmi`)
- Using steroids and certain seizure medications
- Being inactive
- Smoking
- Drinking alcohol excessively
- Eating a diet low in calcium and vitamin D
- Having low testosterone levels (in men)

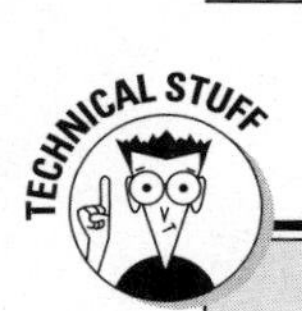

Having your bone mineral density tested

Your doctor may want to screen you for osteoporosis if you've been taking corticosteroids long term (5 mg of prednisone for more than three months), if you have a history of fracture, or if you're a woman over the age of 65 or man over the age of 70.

One of the screening tests for osteoporosis is a bone mineral density test. *Bone mineral density* is a medical term referring to the amount of mineral matter per square centimeter of bone. BMD measures the density of minerals like calcium in your bones using special X-rays or a CT scan. The results are used to estimate the strength of your bones.

There are different ways to measure BMD. The most commonly used test is called the dual-energy-X-ray absorptiometry (DEXA) scan. This scan uses lower doses of X-rays to estimate bone density in your spine and hip. Strong and dense bones allow less of the X-ray beam to pass through them. The amounts of each X-ray beam that are blocked by bone are compared to each other. Results are generally scored as T-scores. Your T-score compares your bone mineral density with the young normal average bone mineral density, and expresses the difference as a standard deviation score. Negative scores indicate lower bone density; positive scores indicate higher bone density. Osteopenia is defined as a score between –1.0 and –2.5. Osteoporosis is defined as a score of –2.5 or lower.

Seeing what Crohn's and colitis can do to your bones

Approximately 30 percent to 60 percent of people with Crohn's or colitis have lower bone density than normal. Several factors in Crohn's and colitis put you at risk for weak bones:

- **Steroid therapy:** Steroids are highly effective anti-inflammatory drugs to help control the symptoms of Crohn's and colitis. But their powerful effect comes with a price of bone loss. More than half of patients who take steroids long term develop osteoporosis. Steroids cause osteoporosis by decreasing the absorption of calcium from food, increasing calcium excretion in the urine, and stimulating the breakdown process of bones. For this reason, doctors try to minimize the use of steroids in Crohn's and colitis as much as possible.

- **Inflammation:** During the process of inflammation, many chemicals called *cytokines* are released. Some of these cytokines can disrupt the process of bone formation and lead to bone loss. This is one reason that keeping your Crohn's or colitis under control is so important.
- **Vitamin D deficiency:** Vitamin D is necessary for the absorption of calcium from the intestines. Both vitamin D and calcium are essential building blocks of your bones. You're at risk of vitamin D deficiency if you have inflammation of the small intestine or if you've undergone resection of the small intestine. Certain medications such as steroid can also result in vitamin D deficiency. Another source of vitamin D is your skin, which makes vitamin D under sunlight. Inadequate sun exposure may also lead to vitamin D deficiency and contribute to bone loss.

Many professional societies and physicians recommend screening for osteoporosis in Crohn's and colitis if you

- Have a history of fractures
- Are a postmenopausal woman
- Are a man over the age of 50
- Have used steroids long term (more than three months)
- Are a man with low testosterone levels

Managing bone loss

If you're at risk for bone loss, you can take some simple steps to keep osteoporosis at bay. And the good news is that if you already have osteoporosis, some of these steps can even *reverse* the bone loss! Work with your doctor to develop a bone-protecting action plan, and follow these suggestions:

- **Get enough exercise.** Many bone specialists recommend people get at least 30 minutes of weight-bearing exercise every day to strengthen their bones and prevent osteoporosis. One of the best weight-bearing activities is walking — it's simple, it doesn't require any special equipment, and you can do it just about anywhere. Other examples of weight-bearing exercise include jogging, hiking, and dancing.

  Note: Swimming and cycling are *not* weight-bearing exercises, but they're great ways to stay in shape. Just make sure if you swim or cycle, you also get plenty of weight-bearing exercise every day.
- **Take a calcium and vitamin D supplement if you're not getting enough through diet alone.** Get at least 800 IU of vitamin D and 1,200 to 1,500 mg of calcium per day. Good sources of calcium and vitamin D include fat-free dairy products; calcium-fortified juices and foods; green, leafy vegetables; and soy products.

- **Quit smoking and don't drink excessively.** Studies have shown that having more than two drinks daily is linked to an increased risk of bone loss. Similarly, cigarette smoking almost doubles the risk of bone loss and fracture (not to mention wreaking havoc on your health in other ways).
- **Drink soda in moderation.** Some studies show that soda drinks, colas in particular, can also contribute to bone loss probably because of extra phosphorus that binds with calcium and prevents its absorption. Caffeinated sodas appear to do more damage than non-caffeinated. And if you're guzzling a soda with dinner, chances are, you probably aren't drinking a glass of milk, thereby increasing your risk of osteoporosis.
- **Take medications for osteoporosis.** If you've been found to be at risk for osteoporosis or you've been diagnosed with osteoporosis, your doctor may want to prescribe medications to treat the condition. These medications either slow the breakdown process of the bones or help form new bone cells.

  Here is a list and description of the medications you may be prescribed:

  - **Bisphosphonates:** Bisphosphonates are the most widely used medications for osteoporosis. They slow the breakdown of the bones. Some commonly used bisphosphonates are alendronate (Fosamax), risedronate (Actonel, Atelvia), ibandronate (Boniva), and zoledronate (Reclast, Zometa).

    Most of these medications come in pill form. Your doctor will recommend taking them early in the morning, on an empty stomach, usually 30 minutes before breakfast and with at least 8 ounces of water to improve the absorption of the drugs. Newer drugs such as ibandronate and zoledronate come in intravenous forms, which bypass potential stomach upset. Ibandronate is usually given once every three months; zoledronate is given once a year.

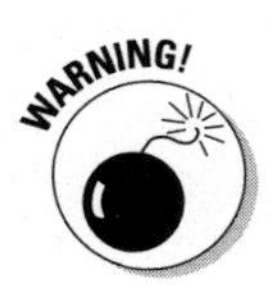

    Taking bisphosphonate for a long time can cause osteonecrosis of the jawbone, which is a rare condition in which a section of the jawbone dies and deteriorates. Even simple dental work can then cause serious problems. So, consider getting any dental work done prior to starting this drug to prevent any risk of osteonecrosis. If you've been on this drug for five years, it may be time to talk with your doctor about whether you should take a break from it.

    If you're pregnant or planning to become pregnant, talk to your doctor before taking bisphosphonate. In animal studies, bisphosphonates have been found to cause defects in babies' bones when taken in larger amounts for a long period of time.

  - **Hormone replacement therapy:** Hormone replacement therapy (HRT) used to be a standard treatment for women with hot flashes and other menopausal symptoms. It has also been shown to have a healthy effect on your bones by stopping the process of bone breakdown. However, some very large clinical trials showed that these drugs may increase the risk of heart disease, stroke, blood clots, and breast cancer. Talk with your doctor about the risks and benefits of HRT before choosing this form of treatment for osteoporosis.

- **Calcitonin:** Calcitonin is a hormone that is naturally produced in the thyroid gland. It's a powerful inhibitor of the bone breakdown process. It comes in a nasal spray and is specially used to treat osteoporosis in women who are at least five years past menopause and can't or do not want to take estrogen products.
- **Denosumab (Prolia):** This is a new drug used to treat osteoporosis in post-menopausal women. It's an antibody that blocks the maturation of cells that are involved in the bone breakdown process. You inject the drug under your skin twice a year.

Screening for Cancers

Having Crohn's or colitis puts you at risk for certain cancers. Colon cancer is the most important cancer associated with Crohn's disease of the colon and ulcerative colitis. Scientists generally believe that it's the persistent inflammation of the colon that triggers the colon cancer. This is one reason that keeping your disease under control is so important. If you're taking immunosuppressive medications, the risk of cervical cancer (in females) is also important to keep in mind.

Colon cancer

Colon cancer is the fourth most commonly diagnosed cancer in the world. It invades the large intestines of thousands of people each year. Most people undergo painful surgeries and invasive chemotherapy/radiation regimens when diagnosed with colon cancer. Colon cancer does not discriminate — even the healthiest people can develop the disease — but certain people, such as those suffering from Crohn's disease of the colon and ulcerative colitis, are at higher risk.

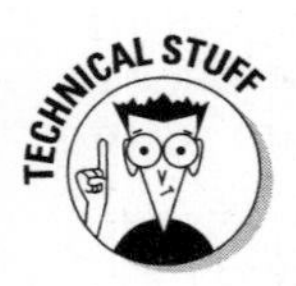

Scientists' understanding about colon cancer and Crohn's or colitis comes mostly from studying people with ulcerative colitis. Less research has been done on the link between Crohn's disease and cancer, but the few studies that have been done suggest the risk for cancer in people with Crohn's disease of the colon is similar to the risk in those with ulcerative colitis. Even so, the things that affect the risk of cancer seem to be similar for both diseases.

Your risk of colon cancer in Crohn's and colitis depends on how long you've had the disease and how much of your colon is affected by inflammation. The risk of colon cancer doesn't start to increase until you've had colitis for eight to ten years. If your disease affects the entire colon, you'll have the highest risk of getting colon cancer (compared to those who have inflammation only in the rectum or sigmoid colon, where the risk of colon cancer is the lowest).

Also, having a family history of colon cancer further increases your risk of getting the disease. Another risk factor is having *primary sclerosing cholangitis* (PSC), which is inflammation and scarring of the bile ducts (see Chapter 2).

Studies have shown that a diet high in fruits and vegetables, whole grains, lean proteins, and healthy fats has been linked to a decreased risk of colon cancer. On the other hand, a diet high in red meats, refined foods, and unhealthy fats has been linked to an increased risk of the disease.

Here is what you can do to reduce your risk of getting colon cancer:

- **Eat a healthy diet.** Consume a diet high in a variety of fruits and vegetables. Limit your intake of red and processed meats because studies have identified *carcinogens* (cancer-causing agents) not only in processed meats, but in a diet that is rich in red meats (beef, pork, lamb, and veal). Replace trans fats (found in cakes, cookies, fried foods, margarine, donuts, pastries, and chips) and saturated fats (found in butter and red meat) with healthy fats called *unsaturated fats* (found in fatty fish like salmon, avocadoes, olive oil, and nuts). Recent studies have suggested a link between trans fats and colon cancer risk. You can read more about trans fats and nutrition in Chapter 9.

  Recent studies have found that if you consume a diet high in refined sugar (such as table sugar), you may have a higher chance of getting colon cancer.

  Lycopene is a red pigment found in tomatoes and other such red-colored produce, such as guava, papaya, pink grapefruit, strawberries, and watermelon. Recently, lycopene has been shown to decrease the risk of developing colon cancer.

- **Consume folate and fiber.** Folate is found in many foods, such as green, leafy vegetables; beans; and citrus fruits. It's also added to grain products. Folate is crucial for the building and repair of cellular DNA. Folate deficiency can damage your DNA and increase your risk of developing colon cancer. Similarly, recent research also suggests that fiber from whole grains, fruits, and vegetables can decrease your risk for colon cancer.

- **Exercise.** Studies have shown that those who engage in regular, moderate exercise — such as brisk walking, jogging, and bicycling — are at a lower risk of developing colon cancer than those who are inactive. Exercise is thought to lower colon cancer risk in part by preventing or reducing excess body weight, another risk factor for colon cancer.

Your colon also acts as a sewage plant — it recycles useful materials and stores the waste for disposal. The longer waste sits in the colon, the more toxic and cancer-producing material come into contact with colon cells. Exercise gets your body moving, which helps move the waste in your body.

Doctors recommend getting at least 30 minutes of moderate to vigorous activity three to five days a week.

- **Follow your doctor's recommendations for screening.** The single best way to prevent colon cancer is to get screened for colon cancer on a regular basis. Scientists believe that active inflammation increases the risk of colon cancer. So, if you have Crohn's or colitis for more than eight to ten years and it's involving more than a third of the colon, your doctor will likely suggest colonoscopy as a screening test. You can read more about colonoscopy in Chapter 6.

Cervical cancer

Recently, studies have shown that women with Crohn's or colitis have a higher likelihood of having an abnormal Pap smear than otherwise healthy women. The risk can become even higher if you're on immunosuppressive medications such as azathioprine. Other known risk factors that can lead to an abnormality in Pap smears include smoking, multiple sex partners, and a family history of cervical cancer.

HPV, which is associated with the development of cervical cancer, has been shown to be present in the abnormal Pap smears of women with Crohn's and colitis. The good news is that the risk of cervical cancer itself does not appear to be any higher. This is probably because those Pap smears that are found to be abnormal are aggressively treated and followed up.

In light of these findings, doctors recommend that women who take certain immunosuppressive medications to control Crohn's or colitis, such as azathioprine and 6-MP, have Pap smears yearly (as opposed to every two to three years, as otherwise recommended). In addition, your doctor may recommend that you get the HPV vaccine (see "The HPV vaccine," earlier in this chapter).

Chapter 11

Alternative and Complementary Therapies

In This Chapter

- Identifying the health benefits of exercise and physical therapy
- Understanding herbal therapy and homeopathy
- Considering traditional Chinese medicine
- Seeing how mind-body intervention helps
- Exploring the use of worms in Crohn's and colitis treatment

Researchers and scientists still need to discover a cure for Crohn's and colitis. Right now, we don't have any drug that is 100 percent effective in controlling the signs and symptoms of these diseases. You may not respond to a particular drug at all (though that happens rarely), or you may have a partial response, controlling some, but not all, symptoms. Even if your symptoms improve with a certain drug today, the drug may not be as effective down the road, and you may end up needing surgery.

In the absence of a cure, many people turn to unconventional forms of treatment, such as herbal therapy, homeopathy, and mind-body intervention, in the hopes of getting better and avoiding surgery. These forms of therapy are known as *alternative* or *complementary therapies.* Alternative medicine is a form of healthcare practice and therapy that typically is not included in *conventional medicine* (the type of medicine taught in medical school). *Complementary medicine* is a type of alternative medicine used *together* with conventional medical treatment with the intention of increasing its effectiveness.

About 30 percent of the Western population uses alternative therapy for their health-related problems. Crohn's and colitis patients are among this group. Studies from the United States and Europe have shown that as many as 50 percent of Crohn's and colitis patients use some form of alternative therapy. Herbal therapy is the most commonly used form.

In this chapter, I discuss and review different forms of these alternative and complementary therapies, describing their potential benefits, indications, and possible side effects.

Different doctors feel differently about alternative and complementary therapies. Personally, I'm not against them, and I even recommend to my patients therapies like mind-body interventions from trained professionals. That said, alternative and complementary therapies should *not* replace anti-inflammatory and immunosuppressive drugs, which are well studied in medical research. Some alternative and complementary therapies, such as herbs, may be helpful, but they can also be associated with serious, unknown side effects such as drug interactions with your mainstay anti-inflammatory drugs. If you're considering an alternative or complementary therapy, talk with your doctor.

For more information, check out the website of the National Center for Complementary and Alternative Medicine (`http://nccam.nih.gov`).

Let's Get Physical: Exercise

There is no question about the health benefits of properly performed exercise. A healthy body can also do wonders for the mind and spirit. Exercise positively affects every part of the body, including the digestive system.

Recognizing the health benefits of exercise

Regular exercise offers many benefits, including the following:

- **Improving digestion:** Studies have shown that regular exercise revs up your intestines by improving blood circulation in your intestines and helping digestion. It also increases body core temperature, which improves enzyme function for digestion and metabolism.
- **Boosting the immune system:** Exercise also has a beneficial effect on your immune system and helps you fight against infections. Exercise helps flush the bacteria out of your lungs, decreasing your chance of getting a cold, the flu, and other airborne illnesses. Studies have also shown that you get rid of *carcinogens* (cancer-causing toxins) through urine and sweat. Physical activity helps move antibodies and white blood cells at a faster rate in your body, which can help them detect illnesses earlier.
- **Keeping the heart healthy:** Exercise can prevent heart disease. If you already have heart disease, proper exercise can prevent further complications. It stabilizes your heart rate, improves blood pressure, and strengthens the heart muscle.
- **Fighting cancer:** Regular exercise prevents certain cancers such as breast cancer and colon cancer. A recent European study showed that men who jogged for at least 30 minutes a day were 50 percent less likely to get any kind of cancer. Newer studies have also shown that

exercise prevents recurrence of cancer. Scientists think that this happens because physical activity and exercise lower the levels of cancer-causing or cancer-promoting chemicals and hormones in your body.

- **Strengthening bones:** Regular exercise helps improve the strength of your bones by making them more dense and preventing fractures.
- **Improving your mood:** Exercise reduces feelings of depression and anxiety. Some people call exercise "natural Prozac."
- **Getting good sleep:** Regular physical activity can help you fall asleep faster and deepen your sleep. (***Note:*** Avoid exercise close to bedtime, because that can have the opposite effect.)
- **Combating health problems:** Regular physical activity can prevent many other illnesses, such as diabetes, asthma, high cholesterol, and obesity.
- **Sparking your sex life:** Regular physical activity can help you look better and feel more energized, which can have a positive effect on your sex life. Studies have shown that men who exercise regularly have less erectile dysfunction. Regular exercise also increases the production of sex hormones such as estrogen, progesterone, and testosterone.
- **Fun:** Exercise and physical activity can simply be a fun way to spend your time. It may give you a chance to unwind, forget about your worries, and enjoy the outdoors. It can also be a source of social connection with family and friends.

Looking at how exercise can help with Crohn's and colitis

Everyone needs exercise to stay healthy (see the preceding section). But if you have Crohn's or colitis, you have even *more* reason to be physically active:

- **Bone weakness:** During active inflammation, chemicals called *cytokines* are released; cytokines have a direct negative effect on your bones. Taking steroids also weakens your bones. Exercise helps strengthen your bones and keep your muscles strong and flexible.

  There are three different kinds of exercises for bones and muscles that can be especially beneficial if you have Crohn's or colitis:

  - **Weight-bearing exercises:** Weight-bearing exercises such as walking, climbing stairs, dancing, and hiking are all good ways to improve your bone and muscle strength. Many experts recommend walking 3 to 5 miles a week to help build your bone health.
  - **Resistance exercises:** Resistance exercises also help strengthen your muscles and build bones. Weightlifting and water exercises are examples of resistance exercise.

- **Flexibility exercises:** Regular stretching and yoga are good flexibility exercises that have a healthy effect on your bones and muscles.

Talk to your doctor before beginning any exercise program. This is especially true if you already have osteoporosis. Running, jogging, and jumping may put stress on your spine and may lead to fractures.

- **Colon cancer:** If you have colitis for more than eight to ten years, you're at a higher risk for developing colon cancer. Studies have shown that getting at least 30 minutes of moderate to vigorous exercise 5 or more days a week helps lower the risk of colon cancer. Moderate-intensity exercise includes walking, dancing, bicycling, or yoga; vigorous exercise includes jogging, running, or swimming.
- **Stress and depression:** Chronic inflammation and persistent symptoms of diarrhea and abdominal pain can affect your mood and cause stress and depression. Exercise helps relieve stress and lifts your mood. It may even help prevent flares in the future. Exercises such as running and yoga are great for stress reduction and improved mood — but the key is to find an exercise that *you* enjoy.
- **Surgery:** After surgery, your wounds will heal quickly if your muscles and tissues are healthy and strong — and they will be if you exercise regularly prior to surgery. Physical activity also improves blood circulation and prevents formation of blood clots, a common but serious side effect of prolonged bed rest (which happens after surgery).

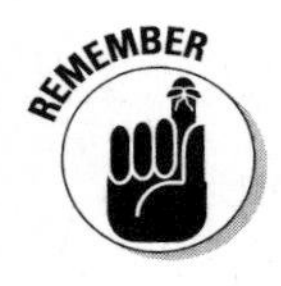

After abdominal surgery, you have to avoid some exercises such as sit-ups and lifting anything heavier than 15 pounds for at least six weeks. Be sure to get the green light from your surgeon before you begin exercising again.

Gathering some useful exercise tips

Before you join a gym and start pumping iron, keep in mind the following tips:

- **If you're worried that a walking, jogging, or running program will take you too far from a restroom, try exercising on a treadmill instead.** Map out the restrooms before beginning your workout.
- **If you have a history of incontinence, avoid running.** Stick with walking instead.
- **Avoid exercising when it's very hot.** Exercising during hot weather will increase your risk of dehydration.
- **Drink plenty of water before and after exercise.** Drink 8 to 10 ounces just before exercising and 4 to 6 ounces every 10 to 20 minutes during exercise. This will decrease your risk of dehydration, especially during

a flare. Try electrolyte-based drinks, such as sports drinks (for example, Gatorade, Powerade, or All Sport). They can help you maintain a balance between dehydration and diarrhea. Because many sports drinks contain a lot of sugar, you may want to dilute them with water.

- **Avoid eating solid food for three to four hours before aerobic exercise.**
- **If you exercise at a gym, use hand wipes to clean shared equipment before you use it, and wash your hands after the workout.** Taking immunosuppressive drugs makes you more susceptible to infections.

Talk with your doctor before starting any exercise program. This is especially true if you have active disease and or just had surgery when only light exercise is all you can do. Vigorous exercises in these situations may increase your risk of dehydration and interfere with the wound-healing process.

Working Over-Thyme: Herbal Therapy

Plants can synthesize a wide variety of chemical compounds that are used to perform important biological functions to defend against attack from predators (such as insects). Many of these chemicals can also have beneficial effects for humans. So, herbs can be used to effectively treat many diseases. Herbs also provide essential nutrients that may be lacking in your diet.

Herbal therapy comes in different forms. It can be dispensed as an oral supplement, a tea, a tincture, or a topical cream or lotion.

To learn more about herbal therapy, check out *Herbal Remedies For Dummies,* by Christopher Hobbs, LAc (Wiley). Also, see if you can find a well-respected herbalist in your area. Ask your doctor for recommendations. Also, check out the Find an Herbalist search tool provided by the American Herbalists Guild: `www.americanherbalistsguild.com/fundamentals`.

Healing with herbs

People around the world have been using herbal medicines for ages. The study of herbs dates back more than 5,000 years to the Early Bronze Age civilization. In 1500 b.c., the Ancient Egyptians wrote the Ebers Papyrus, which contains information about 850 plant medicines such as garlic, juniper, cannabis, castor bean, and aloe. Similarly, in India, Ayurveda medicine has used many herbs since as early as 1900 b.c. Herbal therapy also held importance in Chinese, Greek, and Roman medicinal practices.

Many of the *allopathic drugs* (drugs prescribed by medical doctors today) have a long history of being used as herbal remedies. For example, digoxin, a heart medication, comes from the foxglove plant; taxol, a drug used to treat ovarian cancer, comes from the Pacific yew tree; and the mesalamine drugs used for Crohn's and colitis are derived from salicylic acid, which was originally extracted from willow bark.

Identifying beneficial herbs for Crohn's and colitis — and knowing which herbs to avoid

Many herbs are believed to promote the health of the digestive system. They've been shown to improve the symptoms of acid reflux, nausea, and diarrhea. Some of these herbs have been shown to possess anti-inflammatory properties, which makes them attractive to use in the management of Crohn's and colitis. Here are some of the herbal therapies commonly used to treat Crohn's and colitis:

- **Aloe vera gel:** Aloe vera, also known as the plant of immortality, has been used as a remedy for thousands of years. It has been used to facilitate the healing of wounds and to treat skin problems. Aloe vera gel (a thick, gelatinous liquid present in the leaves of the aloe vera plant) has also been found in clinical studies to have an anti-inflammatory effect. Some herb specialists prescribe oral aloe vera gel for treating colitis, but the scientific evidence for its effectiveness is lacking.
- **Boswellia:** Boswellia is an herb that comes from a tree native to India. Its active ingredient is the resin coming from the tree bark. It has anti-inflammatory properties. Herb specialists have used it to treat colitis.
- **Bromelain:** Bromelain is a mixture of protein-digesting enzymes derived from pineapple stems. It's believed to reduce inflammation. Some animal studies have shown that daily treatment with oral bromelain decreases the incidence and severity of colitis.
- **Curcumin:** Curcumin is an active ingredient of a spice called turmeric. Clinical studies have shown it to have very potent anti-inflammatory effects. Animal and human studies have shown its beneficial effects in controlling inflammation and symptoms in Crohn's and colitis.
- **Ginger:** Ginger has strong anti-nausea effects and has been used to treat nausea during pregnancy. It has also been shown to reduce inflammation. It has very few side effects.

Although many herbs are useful as anti-inflammatory remedies and may have a place in the treatment of Crohn's and colitis, other herbs can worsen the symptoms of Crohn's and colitis. Some of these herbs can lead to interactions with drugs and cause complications. Talk with your doctor before taking any herbal therapy. Here are some herbs to avoid if you have Crohn's or colitis:

- **Black cohosh:** The roots and underground stems of this plant are frequently used for menopausal symptoms. One of the side effects is abdominal pain. It can also cause liver damage.
- **Evening primrose oil:** Evening primrose oil is often used to treat eczema and rheumatoid arthritis. It can also cause some stomach upset and diarrhea.
- **Fenugreek:** Fenugreek seeds are used to increase milk production in nursing mothers. One of the side effects of this herbal therapy is rectal bleeding and increased gas production.
- **Flaxseed and flaxseed oil:** Flaxseed and flaxseed oil are used to lower cholesterol and treat symptoms of arthritis. They can cause nausea, bloating, and abdominal pain. If you have a stricture in your intestines, they can lead to intestinal blockage.
- **Garlic:** Garlic is often used to treat cholesterol and high blood pressure. It also thins the blood. Be careful using garlic when you're gearing up for surgery.
- **Gingko biloba:** Gingko biloba leaf extracts are used to improve memory and sexual function. They can cause abdominal pain and diarrhea. They also cause thinning of the blood, so use it with caution prior to surgery.

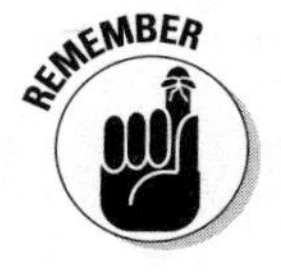

Just because herbs are "natural" doesn't mean they're safe. Be sure to talk with your doctor about all supplements you take, including herbs.

Homeopathy

At the end of the 18th century, the Germans developed an alternative medical therapy known as *homeopathy.* They based homeopathy on a theory of "like cures like," also known as "the law of similar." According to this theory, a disease can be cured by a substance that produces similar symptoms in healthy people. Homeopathic remedies are derived from substances derived from plants, minerals, or animals. They're mostly formulated as sugar pellets, but others forms like ointments, gels, drops, creams, and tablets also exist. Liquid medications are better tolerated than pellets, because pellets are made of lactose, which can cause problem in lactose-intolerant people.

The history of homeopathy

In the late 1700s, Samuel Hahnemann, a German physician and chemist, proposed a new approach to treating illnesses. At this time, truly effective medical therapies didn't exist, and most of the treatments (such as bloodletting and the use of sulfur or mercury) were associated with many side effects and complications. Supposedly, Hahnemann was translating an herbal text and read about cinchona bark as a treatment to cure malaria. When he took some cinchona bark, he developed symptoms very similar to malaria symptoms. This led to a widely popular concept in homeopathy called "like cures like." Dr. Hans Burch Gram studied homeopathy in Europe and later introduced it into the United States in 1825. In 1835, the first homeopathic medical college was established in Allentown, Pennsylvania. In the 1960s, homeopathy became increasingly popular in in the United States. According to a 1999 survey of Americans and their health, more than 6 million Americans had used homeopathy in the preceding year.

Getting help from homeopathy?

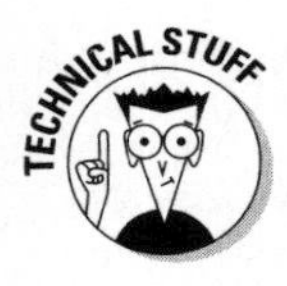

Homeopathic remedies are prepared by serial dilution of a chosen substance in alcohol or distilled water, followed by a forceful striking on an elastic body, called *succession*. Each dilution followed by succession is supposed to increase the remedy's potency. Homeopaths call this process *potentization*. Dilution usually continues well past the point where none of the original substance remains. Most of the time, the homeopathic doctor individualizes the treatment for each patient; it's not uncommon to see people with the same medical condition receiving different treatments.

Homeopathy is a controversial topic in medical research, and many clinical trials and scientific analyses of the research on homeopathy have concluded that there is little evidence to support homeopathy as an effective treatment for any specific condition. Although many homeopathic remedies are highly diluted, some products may not be diluted very much and contain substantial amounts of active ingredients. Like any other drugs, the chemical ingredients of the homeopathic drugs may cause side effects or drug interactions. Negative health effects from homeopathic products have been reported in medical literature.

Only take highly diluted homeopathic remedies, and do so under the supervision of a trained professional.

Homeopathy and Crohn's and colitis

Homeopathy has been widely used to treat symptoms of irritable bowel syndrome. However, use of homeopathic medications for Crohn's and colitis is a bit challenging because you're dealing with inflammation — besides, the exact cause of these illnesses isn't very clear. Nevertheless, people have tried to use homeopathic remedies for Crohn's and colitis in an effort to avoid immunosuppressive medications and surgery.

Homeopathic professionals try to individualize the treatment according to signs and symptoms, as well as the patient's personality. Here are some homeopathic remedies that have been used to treat symptoms of Crohn's and colitis:

- **Aloe:** For urgency and incontinence
- **Arsenicum album:** For sore and burning stomach and rectum, as well as watery diarrhea
- **Mercurius solubus:** For diarrhea, especially bloody stools
- **Nux vomica:** For nausea, abdominal pain, and gas
- **Bryonia:** For nausea, vomiting, and bloody stools
- **Lycopodium:** For bloating abdominal pain and diarrhea
- **Podophyllum:** For crampy abdominal pain, vomiting, and diarrhea with mucus discharge

Talk with your gastroenterologist before taking any homeopathic remedy. There is no strong evidence that homeopathic medications can cure Crohn's and colitis, and most of them control symptoms rather than inflammation. These remedies may also interact with other immunosuppressive and anti-inflammatory drugs. For these reasons, I don't recommend this form of therapy to my patients.

Traditional Chinese Medicine

Traditional Chinese medicine dates back to 1600 B.C. It includes various forms of herbal medicine, acupuncture, massage, exercise, and diet.

Understanding traditional Chinese medicine

Advocates of Chinese medicine usually relate this type of medicine to nature. They believe that just as our planet has a North Pole and a South Pole and a magnetic field, the body also has its own force or energy field, called *qi* (pronounced as *chee*). They believe that *qi* flows through pathways in the body called *meridians,* which connect the internal organs. In order to have a healthy body and mind, they say that *qi* needs to be in abundance and circulating freely.

Chinese medicine practitioners also say that people require balance in their lives. The terms *yin* and *yang* are used to describe balance in health and life. *Yin* pertains to darkness, rest, and cold. *Yang* pertains to light, activity, and heat. The Chinese medicine specialists assess the state of *qi* and *yin* and *yang* in a patient in order to treat illness.

Controlling Crohn's and colitis with traditional Chinese medicine

About 40 percent of patients with Crohn's or colitis in Taiwan use Chinese medicine as the main therapy or combined with other therapies. Similarly, this form of therapy is increasing in popularity in the Western world. In a recent survey of German patients, 30 percent of them were found to use Chinese medicine to manage their Crohn's or colitis.

Assessing acupuncture

In acupuncture, small needles are inserted into the skin and muscles to influence the flow of *qi.* According to Chinese medicine, acupuncture relieves pain and treats or even prevents many diseases. However, scientific reviews of different studies performed to test the effectiveness of acupuncture don't show any good results; higher-quality research is needed before we can say it really works.

When it comes to acupuncture and Crohn's and colitis, only a few studies have been done to study its effects in these illnesses, but they have shown some promising results in controlling various symptoms of Crohn's and colitis. Before we can draw any meaningful conclusions from these trials, we need larger and better-designed studies involving more patients.

In Chinese medicine, the goal of treatment for Crohn's or colitis is to balance the immune system and harmonize the intestinal energy. Chinese medicine addresses the emotions, lifestyle, and eating habits as important factors affecting the intestines. Acupuncture and Chinese herbs are often used to strengthen the immune system. They also help relieve the stress that can cause a disease flare. Some researchers have shown the soothing effect of aloe vera and cinnamon on the intestinal walls.

The following Chinese herbs are commonly used to treat Crohn's and colitis:

- **Atractylodes:** A plant with purple flowers that's native to China. Its roots are used to treat diarrhea, bloating, and nausea. Usually avoided for long-term use. It's also an active ingredient of the Jianpiling formula that has been studied in Crohn's and colitis.
- **Changtai granule:** A formula composed of four different herbs. Purported to have anti-inflammatory and antibacterial properties. Usually avoided during pregnancy.
- **Chinese plum tree:** Thought to have strong immune-stimulating effects. Some small studies have shown that it restores the balance of bacteria in the intestines. Usually avoided during fever and cold. Has some interaction with sulfa-containing drugs.

Mind-Body Intervention

Mind-body intervention is a type of alternative therapy that practitioners use to enhance your mind's capacity to affect your body symptoms and functions.

Many clinical studies have shown that stress can worsen the symptoms of Crohn's and colitis. Similarly, researchers have also found that stress management, moderate exercise, and self-care strategies improve quality of life in Crohn's and colitis. Many mind-body therapies such as breathing exercises, relaxation techniques, and meditation reduce pain symptoms.

Different techniques are used in mind-body intervention and offer numerous benefits to mental and physical health. In this section, I briefly cover some of the commonly used methods.

Aromatherapy

Aromatherapy uses volatile plant materials, known as essential oils, and other aromatic compounds to alter your mind, mood, or health. Essential oils such as tea tree oil and lemon oil are thought to have antibacterial properties. In many parts of the world, lemon oil, jasmine, and peppermint are used to reduce stress and depression.

Although you may benefit from these essential oils, keep in mind that your household pets may not. Some of these oils may be toxic to pets. Be sure to talk with a licensed aroma therapist before bringing such oils into your home.

Hypnotherapy

Hypnotherapy is given to you in the state of hypnosis. Practitioners of hypnotherapy claim that they can influence your mind and thinking, which can then affect your health and disease.

Yoga and meditation

Studies from Harvard University have shown that yoga and meditation have a positive impact on heart rate, blood pressure, brain function, and body metabolism. Yoga and meditation are very popular in Western countries as a form of relaxing and stress-relieving exercise.

For more information, check out *Yoga For Dummies,* 2nd Edition, by Georg Feuerstein, PhD, and Larry Payne, PhD, and *Meditation For Dummies,* 2nd Edition, by Stephan Bodian (both published by Wiley).

Music therapy

In music therapy, a trained music therapist uses music and all its aspects (physical, emotional, and spiritual) to help you improve or maintain your health. Music has been used as a healing therapy for centuries. In the United States, Native American medicine men often use chants and dances as a form of healing their patients.

Support groups

In support groups, the members of the group provide each other with various types of help. This help could be in the form of providing relevant information, relating personal experiences, listening to others' experiences, and establishing social networks.

Talk with your gastroenterologist to see if there's a Crohn's and colitis support group in your area. Or go to `www.ccfa.org/living-with-crohns-colitis/find-a-support-group/` to find a support group near you.

T'ai chi

T'ai chi is a type of Chinese martial art practiced for both its defense training and its health benefits. Recently, many health studies have shown its benefits. It has been studied aggressively at various levels, including research on methods and duration of exercise.

For more on t'ai chi, check out *T'ai Chi For Dummies,* by Therese Iknoian (Wiley).

Worm Therapy

Scientists and researchers have suggested many possible causes of Crohn's and colitis (see Chapter 4). These include mutations in genes, changes in the immune system, and environmental factors. Mutations in human genes take hundreds of years to cause a disease, so the rapid increase in the incidence of Crohn's and colitis has made people wonder if other factors are playing an important role.

Many environmental factors can increase your risk of having Crohn's and colitis. Improved hygiene and sanitization can lead to a change in intestinal bacteria and parasites, shifting a balance from good microorganisms to harmful ones. This is the basis of the hygiene hypothesis that I cover in Chapter 4. Getting exposed to fewer worms and bacteria during childhood may not be a good thing. Exposure to worms and bacteria is one way Mother Nature teaches our immune systems to fight these nasty organisms in the future.

Putting worms to work for your health

Worm infections have emerged as one possible explanation for the low incidence of autoimmune diseases and allergies in less-developed countries and the significant increase of these diseases in industrialized countries. In the 1930s, we started deworming everyone by giving people anti-worming drugs, as well as through improved sanitation. Kids used to run around barefoot and picked up some types of worms through their skin. People who drank out of wells or streams also picked up worms. Today, we wear shoes and have water-filtration systems. In addition, our food is much cleaner.

Worms help to dampen hyper-reactive immune systems. Without worms, immune systems tend to react much faster and may lead the human body to overproduce powerful substances that lead to excessive inflammation of the intestinal tract. Deworming results in a hyperactive immune system.

The hygiene hypothesis triggered the idea of exposing our bodies to harmless worms or their eggs. That, in turn, brought about the concept of worm therapy for different immune-mediated diseases.

Hookworms and whipworms are commonly used parasites in worm therapy. Unhatched whipworm eggs are also used for this purpose. The effectiveness of worm therapy in treating diseases and conditions such as multiple sclerosis, asthma, eczema, hay fever, and food allergies is being studied.

Seeing how worms can help Crohn's and colitis

Scientists and researchers are studying the role of worm therapy for Crohn's and colitis with interest and enthusiasm. The idea behind this therapy is complex, but it makes sense for Crohn's and colitis because these diseases affect intestinal cells that are (or should have been) in direct contact with worms and bacteria since childhood. Clinical studies have shown that eating worms or their eggs reduces inflammation.

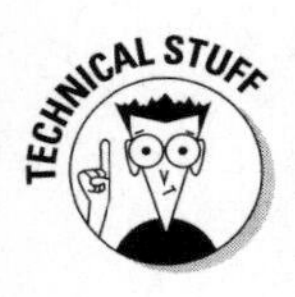

Interleukin-22 is a *cytokine* (a protein produced by your white blood cells) that is involved in healing of the mucosa. It's a good protein that your colon needs when it tries to heal. Eating worms or their eggs increases the level of these cytokines in the mucosa and hastens the healing process. IL-22 also helps your colon cells produce more mucus, a protective layer around the cells.

Worm therapy is only experimental at this stage and is offered only in select centers involved in clinical research. Although the studies done so far haven't shown any worrisome side effects, we currently don't know how safe it is to ingest the worms and their eggs.

Part IV
Living and Coping with Crohn's and Colitis

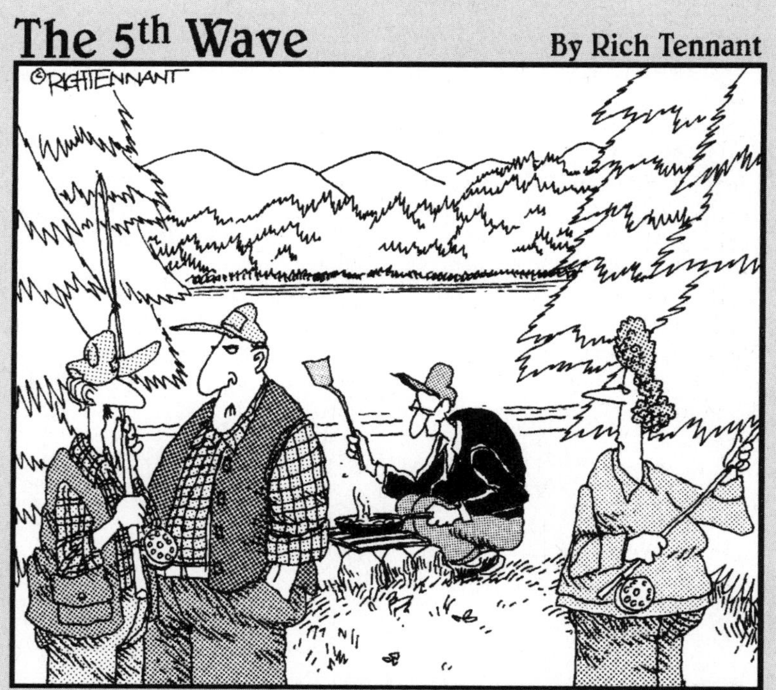

"Don't use that excuse on me, Wayne. Ain't no good reason why a man with Crohn's disease can't help himself to some of Earl's fried mealworms."

In this part . . .

Crohn's and colitis can be embarrassing or make you feel isolated or afraid. But these feelings aren't permanent, and you can live a happy, full life despite your diagnosis. In this part, I give you information on how to do exactly that.

Chapter 12

Living with Crohn's and Colitis

In This Chapter

- Facing the diagnosis
- Discussing the diagnosis with others
- Helping a loved one with Crohn's or colitis

When you're faced with an illness like the flu or a broken bone, you may feel pain, aggravation, or inconvenience, but there's a light at the end of the tunnel. With a disease like Crohn's or colitis, however, that isn't the case. Crohn's and colitis are chronic conditions, which means they're with you your entire life. But the good news is, your life isn't over! You'll have good days and bad days, and this chapter fills you in on how to make the most out of both.

Dealing with the physical aspects of your disease is important, but just as important is learning how to live and cope with your Crohn's and colitis. If you're reading this book because a loved one has Crohn's or colitis, turn to the end of this chapter — there, I discuss how and when you can be most supportive.

Dealing with Your Diagnosis

No matter what the illness, most people handle being diagnosed with a chronic condition in a similar way: They go through the five stages of grief (outlined by psychiatrist Elisabeth Kübler-Ross) — denial, anger, bargaining, depression, and acceptance. Some of these stages may last for days; others may last for months. It doesn't matter how long it takes you to get to acceptance. It doesn't even matter if you skip over one of the stages on the way. The important thing to know is this: These emotions are completely normal, and you are definitely not alone.

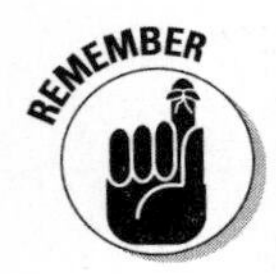

Though there are a lot of different theories about Crohn's and colitis, no one is exactly sure what causes them. There is nothing you could've done to prevent it or avoid it. Developing either of these illnesses is not your fault or anybody else's fault.

Stage 1: Denial

Early on in your diagnosis, you may try to convince yourself that the lab reports were wrong or the doctor had you confused with another patient. Because the symptoms associated with Crohn's and colitis often appear out of nowhere, you may want to believe that your symptoms could be caused by an infection, food poisoning, or stress and that they'll eventually go away on their own. You may even decide you don't need to take your medication or change your diet because you'll start feeling better soon. If any of this sounds familiar, you're in Stage 1, denial.

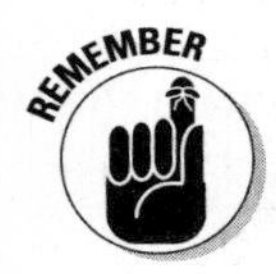

Denial is a self-defense mechanism. Our brains are way smarter than we even realize. When something bad happens the brain has a way of putting off the unavoidable until it knows you're ready to deal with it. There's no set time limit on how long denial will last. Also, different people experience denial in different ways:

- **You may deny that you have an illness altogether.** For example, you may say things like, "I can't be sick — I feel fine."
- **You may deny the significance of the illness.** When asked about your diagnosis, you may downplay it and change the subject.
- **You may simply choose to put off your diagnosis for a while.** Right now, you may feel too busy to deal with your disease. You may even say something like, "I'll change my diet after the holidays," or "I'll start taking my medication after I get back from vacation."

Denial about Crohn's or colitis can be very problematic. You can let the disease progress, and the continuing process of inflammation in your intestines can lead to complications such as strictures or fistulas and even necessitate surgery sooner than you would have needed it otherwise.

If you're going through denial right now, here are some ways to get through this stage:

- **Ask your doctor how he came up with the diagnosis.** Listen closely to all the reasons your doctor lists for knowing you have Crohn's or colitis.
- **Ask for a copy of the lab results or pathology results from your doctor.** Sometimes, just seeing the results in black and white is enough for someone to move beyond denial.

- **Talk with your doctor in great detail about all the findings.** Tell the doctor you're having trouble believing the diagnosis and you just want her to walk you through all the findings one more time.
- **Don't be afraid to ask questions.** The more open and honest your dialog with your doctor, the more likely you are to trust the diagnosis.
- **Educate yourself about Crohn's and colitis.** This book is a great place to start!

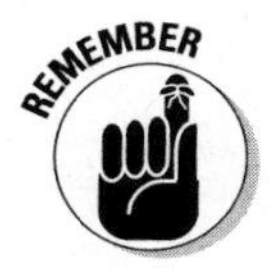

The sooner you deal with your disease, the sooner you'll start feeling better.

Stage 2: Anger

The second stage of grief is anger. Often, after people move beyond denial, they get angry. At this point, the reality of having a chronic disease is sinking in, you're realizing the lifelong difficulties that come with living with Crohn's or colitis, and you're ticked off. You may be angry at the doctor who diagnosed you. You may be angry at the illness itself. You may be angry at people who are healthy, including your family and friends. You may even be angry at the rest of the world for going on like nothing happened. People who are angry about their illness often ask, "Why me?" or "Why not someone else?"

When you're feeling angry about your disease, you may take out your anger on those around you. Family members, friends, co-workers, and even pets can be on the receiving end of your emotion. Depending on the intensity and duration of your anger, you could end up isolating yourself from the very people whose support you need.

Being angry about your diagnosis for a period of time is completely normal. But coping with this disease is easier if you have a strong community of support around you. Besides, there are better ways to let off steam than yelling at your family and friends. Here are some suggestions:

- **Therapy:** If you're feeling angry about your diagnosis, you may want to consider talking to a therapist. A therapist can be helpful in numerous ways, but having someone to talk to about all the emotions you're feeling can be beneficial. A good therapist can give you strategies for dealing with your anger, as well as help you cope with your condition long term.

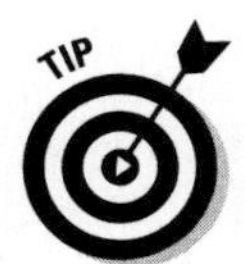

  For help in finding a therapist, start by asking your doctors, family members, and friends if they have anyone they recommend. You can also search for a therapist in your area at `http://therapists.psychologytoday.com`. Choose two or three who sound good to you, and talk to them on the phone before you make an appointment. Sometimes just a simple phone conversation, where you ask some basic questions about their practice or how they help people cope with chronic diseases, can give you a sense of which person you have good chemistry with.

If you go for three or four appointments with a therapist and you're just not getting the right vibe, don't hesitate to try another therapist — you don't want to jump around forever, but you do want to find someone you click with, and it may take a couple tries before you find that person.

- **Exercise:** Not only is exercise a great way to help keep your body healthy, but it's also an excellent way to reduce stress and alleviate feelings of anger. You can choose vigorous exercise (like kickboxing or running) or a more relaxed exercise (like t'ai chi or walking) — what matters is that you find something you enjoy and that your body is able to tolerate. When your disease is active, the most you may be able to do is a few laps around your living room — that's fine. Every little bit helps. (Check out Chapter 11 for more on exercise.)
- **Yoga:** Yoga can be a great way to calm the body and mind — which are key if you're feeling angry. You can take a class at a private studio or your local YMCA. Or if you prefer, you can do a DVD in the privacy of your own home.

  For more information on yoga, check out *Yoga For Dummies,* 2nd Edition, by Georg Feuerstein, Ph.D., and Larry Payne, Ph.D. (Wiley).

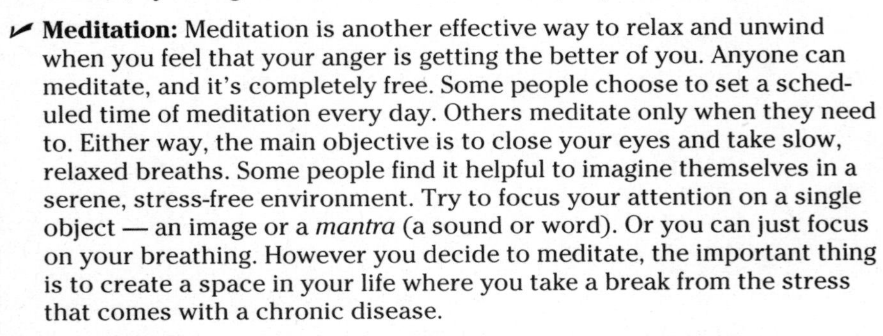

- **Meditation:** Meditation is another effective way to relax and unwind when you feel that your anger is getting the better of you. Anyone can meditate, and it's completely free. Some people choose to set a scheduled time of meditation every day. Others meditate only when they need to. Either way, the main objective is to close your eyes and take slow, relaxed breaths. Some people find it helpful to imagine themselves in a serene, stress-free environment. Try to focus your attention on a single object — an image or a *mantra* (a sound or word). Or you can just focus on your breathing. However you decide to meditate, the important thing is to create a space in your life where you take a break from the stress that comes with a chronic disease.

  For more information on meditation, including a CD of guided meditations, check out *Meditation For Dummies,* 2nd Edition, by Stephan Bodian (Wiley).

- **Journaling:** Writing in a journal can be an excellent way to cope with anger. If you're not big on writing, don't worry — no one will be reading, editing, or critiquing your journal. Unless you want someone else to read it, this journal is just for you. You won't be graded on grammar, spelling, or penmanship. Your journal can be whatever you need it to be. If you need to write "I hate Crohn's" or "I hate colitis" over and over again, go for it. If you need to vent your frustrations with having to take medications, this is the place to let it all out. Write what you feel and use it as a way to openly express what you're going through.

- **Massage:** When you're angry, your body naturally tenses up. Massage is a great way to relax and unwind, and it can help alleviate feelings of anger. Frequent massages at spas can get expensive, but more affordable options are available. If your community has a training program for massage therapists, you may be able to get great-quality massages there for a greatly reduced price.

Stage 3: Bargaining

After the feelings of denial and anger subside, you may start bargaining — trying to make deals with God or the universe or the disease itself. When you bargain, you may find yourself saying things like, "I promise I'll eat better and take care of myself if you just make my Crohn's go away," or "Just keep this colitis thing out of my life for a few more years, until the kids are off to college — then, I swear, I can deal with it." Bargaining is the equivalent of telling a cop, "I swear, I'll never speed again if you just let me off the hook this one time."

The problem with bargaining is, it doesn't work. You may be able to talk your way out of a speeding ticket, but you can't talk your way out of Crohn's or colitis.

Stage 4: Depression

When you get through the bargaining stage, and you realize you can't bargain your way out of your illness, you may start to experience feelings of depression. You may feel sorry for yourself or begin to think remission is beyond your reach. Having to take medications or change your diet or lifestyle can easily get you down. Plus, the symptoms of your disease — including nausea, diarrhea, and pain — can add to the sadness.

Depression is a common reaction to stress. Being told you have a disease that will last forever isn't easy. Sure, you may have periods of remission, but the remission may not last as long as you hope.

Avoid setting unrealistic expectations for your disease. Keep in mind that you will have occasional flares, as well as periods of remission. You can't predict how long either will last.

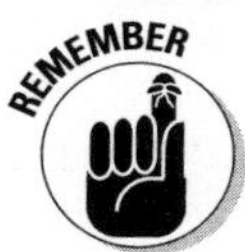

When you feel sad, try to avoid isolating yourself from others. Your family and friends want to support you, but they may not know what you need. Instead of dealing with the diagnosis all by yourself, let your friends and family know how you're feeling. Communication is key!

You may feel like your loved ones can't truly know what you're going through. If so, connecting with others who are dealing with Crohn's and colitis may be helpful. The Crohn's and Colitis Foundation of America (CCFA; www.ccfa.org) has local chapters that offer free support groups where you can meet with other people who are going through what you're going through. If you're not ready to share your feelings face to face, or if you can't find a support group in your area, try an online chat room or message board. Just keep in mind that not everything you read online is accurate, and online chat rooms or message boards can be filled with misinformation. The CCFA has an online support group (www.ccfacommunity.org) that's a great place to start!

If your depression becomes all-consuming, seek professional help right away. You can talk to a licensed therapist or one of your healthcare providers. **If you're having suicidal thoughts, call the National Suicide Prevention Hotline at 800-273-8255 or dial 911.**

Adjusting to being diagnosed with a chronic illness can be difficult and stressful. It can often produce unexpected reactions. The best way to ensure your health — both physical and mental — is to get help from a professional.

Stage 5: Acceptance

Achieving acceptance is highly individualistic and happens in a number of ways. Maybe you've discussed an in-depth a plan for your disease with a healthcare provider that makes you comfortable and confident. Maybe you're finally embracing your new medications or lifestyle changes, and seeing the benefits. Maybe you've just opened this book and you're finally accepting the reality of your diagnosis. No matter what you've done to reach this step, you've come a long way since the day you were told you have Crohn's or colitis! You've worked hard to get to this point, and you should feel good about all you've accomplished.

When you reach the acceptance stage, that doesn't mean you'll never again go through denial, anger, bargaining, or depression. But it does mean that you've finally come to the point where you can accept your Crohn's or colitis and move forward in achieving better health.

People Who Need People . . .: Keeping Your Relationships Going Strong

Your friends and family will provide a wealth of support as you live with Crohn's or colitis. But before they can help, you need to tell them about your diagnosis. In this section, I give you some tips for doing exactly that.

Dating is hard enough without a chronic condition with sometimes embarrassing symptoms. I can't find your soulmate for you, but I can give you some tips to make the dating process at least no more painful than it is for everybody else.

Finally, if you've already walked down the aisle and said your "I do's," your job isn't done. Your spouse, your partner, your better half . . . that's the person who's got your back better than anyone, and it's easy to take that relationship for granted. In this section, I offer some suggestions for keeping your marriage strong when you're dealing with a chronic condition like Crohn's or colitis.

So, what's new with you? Telling people about your diagnosis

Deciding to tell your friends about your condition can be extremely difficult. You probably don't sit around talking about your bowels all the time, so you may be embarrassed to bring up such a delicate subject. That's completely normal — and you don't have to go into all the gory details on your symptoms. But if you can find a way to talk about your disease with your friends and family, they'll be able to offer you support when you need it — and they'll appreciate that you trusted them enough to talk about what you're going through.

Before you decide to talk about your disease, make a plan:

1. **Start by making a list of the people you want to tell.**

   You don't have to inform every acquaintance — or even every friend — that you've been diagnosed with Crohn's or colitis. Your closest friends will probably suspect something's going on with you. You may have had a change in attitude, or you may have had to miss social outings because you didn't feel well. They may even ask you what's going on.

   Anyone you decide to tell about your Crohn's or colitis should be trustworthy enough and have enough respect for you to keep your diagnosis to themselves if you ask them to do so.

2. **Ask yourself why you want to tell your friends.**

   Do you want to tell them for the added support? Do you want them to know why you haven't been spending as much time together? It's important to be honest with yourself about the reason you want to tell them about your condition. That way, you can communicate that reason to them when you tell them about your diagnosis. For example, if you're telling them because you need some support, and you don't tell them what you need, they may not realize what you're asking for, and you could end up feeling disappointed.

3. **Make sure they'll be ready to listen to your problems.**

   Timing is key. If your friends are having difficulties in their own lives, they may not be ready to fully listen to yours. Wait until a time when they can offer the compassion you need. Even though your disease is a major concern for you, be considerate about their struggles.

4. **Pick a place that will be conducive to conversation.**

   You probably don't want to discuss your Crohn's or colitis in a crowded restaurant or a noisy bar. Find a quiet place where you won't be interrupted.

5. **Pick one friend to tell at a time.**

   If you tell a group of people all at once, you may be bombarded with questions and comments, which can get very overwhelming. Telling only one person at a time may be more time consuming, but it'll give your friend the opportunity to give you the attention you need.

6. **Explain what's going on without getting into a bunch of medical jargon, and only discuss as much as you and your friend are comfortable with.**

   Explain that you've been diagnosed with a condition that will affect you forever, and that you'll experience unpleasant symptoms from time to time. There will be times when you'll have less energy and won't feel like doing all the things you normally do. Make sure to explain that you aren't expecting them to do anything — maybe you just need someone to talk to from time to time.

   This may be enough information for some people. Others may ask for more information about the diagnosis. Share with them only what you're comfortable having them know. You don't need to get into the nitty-gritty details of having diarrhea, and they probably don't need a blow-by-blow recounting of your last colonoscopy. Just give them the basics and tell them that you need their support.

   If they want more information, you might steer them to the website of the Crohn's & Colitis Foundation of America (`www.ccfa.org`), or recommend that they pick up a copy of this book! If you're attending a support group, you may want to invite family members or very close friends along for more information.

What you tell your next-door neighbor probably won't be the same level of information you tell your sister. Trust your instincts on how much to share, and pay attention to how the person you're talking to is responding. If she seems uncomfortable, wrap up the conversation. And if she wants more information than you're comfortable getting into yourself, steer her to other resources.

Come here often? Dating with Crohn's and colitis

Dating *without* a chronic illness is difficult enough. Throw a little Crohn's or colitis into the mix, and things can get interesting. The good majority of people with Crohn's and colitis are diagnosed between the ages of 15 and 35, and this also happens to be when most people are dating, so you're not alone.

Here are a few suggestions for surviving the dating scene when you have Crohn's or colitis:

- **Date when you feel comfortable doing so.** If you've just been diagnosed and you're trying to manage the symptoms of a flare, now probably isn't the best time to put yourself out there. Take some time to get familiar with the effects of the disease.
- **Choose a restaurant where you can find something to eat.** Crohn's and colitis are a little different for everyone, so figure out which foods, if any, cause you problems. Then choose a restaurant for your date where you can find something that *doesn't* give you trouble.

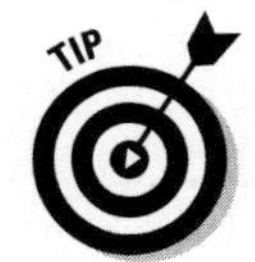

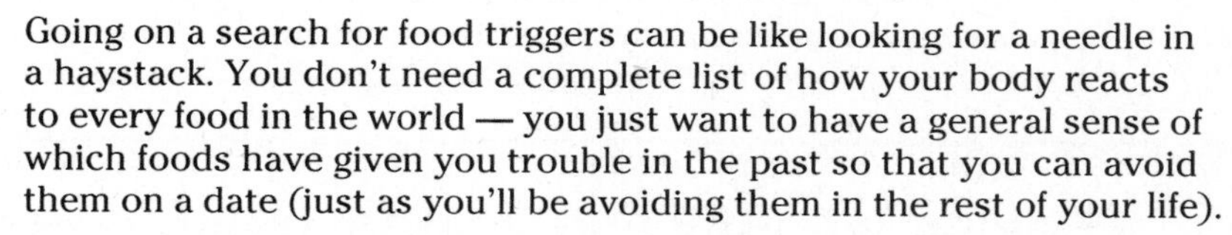

  Going on a search for food triggers can be like looking for a needle in a haystack. You don't need a complete list of how your body reacts to every food in the world — you just want to have a general sense of which foods have given you trouble in the past so that you can avoid them on a date (just as you'll be avoiding them in the rest of your life).

- **Learn the signals your body gives you that a flare may be coming on.** If you're confident that you won't be hit with a flare out of the blue, you'll be more comfortable dating.
- **Don't talk about your condition on your first date.** This information probably isn't even something you'll want to share on the second or third date. Dating is about putting your best foot forward, and also making the other person feel comfortable. The last thing you want to do is make your date squirm as you recount the details of your diagnosis. Besides, if you're dating, you know that not every first date leads to a second, so you don't need to share personal health information until you're sure this is going to last more than a few dates. You'll know when the time is right to talk about your health.

What happens if the person you're dating can't deal with your disease? Not everyone is equipped to deal with having a partner who's struggling with a chronic illness. But you're better off discovering this early in the relationship than finding out after you've invested a lot of time and energy. Besides, just because one person couldn't handle it doesn't mean another person can't.

Like a horse and carriage: Keeping your marriage strong

Crohn's and colitis can put a strain on all your relationships, but it can be especially trying on your marriage. Your partner needs to be knowledgeable about your disease and completely supportive of you. Make sure your partner is aware of everything you're going through. Don't get mad when your partner doesn't know you're feeling bad if you haven't shared your feelings — no one is a mind reader.

One way to help you and your partner get on the same page is to invite him or her to accompany you to your doctors' appointments. This may be the only time you're truly open to share what you're forced to go through on a day-to-day basis. And it may also give your partner some insight into what you're dealing with and how much support you need.

When your Crohn's and colitis are acting up, you may feel awful. Even if you aren't having stomach pains, vomiting, and diarrhea, you may be extremely fatigued. If this happens, your spouse may have to take on more responsibilities than normal. If your spouse isn't used to taking care of the finances, the kids, or the house, this can cause some strain.

Having a happy and healthy holiday season

The holidays are stressful for most people, and increased stress isn't great for someone with Crohn's or colitis. Stress can make your symptoms worse, and you may experience more abdominal pain and make more trips to the bathroom. You may end up missing out on family gatherings, travel, and all that holiday fun! The good news is, you can plan for the holidays and take steps to reduce your stress, and increase your chances of getting through the holidays flare-free. Here are some tips:

- **Get your shopping done early.** You don't want to be rushing around at the last minute, battling hordes of stressed-out shoppers.
- **Make a budget and stick to it.** There's nothing like a huge credit card bill to add to your stress, so figure out how much money you have to spend, and stick to it. Your body will thank you for it.
- **Pay attention to what you eat.** It can be tempting to go hog-wild at the holidays, and load up on all kinds of foods your eyes only see once a year. You don't have to be a Grinch and say no to everything you like — just know your body and your limits.

Remember: With a little bit of planning, you can have a happy and healthy holiday season.

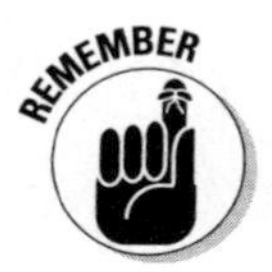

Express your appreciation for everything your partner is doing to help. And recognize that he or she is feeling stress because you're sick. Your partner may feel powerless to do anything about your disease, so let him or her know that even helping with the kids or laundry or mowing the lawn is a huge help.

If you feel like your sex life is suffering because of your Crohn's or colitis, turn to Chapter 16. There, I offer more information on the common problems that people with Crohn's and colitis experience. You may not feel like being intimate during the active phase of your disease, but you will achieve remission again. When the disease is active and you're feeling more pain or less control over your bowel, there are ways to still have intimacy without intercourse. From oral sex, massage, and kissing to cuddling and bathing together, the only limit is your imagination. The best thing to do is keep an open mind and be willing to try new things.

Caring for a Loved One with Crohn's or Colitis

Learning that your loved one has a chronic condition can bring up a wide range of emotions. But the more you know about the disease, the more you can help your loved one control and manage the symptoms, which will give both of you a sense of control and confidence.

Before you tell anyone that your loved one is struggling with Crohn's or colitis, make sure your loved one is okay with your talking about it. If she's still coping with the diagnosis, she may want to keep that information to herself for a while. Later on, she may be more comfortable with her disease and may give you the green light to share her special dietary restrictions or bathroom needs with others.

If your loved one doesn't want you talking to anyone about his disease, and you need a shoulder to lean on for support, consider talking to a therapist. In the privacy of a therapist's office, you can talk about the wide range of emotions you're feeling and get the support you need.

Finding little things that help a lot

No single diet works for every person with Crohn's or colitis. Shortly after diagnosis, your loved one will have to figure out which foods are best to eat. Keeping a daily food diary may be helpful, and this is a great opportunity for you to lend a hand. You can help your loved one remember to keep track of the foods she has eaten and how she felt during the day.

Your loved one may be going to multiple doctors' appointments after being diagnosed. You can help by accompanying him to these appointments (if he's comfortable with that) and taking notes on what the doctor says. When you're the one with the disease, your head is often spinning with all kinds of questions. The minute you get out in the parking lot, you may be thinking, "Wait, what did the doctor say I should do?" If you were there taking notes the whole time, those notes will be a huge comfort to your loved one.

Helping during a flare

Crohn's and colitis symptoms come and go. There will be periods of time when your loved one will experience very few symptoms or disease activity and will be in remission. Other times, she'll experience active disease or *flares.* Flares are when your loved one will probably need you the most. She'll experience symptoms of diarrhea, abdominal pain, fever, fatigue, nausea, weight loss, and urgent bowel movements.

When you're out of the house together during a flare, be sensitive to these issues. If your partner says he needs to go to the bathroom urgently, try your best to accommodate him. Your support can help lessen some of your loved one's anxiety. If he's feeling particularly tired, try helping with chores and responsibilities around the house. If he's having frequent diarrhea or vomiting, encourage him to stay hydrated by sipping fluids (for example, water or sports drinks) throughout the day.

Helping after surgery

After surgery, you can do a number of things to make your loved one comfortable:

- **To make things cozier at the hospital, bring familiar items from home.** For example, you might bring clothing, toiletries, ear plugs, pillows, and phone numbers for friends and family. Ask your loved one what she wants with her.
- **At the hospital, try to be present any time the surgeon or healthcare team comes in to speak with your loved one.** Being a second set of ears may be helpful, especially if your loved one is medicated. Jot down notes about when he can eat, plans for any upcoming testing, discharge instructions, and so on.

- **Serve as the gatekeeper for visitors.** Friends and family mean well, but they often don't understand how much rest someone needs after surgery. You may want to ask people to call you before showing up at your loved one's hospital room. You can manage the flow of people and cut some visits short if needed.
- **While your loved one is still in the hospital, prepare your home for her return.** The first days at home can be draining for both you and your loved one. So, make sure all the essentials — food, clothing, medications, the remote control, and a phone — are within easy reach.

  A shower chair may help if your loved one is too weak to stand for a long period of time in the shower. Check with your insurance company on these items, because they may be covered.

  If your home has stairs, figure out which level would be the best for your loved one to be on. Maneuvering stairs after an abdominal surgery can be very difficult, so you may want to arrange for a bed on the ground floor if possible.
- **Make sure you have all the directions from the healthcare team on what your loved one should eat in the days and weeks after surgery.** After an abdominal surgery, some patients require a special diet. The surgeon should clearly tell you what kind of diet your loved one should be on, and you should follow this diet as directed. If your loved one doesn't have much of an appetite at mealtimes, this can be normal, but try to encourage her to eat a little. Eating can be an important factor for healing and recovery.
- **Keep track of any medications your loved one is taking, especially any pain medications.** It's best to take pain medications before the pain gets severe. If you know when the next dose of pain medication can be administered, you can minimize discomfort and make the recovery much smoother.
- **Make sure you know when your loved one will be able to return to activities like showering, housework, driving, and lifting.** If you can't stay home with your loved one all the time, make sure he has a way to contact someone if he needs help. A home health nurse may be helpful. If your loved one has a new ileostomy or colostomy, a nurse can offer helpful tips about the device. Often, insurance will cover visits from a nurse.

Getting the help you need for yourself

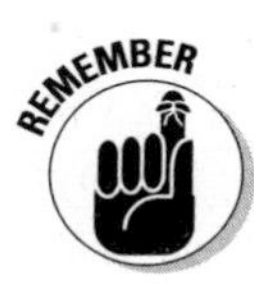

Caring for someone can be draining and stressful. Even though it may not seem like it at the time, your loved one does appreciate the love and support you're providing.

If you begin to have feelings of depression or fatigue, or if you experience changes in your eating, you start drinking alcohol more than normal, or you have a decreased interest in things you used to be interested in, talk with a trusted friend, therapist, or healthcare provider.

Support groups are available for caregivers — see if you can find one in your area. One good resource is your local CCFA chapter (www.ccfa.org/chapters). Most states have local chapters that organize regularly scheduled support group meetings for patients and their caregivers. Some of these chapters are even on Facebook and Twitter. Other useful resources include Lotsa Helping Hands (www.lotsahelpinghands.com), an online community for caregivers and Family Care Alliance (www.caregiver.org), a community-based nonprofit organization that addresses the needs of families and friends providing long-term care at home.

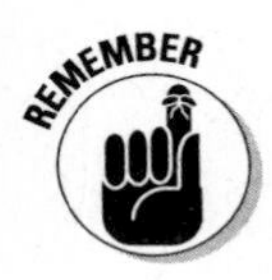

Your loved one needs to be cared for, but you need to be cared for as well. Take time to eat well, get enough physical activity and sleep, and set aside time for yourself each day. Taking time for yourself will also pay off for your loved one.

Chapter 13

Avoiding Triggers

In This Chapter

- Looking at the role of smoking in triggering flares
- Identifying how popular drugs and medications can lead to a flare
- Seeing how stress impacts Crohn's and colitis
- Identifying the foods and drinks that can trigger a flare
- Looking at lack of sleep as a potential trigger

Until we discover a cure for Crohn's and colitis, the main goal is to keep the disease in remission and avoid flares. Taking your medications regularly is one of the best things you can do to keep your disease in remission. But even if you never miss a dose, your disease may become active. Triggers such as smoking, other drugs, stress, food, or lack of sleep — or a combination of these — can contribute to triggering a flare.

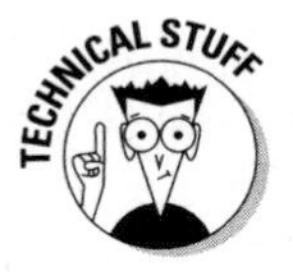

Not all these things will actually trigger a flare in the way that doctors define the term (disease becoming active with increase in the inflammation), but some of these things have the potential to make the symptoms of the disease worse without activating the process of inflammation. For example, certain foods may cause you to have more diarrhea without causing the actual inflammation to become active.

When you know what may trigger a flare, you can do everything in your power to minimize your risk. That's what this chapter is about.

Smoking: Why You Need to Quit

Smoking is one of the leading causes of preventable death in the world. In the United States alone, about 500,000 deaths per year are attributed to smoking-related diseases. Unless you've been living under a rock for the past 40 years, none of this comes as a surprise to you. But what you may not be aware of is this: If you have Crohn's disease, smoking is your worst enemy.

What about colitis?

"What about colitis?" you ask. Well, believe it or not, smoking may actually be protective for people with colitis. Studies have shown that people who have never smoked have a two to three times *higher* chance of getting colitis than smokers do. Scientists think that the nicotine in cigarettes affects the smooth muscle inside the colon and has some anti-inflammatory properties.

Researchers have studied the effect of nicotine patches in patients with active colitis. The studies showed improvement in symptoms of colitis and inflammation in the colon, but patients who wore the patch had more side effects, such as nausea, headaches, sleep problems, and dizziness. Studies done so far have also shown that nicotine patches, when compared to the standard therapy, may not be very effective in keeping someone in remission long term.

If you currently don't smoke, under no circumstances should you start smoking to try to prevent a flare of your colitis. And if you currently smoke and have colitis, you should still quit smoking. The extremely harmful effects of smoking — including cancer, heart disease, and stroke — far outweigh any protective effects nicotine has when it comes to colitis.

If you have Crohn's, you must stop smoking — plain and simple. Research has clearly shown that smoking worsens the disease. It increases the chance that you'll require surgery, and if you've already had surgery, it increases the chance that you'll need surgery again. In addition, some of the medications that are so effective in treating Crohn's disease (such as anti-TNF therapy) may not work as well if you smoke.

If you smoke, I don't need to tell you that it's both a psychological habit and a physical addiction. For most people, quitting is hard, but you can do it! Experts recommend the following mnemonic device as a way to think about quitting smoking:

S: Set a quit date.

T: Tell your family, friends, and co-workers that you plan to quit.

A: Anticipate and plan for the challenges you'll face while quitting.

R: Remove cigarettes and other tobacco products from your home, car, and work.

T: Talk to your doctor about getting help to quit.

There are a variety of approaches to quitting smoking. Some people quit cold turkey; others slowly decrease the number of cigarettes they smoke per day;

and others use nicotine replacement therapy. Support groups also can be a huge help when you're trying to quit smoking.

Smoking cessation medications can help with the withdrawal symptoms. They're most effective when they're used as part of a comprehensive smoking cessation program monitored by your physician. There are two types of medical therapy for smoking cessation:

- **Nicotine replacement therapy:** Nicotine replacement therapy involves "replacing" cigarettes with other nicotine substitutes, such as Nicorette gum or NicoDerm patches. These approaches work by delivering small and steady doses of nicotine to the body to relieve some of the withdrawal. You can buy Nicorette and NicoDerm over the counter at any pharmacy. Possible side effects of the gum can include jaw pain (if you're chewing up a storm), headaches, nausea, and diarrhea. For the patch, side effects can also include itching, burning, or redness at the application site.
- **Non-nicotine medication:** These medications help you stop smoking by reducing cravings and withdrawal symptoms — without the use of nicotine. Examples include bupropion (Zyban) and varenicline (Chantix). Non-nicotine medications require a doctor's prescription. Discuss all possible side effects with your doctor before taking any drug, especially the increased risk of depression, suicidal thoughts, and agitation.

If you're looking for help with quitting smoking, try the following resources:

- **Smokefree** (`www.smokefree.gov`): Smokefree provides free, accurate, evidence-based information and professional assistance to help support the immediate and long-term needs of people trying to quit smoking. Companion websites include `http://teen.smokefree.gov` and `http://women.smokefree.gov`.
- **American Cancer Society** (`www.cancer.org/healthy/stayawayfromtobacco`): The website of the American Cancer Society offers numerous resources on quitting smoking.
- **American Lung Association** (`www.lung.org/stop-smoking`): The American Lung Association's website offers everything from advice on quitting smoking to resources for employers to help employees quit (smoking, that is).

Another great resource is *Quitting Smoking For Dummies,* by David Brizer, MD (Wiley).

Inviting Mary Jane to the party?

Recently, a study from Israel found that after three months of inhaling cannabis (marijuana), patients with Crohn's and colitis reported improvement in *general health perception* (how they perceived their own health), social functioning, ability to work, and physical pain. The study also showed improvement in the symptoms of Crohn's and colitis.

Now, this study was a small one, and it wasn't well designed scientifically. So, medical societies don't recommend the use of marijuana in Crohn's and colitis patients. It may temporarily reduce pain and improve appetite, but currently there is no good evidence that it can control inflammation. And in some patients, it may worsen their symptoms of nausea and vomiting. The harmful effects of marijuana, including possible addiction, may outweigh the potential benefits. Although some states have legalized marijuana for medical use for other medical conditions ,the Food and Drug Administration (FDA) has not approved its use for Crohn's and colitis because of lack of good quality scientific data.

The use of marijuana is an area of controversy in the medical field. If you're considering using it, talk with your doctor.

Drugs: Just Say No?

Drugs — whether they're prescription medications prescribed by your doctor for other health problems or over-the-counter medications you take for something as simple as a headache — can trigger a flare of Crohn's or colitis. Drugs can either directly affect the intestinal inflammation and worsen the disease or simply increase the symptoms of diarrhea and abdominal pain. In this section, I review some of the common drugs that may trigger your Crohn's or colitis.

Non-steroidal anti-inflammatory drugs

Non-steroidal anti-inflammatory drugs (NSAIDs) are used to treat pain and fever. Common NSAIDs available over the counter include aspirin, ibuprofen (Advil, Motrin), and naproxen (Aleve). As the name implies, these drugs are not steroids and they're used to suppress inflammation. You'd think that they would be helpful in reducing intestinal inflammation, too, but this isn't the case. In fact, NSAIDs can worsen the inflammation of your intestines and trigger a Crohn's or colitis flare.

Here's how this happens: NSAIDs work by blocking two enzymes in your body. These enzymes are called cyclooxygenase-1 (COX-1) and cyclooxygenase-2 (COX-2). COX-1 helps in the production of *prostaglandins* (a group of lipids made at sites of tissue damage and involved in controlling processes such as inflammation, blood flow, and the formation of blood clots). Prostaglandins protect your stomach and intestines from acid and help in digestion. COX-2 helps in the production of prostaglandins that are involved in the inflammation process. Blocking COX-1 causes decreased production of protective prostaglandins, causing you to lose the protective effect on the inner lining of the stomach and intestines. This can cause ulcers in your stomach and intestines, which further worsens the existing inflammation of Crohn's or colitis.

Recently, some studies have questioned the link between NSAIDs and Crohn's or colitis flares. Researchers have found that NSAIDs don't trigger flares in everyone, and NSAIDs that block only the COX-2 enzyme (such as celecoxib [Celebrex]) may not be very harmful. However, this group of NSAIDs increases the risk of heart disease; for this reason, many COX-2 inhibitors have been taken off the market.

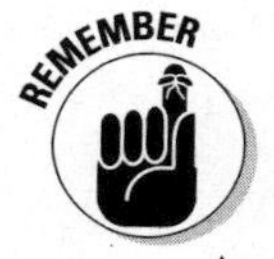

Always discuss the issue of taking NSAIDs with your doctor. You may need these medications for joint pain and other aches, and taking them under your doctor's supervision can be helpful.

If you need a painkiller, you can try something other than an NSAID, such as acetaminophen (Tylenol).

Antibiotics

Your doctor may prescribe antibiotics such as ciprofloxacin (Cipro, Proquin) and metronidazole (Flagyl) to manage your Crohn's and colitis (see Chapter 7). You may also get antibiotics for treatment of infections in other organs such as urinary tract or respiratory tract infections. The problem is, antibiotics can also cause diarrhea as a side effect or may even put you at risk for intestinal infections that can mimic a flare. The diarrhea associated with antibiotics is non-bloody and usually goes away after stopping the antibiotic.

Taking antibiotics also increases your risk of getting *Clostridium difficile* infection in the colon, commonly known as *C. diff.* The risk of getting *C. diff* becomes higher if you're on medications that suppress your immune system, such as prednisone. *C. diff* infection can mimic acute flare. Talk to your doctor about any antibiotics you've taken recently, so that he can rule out *C. diff* infection, which can become serious and require hospitalization if not treated promptly.

Stressing Out

Defining stress is difficult. Everyone has a different definition. Some experts define it as feeling like you have to handle more than you're used to. When you're in stress, your body responds as though you're in danger, producing hormones and chemicals that increase your heart rate, make you breathe faster, and give you a burst of energy. This is also known as fight-or-flight response.

Stress isn't all bad. It can help you work hard and react quickly — for example, when rushing to meet a deadline or winning a race. However, if stress happens frequently or lasts for a longer period of time, it can cause harmful effects. It can cause headaches and sleep problems, and more important, it can weaken your immune system. If you already have a health problem such as Crohn's or colitis, stress can make it worse.

Your immune system's ability to fight infections and other invaders is reduced during periods of stress. One of the hormones produced in your body during stress is corticosteroid, the same steroid you may be given during treatment for Crohn's or colitis flares. Just like the drug, the internal production of the steroid hormone suppresses your immune system. This causes your white blood cell count to become low and predisposes you to infections.

Studies have shown that stress may play a role Crohn's or colitis flares. At the same time, being diagnosed with a chronic illness is stressful in and of itself. This stress can be physical, emotional, or both. The emotional stress can manifest itself in a variety of ways, such as irritability, depression, or panic attacks. Both physical and emotional stress can cause worsening of the symptoms of Crohn's or colitis. You may end up in a vicious cycle of stress causing symptoms and increased symptoms causing stress.

You may not be able to get rid of stress, but you can find ways to reduce or manage it. Here are some strategies for reducing or managing stress:

- **Find ways to manage your time better.** Make a schedule and prioritize things in life. Learn to say no.
- **Take good care of yourself.** Getting plenty of rest, eating well, limiting your alcohol intake, and quitting smoking are all ways of doing this.
- **Let go of things you can't change.**
- **Ask for help.** Studies have shown that having a strong family and social network helps you manage stress better.
- **Talk with a therapist.** Therapy can be a great stress reliever in and of itself, and a good therapist can give you strategies for reducing stress when you're not on the therapist's couch.
- **Speak up.** Not being able to discuss your problems and concerns can create stress.
- **Release some tension by using your imagination to paint, write, draw or play an instrument.**

- **Get some physical activity.** Whether you go for a walk or jog, or take a yoga class, physical activity can help clear the mind.
- **Get a massage.** Very few things in life are as good at reducing stress as a good massage can be.

Food, Glorious Food

Certain foods may give you more trouble than others. There are no set rules or guidelines about food avoidance when it comes to Crohn's or colitis, especially when the disease is in remission. Everyone reacts differently to different foods. Your body usually tells you which foods are giving you trouble and bothering you, and then you can simply avoid those foods in the future.

Sometimes, finding the culprit food that's causing you troublesome symptoms is difficult, because the adverse reactions don't necessarily occur right after eating. It may take hours or even days before a food produces any symptoms. Keeping a food journal can be helpful in these situations. You may want to start writing down what you eat and tracking your symptoms of pain and diarrhea. After a few weeks or months, you can take the journal to your doctor and she can review it with you, helping you identify the foods you should avoid.

In this section, I cover some foods that may give rise to increased symptoms or disease flare.

Artificial sweeteners

Artificial sweetener is a substitute for regular table sugar. It's commonly used in sugar-free or diet sodas and other foods. Commonly used sweeteners are

- Acesulfame potassium (Sweet One)
- Aspartame (Equal and NutraSweet)
- Saccharin (Sweet'N Low)
- Sorbitol
- Sucralose (Splenda)

Artificial sweeteners are commonly used in many processed foods, such as candies, puddings, canned foods, jams and jellies, dairy products, and baked goods. They're good substitutes if you're trying to lose weight or if you have diabetes. Plus, they don't cause dental cavities.

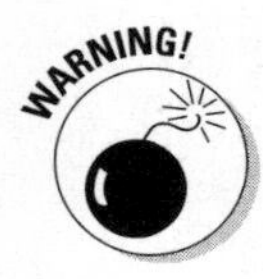

Sugar substitutes are big molecules and don't get absorbed through the intestines. Being bigger molecules, they suck water through the stool and intestinal cells, which leads to diarrhea, further exacerbating your symptoms of Crohn's and colitis.

Some concerns have been raised about artificial sweeteners, including increased risk for cancer and memory loss. However, these concerns haven't been proven by any clinical research studies and artificial sweeteners are currently considered safe to use without any dangerous side effects.

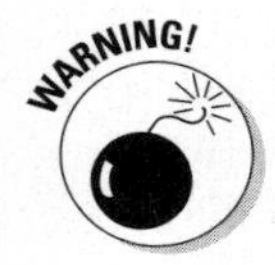

During active inflammation, you may not be able to absorb sugars such as fructose and, just like lactose intolerance (see Chapter 9), you can develop fructose intolerance. In this case, fructose-containing foods may cause increased symptoms of diarrhea and bloating. Corn syrup, strawberries, and tomatoes are examples of foods high in fructose.

Natural sweeteners are sugar substitutes that are obtained from natural sources. They're considered healthier than processed table sugar and other artificial sweeteners. Examples of natural sweeteners include maple syrup, honey, and date sugar. These sweeteners haven't been shown to cause a worsening of intestinal inflammation and may be better tolerated when you have Crohn's or colitis.

High-fat foods

During the process of acute inflammation, your body won't be able to absorb fat. Unabsorbed fat is then excreted out in the stool, producing a nasty smell and causing your stool to stick to the commode. If you eat more fat, you'll experience stinky, high-volume diarrhea.

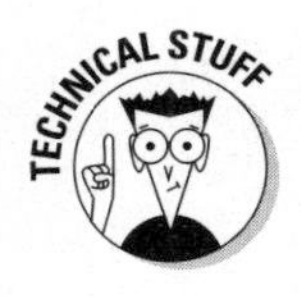

This is not an actual disease flare but an increase in your symptoms of diarrhea because of high fat intake. Keep track of what you're eating — you don't want your doctor to increase the dose of your medications or add new medications when all you need is to cut down on your fat intake.

High-fiber foods

Fiber is very important for your health (see Chapter 9). It helps decrease the risk of colon cancer, regulate your blood sugar, prevent constipation, reduce blood cholesterol, and decrease the risk of heart disease. Fiber doesn't get digested or absorbed by your intestines. However, it's important for the health of your intestines because it helps remove the old cells from the intestinal lining.

You may feel abdominal distention and bloating when you consume a high-fiber diet. This happens because the fermentation of the fiber by the bacteria inside your intestines produces gas. You may want to avoid high-fiber foods, especially foods with the highest fiber content, to prevent bloating and abdominal discomfort. Table 13-1 lists some very high-fiber foods.

Fiber also makes your stool bulkier, and when the intestines contract to push the bulky stools down, the rough surface of the fiber can cause mild scraping of the tissue. When your intestines are inflamed, this can cause pain and further damage to the mucosa.

If you have narrowing of the intestines, such as a stricture, the fiber in your food can cause blockage. Most of the time, this gets better by giving rest to the intestines and taking a break from eating; however, it can sometimes lead to complete obstruction requiring admission to the hospital and possibly surgery.

Table 13-1 High-Fiber Foods

Food	*Amount*	*Fiber*
Cooked spinach	½ cup	7 g
Canned black-eyed peas	½ cup	8 g
Raspberries	1 cup	8 g
Fresh green peas	½ cup	9.1 g
Cooked artichoke	1	10.3 g
All-Bran cereal	½ cup	10.4 g
Dried figs	3	10.5 g
Cooked peas	1 cup	13.4 g
Pinto beans	½ cup	18.8 g

Caffeine

Caffeine is found naturally in chocolate, coffee, and tea. It's also added to a variety of soft drinks and energy drinks. As you probably know, caffeine is a stimulant that many people use to stay up late or wake up early in the morning. In fact, up to 90 percent of adults in the United States consume some form of caffeine daily.

Caffeine stimulates the nervous system and body metabolism. Recent research has also shown that coffee drinkers are less likely to develop diabetes, Parkinson's disease, dementia, stroke, and cancer.

The impact of caffeine intake on Crohn's and colitis is not fully known. Because caffeine produces a laxative effect, making you go to the bathroom more often, it may be best avoided during active disease when diarrhea is already a problem. Caffeine also elevates stress hormones, which can cause digestion problems by diverting blood from your intestines to other organs such as the brain, heart, and muscles.

If you suspect that caffeine may be the culprit behind your frequent trips to the bathroom, you may want to avoid drinking coffee and other caffeine-containing foods.

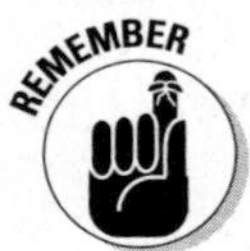

Depending on how much caffeine you get a day, stopping cold turkey can lead to withdrawal symptoms; you may experience nausea, vomiting, and headaches. So, you may want to gradually decrease your caffeine intake to avoid any symptoms of withdrawal.

Dairy products

Many people with Crohn's and colitis are sensitive to dairy products. When they consume milk or other dairy products, they experience symptoms like gas, diarrhea, and even skin rashes or fatigue in extreme cases.

Lactose is one of the primary sugars in cow's milk, and casein is the primary protein in the cow's milk. Both are added to a wide variety of foods. (Lactose is added for flavor and casein is added for breaking down large fat molecules, texture, and as a protein supplement.) Here are some examples of foods that may have casein in it:

- Coffee whiteners
- Fortified cereals
- Ice cream
- Infant formulas
- Salad dressings
- Whipping toppings
- Sour cream
- Nutrition bars
- Processed meats

As you see, casein is found in a variety of foods so the only way to check for the presence of this protein is to carefully read the food labels.

Food allergy versus food intolerance

Sensitivity to a certain food isn't always caused by a food allergy; it could be food intolerance instead. So, what's the difference? Food allergies are reactions that involve your immune system. Typically allergic reactions to casein in dairy products include skin rash or fatigue. If you're allergic to casein, your immune system considers casein a foreign object and mounts an immune response to get rid of it. The chemicals released during this process (such as histamine) alert your body that there is danger, and the process of allergic reaction starts. This immune reaction disrupts the normal functioning of your body.

Unlike allergies, some reactions to food do not involve the immune system. These responses are called *food intolerances.* A classic example is lactose intolerance, which is present in as many as 30 percent of American adults. People with lactose intolerance are sensitive to milk sugar lactose because they don't produce enough of the digestive enzyme called *lactase.* Lactase breaks down the lactose in your small intestine. If the lactose doesn't get digested, it makes its way to the large intestine and produces symptoms of diarrhea and gas.

Whether you have a food allergy or a food intolerance, reactions can occur anywhere from 30 minutes to 2 days after eating the offending food. By that time, you may have eaten other foods, so it may be difficult to identify the food to which you're allergic or sensitive. Keep a food diary and talk with your doctor or a dietitian if you're not sure.

Alcohol

Drinking alcohol can become an important issue for younger patients, especially in societies where drinking is accepted and maybe even expected at social gatherings. Studies have *not* shown that drinking adversely affects inflammation in people with Crohn's and colitis. It does have an irritating effect on the intestines, though, and it can worsen symptoms of diarrhea in some people.

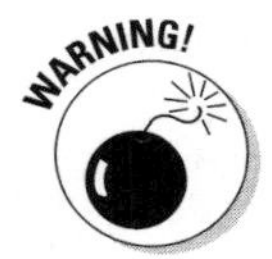

Alcohol can also interact with certain medications you may take for your disease. For example, alcohol may increase the sedation effects of narcotic pain medications. It can also cause abdominal cramps, sweating, and headaches when taken with metronidazole.

Excessive drinking can also damage your liver. If you're taking methotrexate for your Crohn's or colitis, the risk of liver damage becomes even higher and your doctor may suggest that you completely avoid alcohol if you're taking such medications. Otherwise, experts usually recommend occasional consumption of alcohol, such as a glass of wine on the weekends, as long as it doesn't produce any bothersome symptoms.

Mr. Sandman, Bring Me a Dream

Sleep has an important association with your immune system and is important for your overall health. Sleep deprivation leads to many problems, such as heart disease, weight gain, and memory and learning problems. Studies have even shown that poor sleepers die early.

What sleep does for your immune system

Depriving your body of sleep can take a toll on your immune system. A recently published European study showed that white blood cell counts go up if you're sleep deprived at night.

During sleep deprivation, the number of T cells (which defend against ailments) goes down and production of many inflammatory chemicals goes up. Some of these chemicals (such as interleukin-1) make you feel tired and sleepy. In other words, the immune system works to make you sleep, and sleep allows your immune system to work.

There are five phases of sleep: stage 1, stage 2, stage 3, stage 4, and rapid eye movement (REM). Usually, you begin at stage 1 and go through each stage until reaching REM sleep (the stage in which dreaming occurs), and then you begin the cycle again. Each complete sleep cycle takes 90 to 110 minutes. Your brain acts differently in each stage of sleep. REM also allows a complete "battery recharge" of your body, allowing memories to become permanent in the brain and allowing the immune system to repair any damages done to cells and organs. If you have a good night's sleep with sufficient REM stages, you wake up with a sense of clarity and feel rested.

The effect of sleep on Crohn's and colitis

My group from the University of Oklahoma recently conducted a study that showed that poor sleep is associated with active disease, and if you have poor sleep, you have a greater chance of having inflammation in the intestines. My colleagues and I are also studying the impact of poor sleep on disease flares.

As I mention earlier, poor sleep or sleep deprivation is associated with activation of the immune system. Inflammatory chemicals are increased. Chemicals such as interleukin-1 and tumor necrosis factor–alpha (TNF-α) are mostly elevated. These are the exact chemicals that are found to be elevated in Crohn's and colitis. So, it makes sense that there is an association between poor sleep and disease flare. (This has been proven true in other inflammatory diseases as well, such as rheumatoid arthritis and lupus.) Many of my patients acknowledge the fact that after having a poor night's sleep, they feel their symptoms increase.

How to get a good night's sleep

You know that poor sleep is associated with disturbances in the immune system and can activate your disease, so what can you do to get a good night's sleep? Here are few tips I give to my patients:

- **Keep a regular schedule.** If you go to bed and get up at the same time each day, you'll feel much more refreshed and energized than if you sleep the same number of hours but at different times. This holds true even if you change your sleep schedule by only an hour or two.
- **Regulate your sleep-wake cycle.** Melatonin is a natural sleep hormone produced by your brain in response to light. It helps regulate your sleep-wake cycle. Your brain secretes more melatonin in the evening, making you feel sleepy. Spending long days in your office away from sunlight and watching TV at night disturb the secretion of melatonin. So, spend more time outside during the day. Keep curtains and blinds open as well. At night, turn off the TV and computer, and when it's time to sleep, make sure your bedroom is dark.

  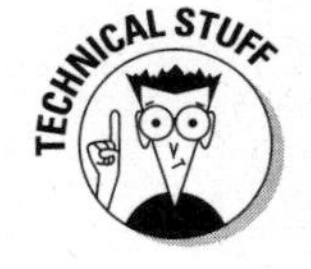

  Recent studies have found beneficial effects of melatonin on the immune system. Many animal studies have found that melatonin suppresses inflammation in the colon. Researchers are currently looking to see if melatonin helps suppress inflammation in people with colitis as well.
- **Make your room sleep friendly.** Keep the noise down. If you can't avoid barking dogs and loud neighbors, try to mask the noise with a fan or some soothing music. Make sure your bed is comfortable. Sleep experts recommend reserving your bed for sleeping and sex. If you associate your bed with answering e-mails and getting work done, you may have trouble sleeping at night.
- **Eat right and exercise regularly.** Diet and exercise habits can impact your sleep. Watching what you put in your body before you go to sleep is especially important. Stay away from big meals and alcohol before bed. Cutting down on caffeine and avoiding drinking too many liquids in the late evening will also help you get a good night's sleep.

  Many people think that having an alcoholic drink before bed will help them sleep well. Although alcohol does make you fall asleep faster, it reduces your sleep quality, waking you up later in the night.

Regular exercise is good for a quality sleep. Early morning or afternoon exercises such as brisk walk, bicycle ride, or even housework helps. Relaxing exercises such as yoga and gentle stretching before bedtime can help with the sleep. But avoid vigorous exercise at night; otherwise, you may find yourself counting sheep.

- **Know when to see a sleep doctor.** If you've tried all these tips and you're still struggling with sleep problems, you may have a sleep disorder that requires professional treatment. Many doctors are trained in sleep medicine. If you don't have a sleep specialist in your area, talking to your primary-care physician will also help.

  Consider seeking medical help if you have one of the following symptoms:

  - Persistent daytime sleepiness
  - Loud snoring accompanied by pauses in breathing (called *sleep apnea*)
  - Unrefreshing sleep
  - Frequent morning headaches
  - A crawling sensation in your legs or arms at night
  - Falling asleep at inappropriate times

Discovering your optimal amount of sleep

The sleep experts will tell you that there is no magic number for an optimal amount of sleep. Not only do different age groups need different amounts of sleep, but also sleep needs are individual. The amount of sleep you need may be different from the amount needed by someone else of the same age and gender. You may feel rested after seven hours of sleep, but someone else may need nine hours of good sleep to have a productive day.

Scientists are also learning that besides *basal sleep* (the amount of sleep your body needs for optimal function), there may also be a *sleep debt* (the accumulated sleep that you may have lost because of poor sleep habits, sickness, and other reasons). The good news is, you can pay off these sleep debts. School-age children need about 10 to 11 hours of basal sleep time, compared to teenagers, who need 8½ to 9½ hours, and adults who need 7 to 9 hours.

Chapter 14

Working and Traveling with Crohn's and Colitis

In This Chapter

- Managing work with Crohn's and colitis
- Hitting the road with Crohn's and colitis

I don't need to tell you that when you have Crohn's or colitis, it affects all aspects of your life in one way or another. Working or traveling can be complicated, especially by active disease. The good news is, you can take steps to minimize any difficulties that Crohn's or colitis may cause. This chapter offers tips on minimizing disruptions and coping with Crohn's and colitis at work and on the road.

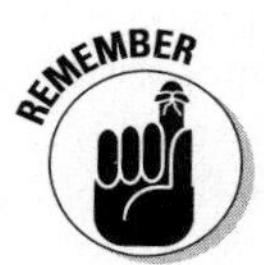

You can lead a full life with Crohn's and colitis — including travel and a rewarding work life. Don't let anybody — least of all yourself — tell you otherwise.

Working with Crohn's and Colitis

Most people with Crohn's and colitis are able to work. (If you were looking for a way to get out of your job, sorry I don't have better news!) But when you have Crohn's or colitis, your entire life — including your work life — is affected, so you need to take some steps to minimize that impact.

In this section, I walk you through job hunting, telling your employer about your condition, managing the day-to-day aspects, anticipating challenges, and dealing with sick days.

Working your job hunt around your disease

If you're looking for a job, try doing so during a time when your disease is inactive. If you're job hunting (or starting a new job) during a flare, your symptoms may make it difficult to jump through all the hoops — job interviews, orientation sessions, and training. If stress triggers your disease, try to reduce your anxiety during your job search (see Chapter 12 for ways to manage stressors).

If possible, consider your disease when choosing your next job. Some occupations may not be as conducive to someone with Crohn's or colitis. For example, you may often feel very fatigued, so an extremely physical job may not be ideal. Also, consider proximity to the restroom. If you often need to go to the restroom many times throughout the day, make sure this is feasible in the job you're considering.

You aren't required to tell a potential employer about your Crohn's or colitis. And during the interview process, potential employers aren't allowed to ask you about your health or if you have any specific illnesses.

An interviewer can ask if you have a physical condition that may hinder your job performance, but this relates only to the specific duties that are discussed in the job description. A potential employer is allowed to make a job offer that's conditional on the employee passing a medical exam. But the medical exam can't be a condition of employment unless it shows the employee is physically unable to perform the job or if hiring an applicant would cause undue hardship on the business. (For example, a firefighter must be able to climb ladders. If an individual is unable to climb a ladder, the fire department can refuse to hire him for that position.)

Telling your employer and co-workers about your condition (or keeping it to yourself)

One of the biggest decisions you'll be faced with is if and when to discuss your disease with your employer and co-workers. In the United States, laws are in place to protect you from being discriminated against because of your medical condition. But these laws don't protect you from opinions or misconceptions about your disease.

Your employer and co-workers can react one of two ways:

- **They may be extremely supportive.** They'll look out for you when you aren't feeling well and cut you some slack when you need it.
- **They'll view you as a bad employee because you're sick.** They may assume you'll be on expensive medications or have frequent hospitalizations, both of which will cost the company in high-priced medical insurance and loss of productivity. These employers may also believe your job performance will suffer because of your illness. Some co-workers may resent having to pick up the slack when you're out sick.

If you have a feeling your boss or co-workers won't be supportive of your diagnosis, there's nothing wrong with keeping your illness to yourself.

The Americans with Disabilities Act and you

In the United States, in the workplace, you're protected by the Americans with Disabilities Act of 1990 (ADA).The ADA defines a person with a disability as one who has a physical or mental impairment that limits one or more major life activities, has a record of this impairment, or is regarded as having this impairment. Crohn's and colitis fall into the category of physical impairment. To be considered for a disability, the physical impairment must substantially limit a major life activity when compared to an average person.

If you qualify for disability, the ADA protects you from any discrimination. Regardless of your disease activity, your employer cannot discriminate against you. The protection of the ADA goes into effect the moment your employer becomes aware of your condition.

Those who are protected under the ADA are also eligible for reasonable accommodation. This rule applies to individuals who are qualified for the job, but who are unable to perform a responsibility because of their impairment. In this situation, the employer must make accommodations so the employee is able to complete the responsibility. For someone with Crohn's or colitis, this may include allowing extra time for restroom breaks.

If you believe you're a victim of discrimination, the first thing you should do is determine the chain of command at your place of employment. Then put your recollection of the discrimination in writing. List the problems you have with the situation, and offer potential solutions. Make sure to take note of any issue you've had and the date in which it occurred. This documentation may be helpful in the future. If your place of employment doesn't take your complaint seriously or if you're displeased with the outcome, you can always contact the Equal Employment Opportunity Commission (`www.eeoc.gov`) or the Department of Fair Employment and Housing in your area. They'll perform an investigation (but it could take weeks or months for the investigation to be finalized).

For more information on the ADA, visit `www.ada.gov`.

Starting your day off right

Some people with Crohn's or colitis experience more symptoms in the morning. You can take steps to get your day off right, paving the way for a good day at work:

- **Give yourself plenty of time in the morning.** That may mean getting up several hours before you actually have to walk out the door. You know your body best — just allow yourself enough time so that you aren't rushed and stressed.
- **Eat a well-balanced breakfast soon after you wake.** You may need to have a bowel movement soon after eating. If this is the case, get your breakfast in first thing, to allow yourself plenty of time to have a bowel movement before you leave. This helps prevent accidents during your commute (see the next section).
- **Avoid caffeine in the morning.** Caffeine is known to stimulate the bowels and generally cause a laxative effect. Although some people may be able to tolerate caffeine, others experience worsening symptoms after consuming caffeine. Try to avoid caffeine — including coffee, tea, soda, and chocolate — before having to get in the car and commute to work.
- **Create a routine.** Creating a routine can help alleviate some of the stress you may experience in the morning, and your body will adapt to it. This can also help you remember to take any morning medications.

Planning your commute

With proper planning in the morning, you can decrease the likelihood of an accident during your commute. If you're starting a new job, map out your commute before your first day. Familiarize yourself with conveniently located and clean restrooms on your drive. Get to know the traffic patterns in your area — knowing the busiest times and heavy traffic spots during rush hour can alleviate some of your fears about having an accident. If you know that leaving 15 minutes earlier means you'll experience significantly less traffic, maybe you can leave home earlier and sit in your car listening to the radio or reading a book before your workday starts.

If you're afraid of having an accident during your commute, pack a change of clothes in your car or use a disposable undergarment.

Packing an emergency kit

Because of the nature of Crohn's and colitis, flares are inevitable, and the likelihood of your experiencing some of the symptoms at work is high. The best thing you can do is prepare for an attack at work before it actually happens. Have a game plan in place for how you're going to deal with the situation. Start by packing an emergency kit to keep at your desk for these episodes.

Here's what to include in your emergency kit:

- A change of clothes
- Disposable undergarments
- Soothing wipes
- Ointments
- Toilet paper
- A heating pad for pain

If you've disclosed your condition to your employer and co-workers, dealing with the attack may be easier for you. At the very least, you'll face fewer questions about why you're taking more frequent restroom breaks.

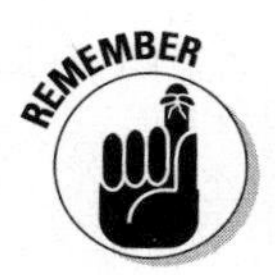

During an attack or flare, your first call should be to your healthcare team. Depending on the severity of your symptoms, they may want to see you right away. Also, the sooner you call, the sooner you can be seen — don't let yourself be miserable for no reason. Your doctor will want to know what's going on.

Speed bumps ahead: Coping with job-related challenges

Part of living with a chronic condition like Crohn's or colitis is being prepared for the challenges that lie ahead. If you know what's coming, you'll be able to handle it better, and your anxiety will be reduced (which, in turn, is beneficial for your symptoms).

In this section, I walk you through handling your own response to an attack, as well as handling your co-workers' responses.

Responding to symptoms when they get in the way

When symptoms get in the way of your ability to perform at your job, try not to be frustrated. I know this is easier said than done, but keep in mind the cyclical nature of your disease. You'll have good days and bad days. And the key is to make the most of the good ones, and do the best to limit the bad ones.

When your disease is in remission, take advantage of your extra energy. This could be a great time to volunteer for more responsibility at work. You don't want to overdo it or put undue stress on yourself, but it can help make up for the times when you need other people to pick up some of your slack.

When you're having a flare or an attack, you may have to rely on co-workers to help you complete some of your tasks. If you have a physical job, your energy level may not be where it usually is. You may have to take more breaks or ask if you can be on light duty for a short period of time.

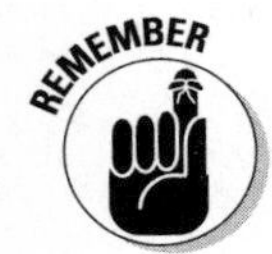

The best thing you can do is conserve your energy during times of active disease. Nothing good will come from overdoing it.

Handling your co-workers' less-than-understanding attitudes

If your co-workers are unaware of your condition, they may have a negative attitude toward you if they feel like they're doing more than their fair share. If you feel comfortable talking with your co-workers about your situation, some basic education about Crohn's and colitis can help.

Don't just assume they'll cover for you when you're having a flare. Let them know you appreciate how much they're doing for you. Also, tell your co-workers that you fully intend to take over your responsibilities and then some as soon as you feel up to it — and be sure to live up to that promise.

Sometimes, even if a co-worker is well aware of your condition, he may still have a negative attitude. If so, there may be nothing you can do to change his opinion. In this case, the best approach is to have a good attitude and do what you can. Getting angry won't help your situation, so you may as well stay positive and focus your energy on feeling better.

Taking advantage of the Family and Medical Leave Act

After getting your diagnosis or after starting a new job, find out how you acquire sick days with your employer. Some companies require you to work for a certain amount of time before you're eligible for benefits or before you're eligible to take any time off.

There are laws in place that protect you against being terminated while you're out sick. The Family and Medical Leave Act (FMLA) was put into place in 1993. Many people use this act for maternity leave, but it can be used for any serious illness or hospitalization lasting more than three days. You can use it for your own illness, or for the illness of a family member (for example, to care for an ailing spouse).

The FMLA protects an employee's job and benefits while he's out. During your absence, your employer must continue to provide you with insurance benefits if you were eligible for them before you left. Also, when you return, your employer must allow you to return to your original job, or a job that is equivalent (meaning similar pay and benefits).

To determine if you're eligible for FMLA leave, check out the following requirements. According to the Department of Labor, the FMLA applies to all

- Public agencies, including state, local and federal employers, and local education agencies (schools)
- Private-sector employers who employed 50 or more employees for at least 20 workweeks in the current or preceding calendar year

To be eligible for FMLA leave, an employee must work for a covered employer and meet all the following conditions:

- Have worked for that employer for at least 12 months
- Have worked at least 1,250 hours during the 12 months prior to the start of the FMLA leave
- Work at a location where at least 50 employees are employed at the location or within 75 miles of the location

The FMLA entitles an employee to 12 weeks of leave to tend to his own serious medical needs or those of a family member. The 12 weeks can be taken all at once, or the time can broken up into smaller segments. The smaller segments can be done numerous ways. Options include shortening your workweek by one day for a long period of time or taking individual days off when needed — the latter may be the better option for those with Crohn's or colitis who experience occasional flares and only need one or two days off at a time or for those who need one day off every so often. If you're considering surgery, the longer stretch of time may be a better option for you.

Employees are only eligible to take off using FMLA for 12 weeks during a 12-month period. The employer determines the 12-month period. The 12-month period could begin at the start of the leave or the end of the leave; some employers choose to use a specific calendar period.

Whether you'll get paid for your time off is determined by your employer as well. Most employers allow employees to use their earned vacation days during leave. The terms of how you'll be paid should be very clearly stated in the company policies, usually found in the employee handbook or available through the human resources department.

Another option for getting paid during your time off is short-term disability or long-term disability through your insurance provider. For more information on disability insurance, check out *Insurance For Dummies,* 2nd Edition, by Jack Hungelmann (Wiley).

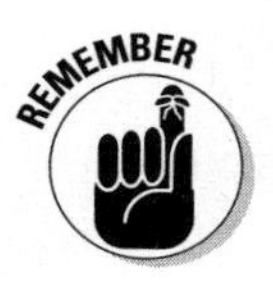

Plan ahead. Some employers require a 30-day notice for leave. Others require certification of illness from your healthcare provider. Your employer may also ask for a second or third opinion. You can obtain the necessary FMLA paperwork from your employer.

Note: Each state's FMLA laws may vary slightly. Look into your state's employment act before filling out your paperwork.

On the Road Again: Traveling with Crohn's and Colitis

Vacations can be great for stress relief and relaxation. However, if you suffer from Crohn's or colitis, a vacation may be a huge source of anxiety for you. But it doesn't have to be. With proper planning and preparation, your next vacation can be the relaxing experience you hope for.

Timing is key when it comes to vacation planning. Predicting a Crohn's or colitis flare may be impossible, but the best time to travel is when your disease is in remission. For this reason, you may want to consider purchasing travel insurance for your trip — it adds to the expense of the trip, and there's a chance you won't need it (as is the case with all insurance), but the piece of mind may be worth the extra cost.

Discuss your upcoming travel plans with your healthcare providers to make sure you're in the best possible health at the time of your trip.

Assembling a vacation survival guide

Before you take a trip, create a vacation survival guide. This guide should include the following:

- The names and contact information of all members of your healthcare team
- A photocopy of your health insurance card
- A photocopy of your driver's license
- A photocopy of your passport if you're traveling internationally
- A summary of your medical records describing your illness, the disease location, any previous surgery, a recent endoscopy report, medical treatment history, and current medications, in case you need to be seen by a doctor while you're away

Do some homework and figure out who to call if you have any kind of problems while you're gone. If you're traveling abroad, the International Association for Medical Assistance to Travellers (`www.iamat.org`) can provide you with a list of English-speaking doctors in the area where you're traveling. It also locates hospitals in the area, just in case.

Getting immunized before you travel abroad

Some of the diseases no longer seen in the United States are quite common in other parts of the world. So, before traveling to certain countries, you'll need to be vaccinated. Make an appointment with your primary-care provider four to six weeks before your trip to discuss any needed vaccinations. If you aren't being treated with immunosuppressive medications, you should generally be immunized as any other traveler would be. But talk with your doctor and see what she recommends for your specific situation.

The only vaccination required by the World Health Organization's International Health Regulations is yellow fever for travel to certain countries in sub-Saharan Africa and for travel to tropical South America. Also, if you're making an annual trip to Saudi Arabia during the Hajj, the Saudi Arabian government requires you to receive the meningococcal vaccination.

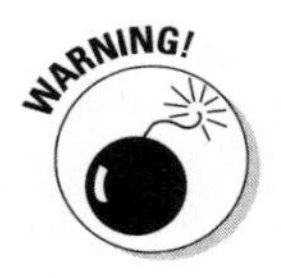

If you're taking immunosuppressive medications such as anti-TNF drugs, do not take live vaccines, such as Bacille Calmette–Guérin, measles, Ty21a, varicella, and yellow fever. Avoid travel to any parts of the world where these vaccinations are required or recommended. You may be able to receive live vaccines if you're on low-dose steroids and standard doses of azathioprine or 6-MP, but talk to your doctor before receiving any live vaccine.

For information regarding vaccinations that are recommended for travel, visit `wwwnc.cdc.gov/travel/destinations/list.htm`. As always, talk to your doctor if you have any questions.

Packing for your trip

To stay organized (and reduce your stress), make a list of everything you want to bring. If you're flying, determine if you're going to check a bag, take a carry-on, or do both. This will make a difference in how you pack and how much you take with you.

Make sure to pack everything you'll need to manage your disease. This includes medications, both prescription and over the counter.

The Transportation Security Administration (TSA) has numerous, constantly changing rules about what you can bring on a plane. As of this writing, all medications must be packed in their original bottles. If you're checking a bag and taking a carry-on, pack medication in both bags, in case one gets lost.

Before your trip, visit the TSA's website (www.tsa.gov) to make sure you're aware of current regulations. Make sure you have plenty of medication to get you through the entire trip, plus some extra (in case you run into a travel snafu).

If you have an ostomy, make sure you have extra supplies available, including appliances, adhesives, and plastic bags. Currently, scissors with blades less than 4 inches are allowed on planes, so you may be allowed to bring your ostomy scissors. If not, cuticle scissors work well.

On road trips always bring toilet paper, soothing wipes, ointments, and a change of clothes just in case. Hand sanitizer is also a good idea.

Maintaining the same diet you would eat at home while on your vacation is important. So, pack nonperishable foods like oatmeal or nutrition bars. On the plane, you may be able to request a special meal or diet. If you're driving to your destination, pack a small cooler full of sandwiches and snacks. Avoid and limit your fast-food intake as much as possible.

I can't wait! Getting the card that says it all (plus more resources)

The Crohn's & Colitis Foundation of American (CCFA; www.ccfa.org) offers members the **I Can't Wait card** that you can carry while traveling; it helps you explain your Crohn's or colitis to laypeople who may not know anything about the condition. The CCFA also offers an **Air Travel Talking Points card** (www.ccfa.org/assets/pdfs/TSA_card.pdf) that provides more information as well (you don't have to be a member to print it out).

Another beneficial item is the TSA's **Disability Notification Card for Air Travel** (www.tsa.gov/sites/default/files/publications/disability_notification_cards.pdf). You can present this card to TSA officers at security checkpoints. It doesn't excuse you from being screened at security, but it does alert them that you have a medical condition and you may have medical devices. It can also help you discreetly communicate about your disease. The TSA also offers a help line for travelers with disabilities and medical conditions called TSA Cares (855-787-2227).

More resources to check out include the following:

- **CCFA Information Resource Center:** 888-694-8872 (available Monday through Friday 9 a.m. to 5 p.m. Eastern time)
- **Air Travel 101–TSA FAQ, from the CCFA:** www.ccfa.org/resources/TSA-air-travel-101.html
- **Travelers with Disabilities and Medical Conditions, from the TSA:** www.tsa.gov/traveler-information/travelers-disabilities-and-medical-conditions

Avoiding travelers' diarrhea

Travelers' diarrhea is the most predictable of all the travel-related illnesses. High-risk destinations are the developing countries of Latin America, Africa, the Middle East, and Asia. Because of poor hygiene in local eating establishments, travelers' diarrhea is often tough to avoid.

Bacteria is often what causes travelers' diarrhea. The number-one cause is *E. coli.* Viruses or protozoa are also known causes of travelers' diarrhea. People affected often experience both vomiting and diarrhea, and symptoms can last up to five days.

Travelers' diarrhea can ruin an otherwise wonderful trip, so the best thing to do is prevent it from ever occurring. There are many things you can do to help reduce your chances of developing travelers' diarrhea:

- **Practice good hygiene.** Before eating, wash your hands, ideally with soap and water. If soap and water aren't available, an alcohol-based hand cleaner is good. Make sure the hand cleaner is at least 60 percent alcohol, and use it before every meal.
- **Choose your food and drink wisely.** Foods that are freshly cooked and served hot are generally safer than foods that may have been sitting for an extended period of time in the kitchen or on a buffet line. Avoid any drinks that may have been diluted with nonpotable water (such as reconstituted fruit juices, ice, and milk) or any foods that may have been washed in nonpotable water, such as fresh fruits or vegetables. Other foods that may pose a risk for you include raw or undercooked meat and seafood. Bottled and sealed or carbonated beverages are generally considered safe. Boiled beverages and those appropriately treated with iodine or chlorine are also safe.

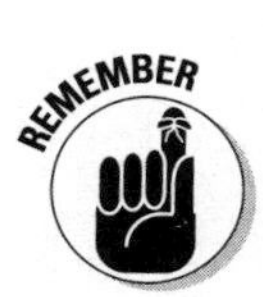

  Tap water and ice have not been properly treated. This is important to keep in mind when brushing your teeth and ordering drinks at restaurants.

- **Take Pepto-Bismol as a preventive.** Bismuth subsalicylate, which is the active ingredient in Pepto-Bismol, can be used to prevent travelers' diarrhea. Studies show that it can reduce the likelihood of developing travelers' diarrhea from 40 percent to 14 percent. If you decide to use bismuth subsalicylate, don't be alarmed if you experience blackening of the tongue and stool — this is a common side effect.
- **Take antibiotics as a preventive.** Antibiotics are effective in preventing travelers' diarrhea. Studies have shown that they can reduce diarrhea rates from 40 percent to 4 percent. The antibiotic of choice has changed many times over the years. A newly approved antibiotic, rifaximin (Xifaxan), is very effective. In one study, rifaximin reduced the risk for travelers' diarrhea in travelers to Mexico by 77 percent.

International names of commonly used medications

If you're traveling abroad, and you need medication, it helps to know the name of the drug where you're traveling. The following list can help.

- **Sulfasalazine:** In the United States, the brand name is Azulfidine. In Mexico, it goes by Azulfidina. In the United Kingdom, it's Salphasazine. And in France, Italy, and Australia, it's Salazopyrin.
- **Mesalamine:** In the United States, the brand names are Apriso, Asacol, Asacol HD, Canasa, Lialda, Pentasa, and Rowasa. In Canada, it goes by Mesasal, Mezavant, and Salofalk. In Mexico, it's Lazar. In the United Kingdom, it's Mesren and Octasa. In Brazil, it goes by Asalit. And in Italy, it's Claversal, Mesaflor, and Pentacol.
- **Metronidazole:** In the United States, the brand name is Flagyl. In Canada, it goes by Florazole. And in Mexico, it's Amebidal.
- **Loperamide:** In the United States and throughout Western Europe, the brand name is Imodium (except in Spain, where it's known as Fortasec).
- **Azathioprine:** In the United States, the brand names are Azasan and Imuran. In Canada, the United Kingdom, and Australia, it goes by Imuran. In Ireland, it goes by Imuger and Imuran. In Finland, it's Azamun. In Scandinavia and France, it's Imurel. In Germany, it's Azafalk, Azamedac, and Imurek. And in Italy, it's Azafor.
- **6-mercaptopurine (6-MP):** In the United States, Canada, the United Kingdom, France, and Italy, the brand name is Purinethol.
- **Prednisone:** It's known in most countries under its generic name, but there are several foreign brands.

If, despite your best efforts, you end up getting travelers' diarrhea, the best treatment is an antibiotic. Seek proper medical care, and stay well hydrated.

Finding a bathroom . . . fast!

When traveling abroad, one of the most beneficial things you can do is figure out the language that's spoken in the region and learn how to say, "Where is the bathroom?" or write the phrase down on a piece of paper that you can show to people.

Be patient with anyone who's trying to help you. Also, look for signs. Different countries have different signs for their restrooms. Finally, don't be alarmed if you find yourself in a restroom with both men and women — restrooms in the country you're visiting may be co-ed. (A good guidebook to the area should give you the information you need ahead of time.)

I don't have room to list all the languages and the translations of "Where is the bathroom?" but a great resource is Google Translate (`http://translate.google.com`). It offers translation into more than 60 languages, from Afrikaans to Yiddish.

Part V
Considering Special Populations with Crohn's and Colitis

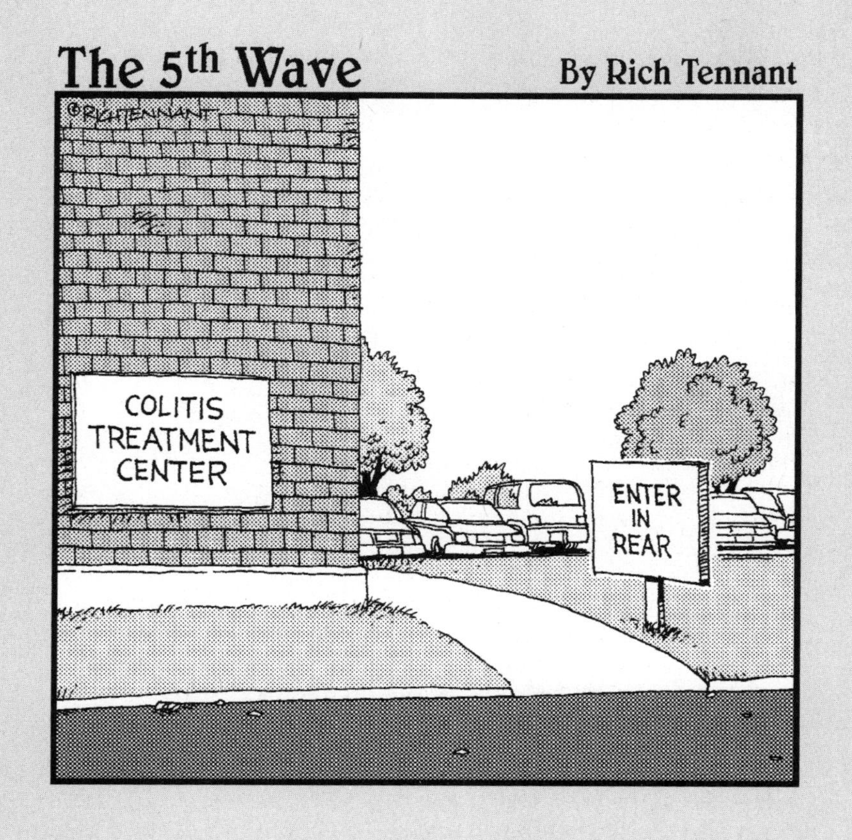

In this part . . .

Being a kid or teenager is tough enough without a disease like Crohn's or colitis. This part offers some important tips that can help make life easier for kids or teens with the disease.

If you have Crohn's or colitis and you're trying to get pregnant (or avoid getting pregnant), you face some special issues as well. In this part, I give you tips on everything from sex to contraception to fertility. I also tell you how Crohn's or colitis may affect your pregnancy.

Chapter 15

Kids with Crohn's and Colitis

In This Chapter

- Appreciating the differences among kids and adults
- Knowing the effects on kids' growth and nutrition
- Understanding management issues related to kids
- Surviving school and transitioning to adult care

Twenty-five to 30 percent of patients with Crohn's and 20 percent of patients with colitis are diagnosed before the age of 20. Although the peak age of onset is late adolescence, 4 percent of kids with Crohn's and colitis are diagnosed in very early childhood (before the age of 5).

Many of the signs and symptoms of Crohn's and colitis are the same in kids as they are in adults, but kids may not be able to describe their symptoms the way adults can. Here's a list of some issues specific to kids with these illnesses:

- **Stomach pain is common.** Because stomachaches aren't unheard of in kids, it may be tough for kids and parents to know when the stomach pain could be a sign of something more serious, like Crohn's or colitis.
- **The only signs of Crohn's or colitis in a child may be fever, weight loss, or simply failure to grow.**
- **Stress can also trigger symptoms in kids.** "What do kids have to be stressed about?" you may be thinking. But everything from just being upset emotionally to experiencing severe trauma can cause stress. (Next time you're tempted to blow off stress in children, ask yourself how eager you'd be to be a kid again.)
- **As in adults, medication is very important in order to keep the disease in remission and prevent it from progressing.** Kids may not like to take medications or find it difficult to swallow pills. They may even experience more drug intolerance and side effects than adults.

- **Kids may be embarrassed about bodily functions, making it difficult for them to talk about the condition.** Sometimes kids (particularly as they get older) don't tell their parents about the symptoms they're having, because they're too embarrassed to talk about it, which can make getting the proper treatment more difficult.
- **No kid wants to be different — all they want is to be like everybody else.** When a kid has Crohn's or colitis, he may feel embarrassed and may even be teased or bullied at school because he has to leave the classroom for urgent bathroom breaks. Kids may not want anyone, especially their teachers or classmates, to know about their condition.

As a parent, you just want your child to be happy and healthy. And in this chapter, I give you the tools you need to help make that a reality for your child, even if she has Crohn's or colitis.

Identifying How Crohn's and Colitis Are Different in Kids Than They Are in Adults

Crohn's and colitis aren't *completely* different in kids than they are in adults. For example, the causes (or possible causes) of the conditions are the same (see Chapter 4). But there are some ways that the diseases differ in kids, and that's what I cover in this section.

Gender

In adults, Crohn's and colitis occur almost equally in men and women. When it comes to children, though, Crohn's is slightly more common in boys than in girls. (Colitis is diagnosed in just as many girls as boys.) Scientists are trying to learn why Crohn's is more common in boys than in girls. Today, the thinking is that it may be related to differences in sex hormones, but we don't know for sure.

Symptoms

The symptoms of Crohn's and colitis in kids can be very similar to the symptoms in adults (see Chapter 2). Just like adults, kids can experience weight loss, abdominal pain, diarrhea, blood in the stool, and fever. However, there are some differences that may require different approaches to the treatment and management of the disease in children.

For example, some studies suggest that colitis may present with more extensive disease in children than in adults. Abdominal pain is found to be a more common symptom of colitis in children than in adults; conversely, rectal bleeding, which is a common symptom of colitis in adults, isn't as common in kids. Another difference among kids with colitis is the rate of progression from *proctitis* (inflammation of the rectum) to *pan colitis* (inflammation of the entire colon); in kids, there is a 65 percent chance that proctitis will progress to pan colitis (compared to only a 30 percent to 40 percent chance of progression in adults). The rate of surgery in kids with colitis is similar to adults (reaching 20 percent to 30 percent 20 years after diagnosis).

In older kids, the location of Crohn's is similar to that found in adults; the majority of kids have the disease involving the terminal ileum and cecum (called *ileocolitis*). On the other hand, younger kids (under 5 years of age) tend to have significant large intestine involvement (called *colitis*). Similarly, kids with Crohn's disease may present with growth failure before the onset of intestinal symptoms such as abdominal pain, nausea, fatigue, or diarrhea.

Effect on growth and development

Growth failure is a very common non-intestinal complication of Crohn's and colitis among children. In this section, I fill you in on the causes and effects, as well as how to manage growth failure in kids with Crohn's and colitis.

Causes

There are many causes of growth failure, including the following:

- **Malnutrition:** The condition that occurs when the body doesn't get enough nutrients. Malnutrition can be the result of many things. Children with Crohn's and colitis often eat less because they have a decrease in appetite as a result of active disease. They may also have learned to associate food with abdominal pain or diarrhea. In addition, kids may have an altered sense of taste because of zinc deficiency. Finally, some medications, such as metronidazole (Flagyl), also play an important role in reduction of nutrients.

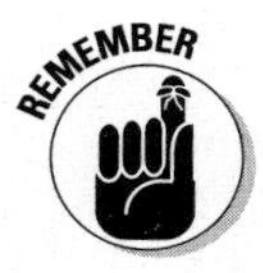

  Studies have shown that children with active disease may consume 20 percent to 60 percent less nutrients than they do when their disease is in remission. Inflammation of the mucosa during active disease also interferes with the normal process of absorption.

- **Steroids:** Treatment with steroids — particularly when used during puberty — may contribute to growth failure. Steroids interfere with the body's production of growth hormones. They also have a negative effect on the process of bone formation.

- **Inflammation:** The process of inflammation itself affects the growth of children. The different inflammatory proteins released during the process of inflammation affect the functions of growth. This association has been proven by many clinical studies where treatment of inflammation with drugs and surgery led to improvement in the growth of children.

Effects

Growth failure in children with Crohn's and colitis produces many effects:

- **Short stature:** Growth failure may lead to short stature, especially in young males who are diagnosed with Crohn's or colitis at an early age. Steroid use is also associated with short stature.
- **Delayed puberty:** Delayed puberty is very common in Crohn's and colitis. Studies have shown that there is an average one-year delay in the onset of puberty in boys; one and a half years in girls.
- **Low weight:** Growth failure in kids can lead to low body weight. About 25 percent of children with Crohn's and 10 percent of children with colitis are underweight at the time of diagnosis.
- **Psychosocial stress:** Growth failure can lead to decreased self-esteem and lower school and social performance. It can also lead to anxiety and depression.

Most of these side effects are reversed if the inflammation is controlled in a timely fashion with medical or surgical therapy.

How to manage growth failure

Treatment of active disease and optimizing nutrition are important steps in managing growth failure in kids with Crohn's or colitis. Children with growth failure have higher energy requirements in order to catch up. Active disease adds fuel to the fire and increases their energy requirement even more. Kids with Crohn's or colitis usually require a high-protein diet (2.5 g to 3 g per kilogram [2.2 pounds] of body weight) to meet their energy requirements and growth. This requirement increases if the disease is active.

Because they don't want to reduce kids' energy intake, doctors and nutritionists hardly restrict the diets of kids with Crohn's and colitis unless there is clear evidence of food intolerance.

Sometimes liquid nutritional supplements are needed to increase kids' energy intake. These supplements can be added in the form of high-calorie drinks such as PediaSure or by feeding kids at night with a *nasogastric tube* (a tube that passes through the nose into the stomach). This help kids gain weight and improve their nutritional status; it also strengthens their muscles and bones.

Treatment of active inflammation is also critical in restoring growth. Your doctor will try to avoid steroids as much as possible when treating your child, to prevent steroids' harmful effects on growth. Treatment with immunosuppressive drugs (such as azathioprine [Azasan, Imuran] and 6-MP [Purinethol]) and biologic therapy may be required to effectively treat the inflammation.

Few studies have shown the benefits of growth hormones injections in kids with severe growth delay. However, we don't have good evidence to use these hormones for Crohn's and colitis patients. Until we get more information about the safety and effectiveness of growth hormones, doctors usually consider this therapy only if growth failure persists *after* a child's Crohn's or colitis has been properly managed and his nutritional needs have been adequately met and failed.

Getting a Diagnosis

Sometimes diagnosing Crohn's and colitis can be tricky in kids, because many other medical conditions cause stomachaches and loose stools in children and are far more common than Crohn's and colitis. Diagnosing kids with these illnesses also can be difficult because they may feel shy or embarrassed describing their symptoms or simply may not know *how* to describe their symptoms.

Some kids develop symptoms of severe abdominal pain and bloody diarrhea, undergo quick evaluation with endoscopy and other tests, and get the diagnosis of Crohn's or colitis in a few weeks. In other kids, symptoms can be less severe, and it may take months or even years before they get the actual diagnosis.

Here are some common symptoms of Crohn's and colitis in kids (for more on the symptoms of Crohn's and colitis, see Chapter 2):

- **Abdominal pain:** Abdominal pain is the common first symptom in about 80 percent of kids. However, abdominal pain is also a common symptom of many other health problems, such as constipation, irritable bowel syndrome, muscle pain, acid reflux, viral infections, and food intolerances. Kids with appendicitis, gallstones, and kidney stones also experience abdominal pain.
- **Diarrhea:** Like abdominal pain, there are many other reasons for diarrhea in kids. Medications, foods, infections, and food intolerances can also cause diarrhea.

Bloody diarrhea usually is a sign of a more serious problem, but certain infections like salmonella and *E. coli* can cause bloody diarrhea as well. If the stool studies show no sign of infection and the bloody diarrhea persists, your doctor will start testing for Crohn's and colitis.

- **Other signs and symptoms:** Kids can also have with low-grade fever and weight loss. Other common signs (like slow growth and late puberty) are covered earlier in this chapter.

  Just like adults, kids can have other organs (like the liver and pancreas) involved, as well as bone and joint problems. Turn to Chapter 2 for more on these symptoms.

As a parent, you have no way of knowing if the stomachache or diarrhea your child is complaining about is just a run-of-the-mill bug, or something more serious, like Crohn's or colitis, so your best bet is to talk with your pediatrician or family doctor.

When a doctor suspects a kid may have Crohn's or colitis, she'll run the same diagnostic tests as are done for adults (see Chapter 6).

Managing Crohn's and Colitis in Kids

For the most part, the treatment of kids and teenagers with Crohn's and colitis is similar to adults. The primary aim of medical therapy (see Chapter 7) is to bring the disease to *remission* (an inactive state without any symptoms). When medical therapy fails, surgery is the next step (see Chapter 8).

In this section, I focus on the aspects of disease management that are unique to kids.

Monitoring medications

Most of the drugs used to treat adults with Crohn's and colitis are also used to treat kids. However, there are certain factors that doctors consider while starting and monitoring drug therapy in children. They have to take into account the child's age, height, and weight when prescribing medications. Drug doses will change as the child grows and gains weight.

Kids aren't just growing physically — they're also growing emotionally. Doctors and parents have to keep in mind how kids are adapting socially and psychologically. Finally, they need to keep in mind potential side effects of the medications and issues of compliance with the prescribed drugs.

Which medications your child may take

Almost all the medications used for adults with Crohn's and colitis are used for children. Chapter 7 offers a detailed review of medical therapy. In this section, I address some special issues and considerations when these medications are prescribed to children and teenagers.

Aminosalicylates

Aminosalicylates (5-ASA), such as mesalamine (Apriso, Asacol, Canasa, Lialda, Pentasa, Rowasa), are one of the the initial therapies for treating Crohn's and colitis. These drugs may be taken orally or through the rectum. Weight-based formulas are used to calculate the doses of aminosalicylates for children.

The number of pills (as many as 10 to 16 pills a day) and frequency of administration (as often as three to four times a day) are important issues when it comes to kids taking pills. You may want to discuss these issues with your doctor.

Some newer, longer-acting formulations, such as Apriso and Lialda, are given once or twice daily and are easier to take. Some drugs, such as balsalazide disodium (Colazal), come in capsules that may be opened and sprinkled on food (such as applesauce). Other drugs are pH released and have to be taken in a capsule or tablet as a whole so that they can reach the site of inflammation.

If kids are unable to take a tablet, a liquid preparation can be used as alternative. Only sulfasalazine (Azulfidine), an older mesalamine drug, is available in liquid form.

Here are some pill-swallowing tips for kids:

- **Have the child put the pill in his mouth and then drink a glass of water through a straw.** With this method, many kids concentrate on the straw and don't think about the pill, so it goes down easily.
- **Consider slipping the pill in ice cream, yogurt, or another soft food to improve the smell and taste of the pill.**
- **Reward your child for both the effort of trying and success of swallowing pills.** Setting up a sticker chart can be helpful.

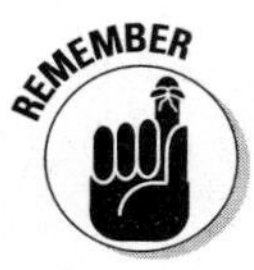

Don't crush or break the pills unless you're told by your doctor that this is okay. Some pills won't work as effectively if they're crushed.

For kids with left-sided colitis (see Chapter 3), topical therapy with enema or suppository is used. Enema therapy can be a daunting endeavor in the beginning, but with education and support, many kids and families adapt readily to this treatment.

Steroids

Steroids are used when active Crohn's or colitis fails to respond to conventional therapy, such as aminosalicylates, and kids have worsening symptoms such as abdominal pain, diarrhea, or blood in the stool. Steroids can be taken orally (as pills) or intravenously (which may be required for severe symptoms and kids who are hospitalized). Dosages are usually determined based on body weight.

When remission is achieved, the dosage is usually tapered gradually, with the goal of discontinuing the steroids altogether. Some kids may not be able to taper off the steroids. Their symptoms recur or worsen each time the steroid dose is tapered or they're taken off the drug. This may require more potent immunosuppressive drugs such as azathioprine or anti-TNF drugs.

The cosmetic side effects of steroid use may be very disturbing to kids and teenagers. Side effects such as facial swelling, weight gain, hair growth, and acne can cause emotional and psychological problems for kids. Reassure your child that these side effects are temporary and will disappear when the dose is lowered or the drug is stopped.

Physicians try their best to avoid repeated courses of steroids in kids because of its long-term negative effects on bones and growth. Taking medications regularly can help kids to have fewer flares and less of a need for steroids. But some flares are unpredictable and come without warning (or with very little warning), and steroids may have to be used.

If a child is having several flares in a year without any obvious reasons, it may be time to step up his therapy and introduce more potent drugs, such as immunosuppressive drugs and biologics.

Immunosuppressive drugs

Immunosuppressive drugs such as azathioprine (Azasan, Imuran) and 6-MP (Purinethol) have been widely used as maintenance therapy in kids with Crohn's and colitis. These drugs have been shown to reduce the need for steroids, protecting kids from the harmful side effects of steroids. Because these drugs suppress the immune system, they're associated with side effects such as increased infection risk. Be sure to discuss the risks and benefits of these drugs with your doctor.

Methotrexate (Rheumatrex, Trexall) and tacrolimus (Prograf) are other immunosuppressive drugs that are less frequently used in kids. (See Chapter 7 for more on these drugs.)

Biologics

Biologics are the most recent drugs developed for the treatment of Crohn's and colitis. Anti-TNF drugs are the most commonly prescribed biologics. These drugs block the tumor necrosis factor–alpha (TNF-α) protein, which is involved in the process of inflammation. Three anti-TNF drugs are used in Crohn's and colitis: adalimumab (Humira), certolizumab pegol (Cimzia), and infliximab (Remicade).

Chapter 7 gives a detailed review of how these drugs work and what the side effects of these medications are.

Antibiotics

Antibiotics are frequently used in Crohn's and colitis, especially in colitis and perianal disease. Metronidazole (Flagyl) and ciprofloxacin (Cipro, Proquin) are two commonly used antibiotics. The dosage is based on body weight, and they're typically given with meals.

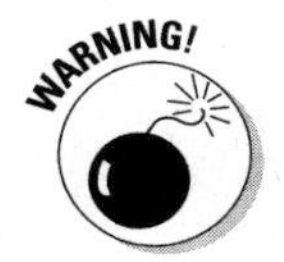

Teenagers should be informed about the interaction between alcohol and metronidazole. Alcohol use can result in severe nausea and vomiting when a person is on metronidazole.

Ciprofloxacin may cause problems with bones, joints, and tissues around joints in children. It has been associated with spontaneous tendon rupture. Your doctor will discuss these potential side effects with you.

Sticking with the medications

Nobody likes to take medicines, but kids may have even more objections than adults do. They may not like the taste of the medication, they may have trouble swallowing pills, the side effects may be unpleasant, or they may just stubbornly resist taking daily medicines. Some kids are embarrassed by having to take medications in front of other kids. Some kids may be fine taking medications when they're feeling lousy, but once their disease is in remission, they may not understand why medication is necessary.

As I explain in Chapter 7, following your doctor's orders when it comes to taking medications is essential to keeping the disease in remission and putting off the need for surgery. Even after surgery, a person may require medications for Crohn's to prevent its recurrence. Forgetting to take or intentionally stopping medications may lead to disease activation and more flares. Active disease and flares will lead to more frequent clinic and hospital visits, more laboratory tests, and possible admissions to the hospital. Having active disease or more frequent flares can interfere with a child's nutrition and growth.

Here are some tips for explaining to your child why taking the medications the doctor prescribed is so important:

- **Listen to your child's concerns and avoid opposing them immediately.** If your child feels like she's being heard, she'll be more likely to listen to you in return.
- **Explain to your child in simple words why taking the medicines is necessary and what its benefits are.** Use the information in this book,

as well as the advice of your doctor, to outline some of the reasons why medicine is important. You don't want to scare your child, but even something as simple as the following can work: "I know you feel better now, and that's great! But in order for you to continue feeling better, you need to keep taking your medicine. If you stop, you'll start feeling bad again, the way you used to. And you don't want that, right?"

Communicate with your physicians, school staff, pharmacists, and teachers about the medications your child needs to take and when. If your child is missing doses, talk with your doctor to see if the medication can be simplified. Once- or twice-daily dosing is the most comfortable regimen for school-age children because parents can remind them to take their medications or watch them taking their medications.

As kids get older, they're able to participate in the management of their disease and goal setting. Be sure to empower your kids to learn to take their own medications and be responsible for caring for their own health.

You may need to get creative with teenagers. Contracts, rewards, and peer support groups can be very helpful.

Finally, technology can also help improve your child's compliance with medications. You can send text messages and set alarms for reminders. There are even electronic monitors such as Medication Event Monitoring Systems (MEMS) available for doctors and parents to measure adherence. They detect actions necessary to administer medication such as removing the cap from the pill bottle. You can later download the information to check frequency and timing of dosing and patterns of adherence. Ask your doctor about MEMS if you're interested.

Paying attention to nutrition

Nutrition is involved with two important tasks:

- **It provides energy.** This amount of energy is measured in calories. Without enough food, you won't have enough energy.
- **It provides your body with chemical substances, called nutrients, to help build, maintain, and repair your body organs.**

Kids constantly grow and develop. They need adequate nutrition to meet the demands of their growing bodies. Childhood growth isn't just about their height and weight — it's also about the growth of their internal organs. Because of all this growing they need to do, kids' energy requirements are very high and any deficiency of nutrients — like the kind often seen with Crohn's and colitis — can have a profound effect on their growth and development.

Kids with Crohn's and colitis need about 20 percent to 40 percent more energy than those without the disease. However, studies have shown that kids with Crohn's and colitis consume only about *half* the calories they require for their age. Boys with Crohn's or colitis need about 2,300 to 2,600 calories every day; girls need about 2,000 to 2,200 calories every day. Talk with your doctor about your child's calorie requirements. Your doctor may refer you to a dietitian for help selecting foods that will help your child meet the energy requirements.

Apart from overall adequate caloric intake, you need to ensure your child is getting enough individual nutrients. Turn to Chapter 9 for more information on the nutritional deficiencies that can happen in people with Crohn's and colitis, and work with your doctor or dietitian to make sure your child is covered.

Some kids will have temporary lactose intolerance because of small intestinal inflammation from Crohn's. They may experience abdominal cramps, bloating, and diarrhea. Changing to soy-based products or adding Lactaid (to help with the digestion of lactose) may help in the short term until the Crohn's is better controlled.

Vaccinating your child

Vaccines, which protect against infectious diseases, are especially important for children with Crohn's and colitis. Infections can occur because kids are taking immunosuppressive drugs and, in turn, infections can cause disease flare. Children with Crohn's and colitis should receive their vaccines on the same schedule as other children *unless they're taking certain immunosuppressive medications.*

If your child is taking immunosuppressive medications (especially biologics such as anti-TNF therapy), she should not take live-virus vaccines. In order to understand why, a brief primer on vaccines may help: Vaccines consist either of live or killed microorganisms. When you get a vaccine, your immune system develops antibodies against those microorganisms, which protects you from the real thing. If your immune system is suppressed, however, it won't be able to mount the proper immune reaction to the live vaccine, and you could actually become infected by that live virus.

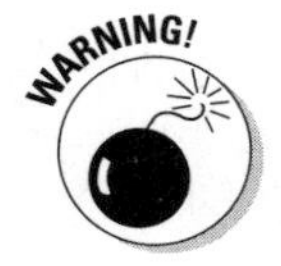

Here's a list of live-virus vaccines that your child needs to avoid when on immunosuppressive drugs:

- **Rotavirus:** Two or three doses of live rotavirus vaccine are given to children at 2, 4, and 6 months of age. This is not a common age for Crohn's and colitis, but if a mother is taking anti-TNF drugs during pregnancy, her baby should not get live vaccines during the first six months of life.

- **Measles, mumps, and rubella (MMR):** These vaccines are usually given at around 1 year of age, and again between ages 4 and 6.
- **Polio:** There are two types of polio vaccines: inactivated polio vaccine (which is the type commonly given in the United States) and live oral polio vaccine (given in many other countries). The live oral polio vaccine should be avoided if the child is taking immunosuppressive medications.
- **Influenza:** Children are given inactivated influenza vaccine (the flu shot) as early as 6 months of age. There is a live influenza vaccine known as FluMist in the United States, which is usually administered in children older than 2 years of age. Because it's a live vaccine, it should be avoided when a child is taking immunosuppressive drugs. Regular flu shots are safe to be given to kids taking immunosuppressive drugs, however.
- **Chicken pox (also known as varicella):** This vaccine is usually given around 12 to 15 months of age with a repeat dose around 4 to 6 years.

For more information on live vaccines that are often given to people traveling outside the United States, see Chapter 14.

People who are in close contact with someone whose immune system is suppressed can also pass on a disease to them after being vaccinated with a live virus vaccine. Therefore, always tell your doctor that your child is taking immunosuppressive medicines such as anti-TNF drugs before any vaccine is administered to your child or any other family members.

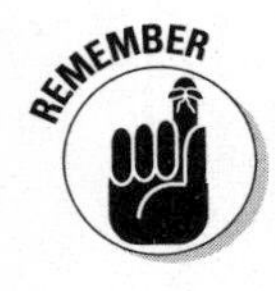

Children are considered immunosuppressed if they're taking drugs such as moderate- to high-dose steroids, azathioprine, 6-MP, methotrexate, and biologic therapy. Severe malnutrition that sometimes can happen with severe Crohn's and colitis is also considered a state of immunosuppression. Before vaccinating your child, talk to your child's doctor about any medications she's taking and whether the vaccination is safe.

Growing Up with Crohn's and Colitis

Living with Crohn's and colitis can be difficult for someone of any age, but unpredictable flares, chronic abdominal pain, diarrhea, and low energy may be especially rough on kids. Plus, kids may face problems because of malnutrition, slow growth, and delayed puberty. Most kids go through a period of adjustment when they get the diagnosis and may experience periods of anger and depression. As they grow up, they mature and can understand their disease better. At any stage, support from parents and siblings are critical and have long-lasting effects.

In this section, I walk you through the various stages of a child's life and offer tips on helping your child cope with Crohn's and colitis.

Preschool: C is for Crohn's and colitis

Not many kids get Crohn's and colitis in preschool, but some do. At this age, your child is being toilet trained and gaining independence and language skills. A chronic illness such as Crohn's or colitis can hinder a child's normal development. The active inflammation can affect his physical growth, and emotional and psychological stress can affect mental growth. Some kids start showing signs of regression and lose the skills they've already learned, such as toilet training.

At this age, kids may express their feelings of stress through behavior instead of words. They may relate their symptoms of Crohn's and colitis with other events and may feel as if it's their fault that they're sick. They may also think taking medications and going to the hospital are forms of punishment.

The more you and your family can comfort and reassure your child, the more you can prevent guilt, anxiety, and depression. You can greatly help your child by encouraging him to talk about his Crohn's and colitis and answering all his questions in simple language. Talking with the child's doctor and consulting with a mental-health professional can help kids and parents develop skills to adjust and cope with these illnesses when needed.

Surviving school

One of the main challenges for kids who have Crohn's or colitis is how to deal with their disease at school. The effects of the illness — and the side effects of the medications — can be considerable. Having frequent bowel movements and needing to go to the restroom urgently and with little warning may be particularly embarrassing. Having to miss school (and missing out on class time, not to mention sports and other social activities) can be frustrating. In this section, I offer important tips that kids and their parents can use to make dealing with Crohn's or colitis easier.

Informing the school about your child's illness

When your child is diagnosed with Crohn's or colitis, let your child's school know about the diagnosis as soon as possible. The school nurse can be your best ally in ensuring that other school staff understand the disease and the problems related to it. Your child's classmates and other teachers should be given at least a little information about the nature of the problem to minimize the feeling of isolation and the risk of teasing and bullying. A science or health project about Crohn's and colitis may be a way to involve classmates and school staff.

Every year, talk to your child's current teacher(s) about the illness. Important topics that you may want to discuss include the following:

- **Bathroom breaks:** Diarrhea and an urgent need to go to the restroom are inevitable for kids with Crohn's and colitis. Ask the teacher and staff members to allow your child to go to the restroom as frequently as needed to avoid any accidents. You may want to come up with a plan to allow your child to sit close to the door so she can leave without disturbing the rest of the class.
- **Missing school:** Crohn's and colitis can ebb and flow. Sometimes the disease may become active or your child may have to be admitted to the hospital for intravenous fluids and medications. Your child may not be able to attend school for an extended period of time. Make sure your child's teacher(s) know the reason for your child's absences. Talk with them about flexible homework arrangements.

  Encouraging classmates to stay in touch by phone or e-mail, or by sending cards, can help your child feel less isolated.
- **Field trips:** School field trips can be problematic for a kid with Crohn's or colitis, because of limited access to restroom facilities. You may want to ask to have your child excused from some of these activities, especially when his disease is active.
- **Taking medication:** Your child's school may have a policy about carrying and storing medications. Talk with the school staff or nurse about it.

  It may not be a bad idea to have the school nurse monitor your child when she takes her medications. This may be another way to ensure that she's really taking the medications when she's supposed to.
- **Physical education and sports:** During the period of active disease or flare, avoiding strenuous physical activities is important. Your child should be given permission to sit out of gym class and be able to miss athletic practices. Talk to his coaches and make sure they're aware of his illness.

Turning 18: Adulthood begins (at least in theory)

Kids are typically cared for by *pediatricians* (physicians trained to manage the particular medical issues of children). Pediatricians who have the expertise to care for kids with Crohn's and colitis are known as *pediatric gastroenterologists.* Because Crohn's and colitis are usually chronic and up to 25 percent of patients are diagnosed before the age of 18, *transitional care* — switching over to being cared for by a gastroenterologist who specializes in caring for adults — is an important consideration for adolescents and young adults.

The transition from adolescence to adulthood can be challenging. They're achieving more self-reliance and independence, and this time of growth and change causes frustration about the present and anxiety about the future — even in the healthiest kids. For kids with chronic illnesses such as Crohn's and colitis, the transition to adulthood is additionally stressful not only for them but also for their families and doctors.

Many obstacles can get in the way of this process of transition. A teenager may be reluctant to move to an adult healthcare system, which is totally new and unfamiliar. Parents may be reluctant to leave the pediatric caregivers with whom they've bonded. Parents may have been intimately involved with the care of their child and may feel ignored when adult healthcare providers involve them only with the permission of their son or daughter. Pediatric gastroenterologists may not feel comfortable letting a kid go to the adult healthcare system, and adult gastroenterologists may not be ready to take care of young adult patients.

The goal of a transition program is to maintain a continuity of care with little interruption and let kids acquire independent living skills. Here are some important tips to improve the transitional care of your teenager:

- **Let your kid start visiting his pediatric gastroenterologist without you.** He may be able to drive himself to his appointments, for example. Or, if he needs a ride, you can wait in the waiting room while he's seen by the doctor. This approach promotes independence and self-reliance, making the transition to an adult gastroenterologist easier.
- **Start an early search for an adult gastroenterologist who is knowledgeable about caring for young adults.** Your pediatric gastroenterologist should be able to refer you to colleagues she recommends and has worked with.
- **When you're ready to make the switch, make sure the adult gastroenterologist has copies of all medical records.** You may want to ask your pediatric gastroenterologist to write a letter summarizing your child's medical history.

Going off to college

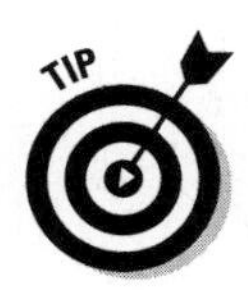

Parents can help a lot when it comes to grade school, middle school, and high school, but when you go off to college, you'll be managing your health problems on your own. Here are some tips for making the move to college when you have Crohn's or colitis:

- **If you'll be living in a dorm, explore the possibility of having a private room with your own restroom.** You'll always want to have a refrigerator in your room to keep your medications such as biologics. Most schools have no problem with students having mini fridges.
- **Look at the dining hall food menu, and make sure it has a menu that works for your Crohn's or colitis.** See what kinds of accommodations it's able to make for your condition.
- **Before you move to campus, explore the health-clinic services like labs, pharmacies, and physicians.**
- **Make sure your disease is under full control and that you have enough medication on hand.** You and your parents can talk to your school's health center before you arrive, to make sure you'll be able to refill your prescriptions without trouble.
- **Make sure your vaccinations are up to date.**
- **Get copies of your medical records from your doctor.** You'll need recent clinic notes, discharge summaries, operative reports, endoscopy reports, imaging results, pathology reports, and recent lab work. You can keep a copy for your personal record and give another copy to your school health center.
- **Identify a local gastroenterologist near campus, and schedule an appointment before classes start (or as close to the start of the semester as possible).**
- **Talk with your gastroenterologist from home about how you can remain in contact with him if the need arises.**

Chapter 16

Having Sex and Getting Pregnant with Crohn's and Colitis

In This Chapter

- Considering how sex and fertility are affected by your disease
- Looking at pregnancy if you have Crohn's or colitis

Crohn's and colitis can affect your sex life in a variety of ways. Whether you want to get pregnant or not, your disease may leave you feeling anything but sexy. If you're trying to prevent pregnancy, you need to know which birth control options are safe if you have Crohn's or colitis. In addition, your menstrual cycle and fertility can be affected by the disease. Finally, if you want to get pregnant, you need to know how your Crohn's or colitis may affect your pregnancy — and vice versa — as well as what to expect after you give birth. In this chapter, I walk you through all these issues.

Think of this chapter as a jumping-off point for conversations with your doctor about sex and pregnancy. Many people are embarrassed to bring up these issues when they're sitting on an exam table in a flimsy paper "gown," but trust me: Your doctor has heard it all before. Sex and pregnancy are important parts of many people's lives, and you don't want to be in the dark about them just because you're embarrassed. Talk openly and honestly with your doctor about your questions and concerns. You — and your doctor — will be glad you did.

Sex and Fertility

When you have Crohn's or colitis, sex can be . . . well, worrisome. You may be unhappy with the toll the disease has taken on your body, and the only way you want to get between the sheets with your partner is if you're covered head to toe. Even if you don't have any problem with body image, you may experience pain during intercourse. Maybe you're not sure how your disease will affect your ability to get pregnant — or, on the flip side, the last thing you want right now is a baby, and you want to know how you can safely prevent pregnancy when you have Crohn's or colitis. This section covers all these concerns.

Sexual activity

Your disease may have wreaked havoc with your body — or your self-image. When your disease is active, you may feel tired, and the last thing on your mind is sex. Fatigue can also set in if you develop anemia (because of bleeding, because of a nutritional deficiency, or because of low testosterone levels). Having to get up to go to the bathroom frequently or fear of incontinence may add to your stress.

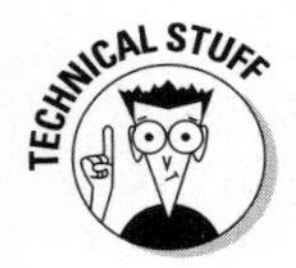

Testosterone is a sex hormone made from cholesterol. Active disease may lead to lower levels of cholesterol, which causes the body to become low on testosterone. Talk with your doctor about having your testosterone levels tested. You may be able to get a testosterone patch to help improve your sex drive.

Other problems you may face during sex include the following:

- Abdominal pain
- Pain in the *perineal area* (the area between the vagina and rectum in women or between the penis and rectum in men)
- Rectal pain
- Feeling like you have to have a bowel movement
- Embarrassment caused by having a stoma
- Passing gas or stool

Some women with Crohn's disease involving the rectum develop *recto-vaginal fistulas,* which are abnormal tracts between the rectum and vagina that allow stool to travel into the vagina, where it doesn't belong. This condition causes pain during sexual intercourse.

Be sure to talk to your doctor if sex is painful for you — it may be a sign that your disease is getting worse.

If you're having *any* sexual issues — not just pain — talk to your doctor. He may be able to make some changes in your treatment plan to help you feel better and help with your sex life. For example, steroids, which are often used during disease flares, may cause weight gain, acne, and mood swings (none of which do much to improve your sex life). But you and your doctor may be able to work together to keep your disease in steroid-free remission, and that can prevent or solve many of these problems.

Thong underwear and bikinis can cause irritation and pain in the anal area, especially if you have a fissure or fistula. You don't have to stick to granny panties — there are plenty of alternatives to thongs that won't leave you feeling like you were born in the horse-and-buggy days.

If you have an ostomy bag and it causes you embarrassment during intimacy, you may find wearing crotchless underwear or teddies with snap crotches useful.

Men with Crohn's or colitis may be concerned more about issues related to performance. Here's the good news: If you have Crohn's or colitis, you aren't at any greater risk for erectile dysfunction than any other guy. The only clinical scenario in which you can have some problem is after pouch surgery (for colitis), when some men have erectile dysfunction or suffer from retrograde ejaculation.

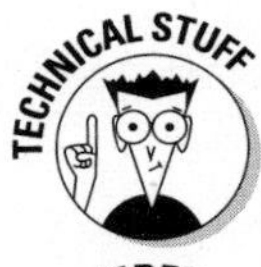

Retrograde ejaculation is commonly known as "dry orgasm." Basically, when you ejaculate, the semen goes into your bladder (with your urine) instead of coming out through the urethra. You still experience orgasm, but you may not ejaculate. This obviously causes problems with fertility, but it may not be a problem for you if fertility isn't a concern.

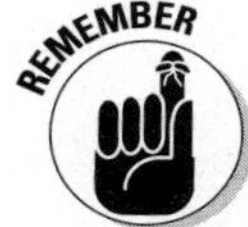

Undiagnosed or untreated depression is what leads to most of the erectile problems in men with Crohn's or colitis — not the disease itself.

A small European study showed that Viagra may help with Crohn's disease. Talk to your doctor to see if this drug is right for you.

Contraception

Whether you want a baby or not someday, contraception is critical when you have Crohn's or colitis. If you *do* want to get pregnant, you want to make sure you wait to conceive until your disease is in remission. And if you *don't* want to get pregnant, well, then you know why contraception matters.

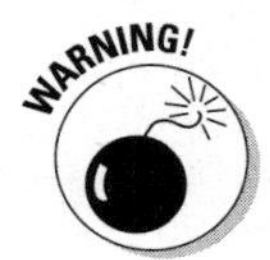

Don't get pregnant if any of the following apply:

- You have active disease.
- You're taking drugs that are associated with birth defects.
- Surgery is being planned.

Birth control pills are absorbed in the small intestine. Inflammation of the small intestine or ileostomies may interfere with the absorption of birth control pills, making them ineffective. Be sure to discuss these issues with your doctor and your partner.

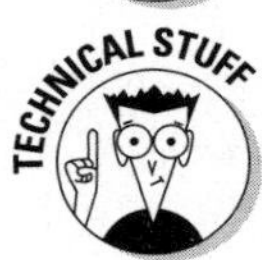

Certain drugs can also interact with birth control pills and decrease their efficiency. However, none of the medications (including antibiotics) commonly used in Crohn's and colitis have been associated with this interaction.

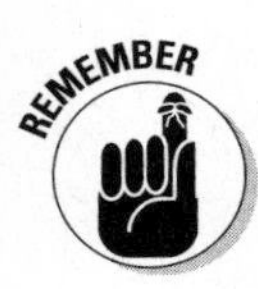

Although generally an effective form of birth control, oral contraceptives sometimes fail. So, if you want to prevent pregnancy, you should use more than one form of birth control, especially during a flare or after a recent surgery. If you're on certain medications, such as methotrexate (luckily not frequently used), your doctor will direct you to be on at least two forms of birth control because of a high risk of birth defects associated with those medications.

You may have heard that birth control pills may be risky for women who have Crohn's or colitis. Unfortunately, few studies have looked into the link between birth control pills and an increased risk of flares. Some studies have found an increase risk of disease flare, especially in Crohn's disease, but others have not shown any increased risk. Your best bet is to talk with your doctor before choosing an oral contraceptive.

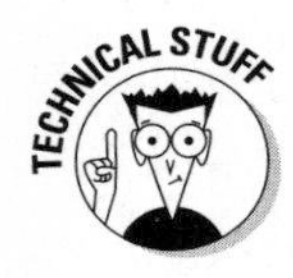

You may have heard that birth control pills *cause* Crohn's or colitis. Some studies have shown an association between contraceptives and the risk of developing Crohn's or colitis. A few studies from Europe showed that high-estrogen birth control pills were associated with increased risk of Crohn's disease. However, many larger studies have failed to show this association. The majority of the studies from the United States have failed to show any increased risk with birth control pills.

There is increased risk of blood clot formation, stroke, and heart disease with the use of birth control pills. The risk increases even more if you smoke and are over the age of 35.

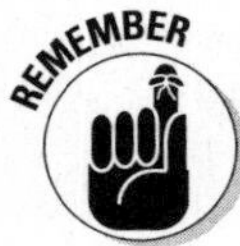

Birth control pills aren't the only option. If you can't or don't want to use oral contraceptives or if you're advised to use two forms of contraception, look into the following commonly used methods of birth control:

- **Condoms:** Both male and female condoms are effective methods of birth control. However, they're associated with failure risks because of condom breakage and slipping, or simply because people forget to use them.
- **Intrauterine devices (IUDs):** IUDs, which are implanted in a woman's uterus, are highly effective methods of birth control. Keep in mind, though, that IUDs can cause irritation or infection (in any woman, not just those with Crohn's or colitis). If you have an IUD, these issues can be mistaken for active Crohn's or colitis, so be sure to inform your doctor that you have an IUD, especially during a flare.
- **Contraception patch and birth control shots:** The advantage of these forms of birth control is that they don't have the issues with absorption during inflammation that oral contraceptives have.

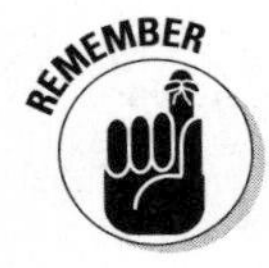

You want to make sure that your choice of birth control method not only works for you and your partner, but also is as effective as possible.

Your menstrual cycle

Chronic inflammation and poor nutrition can affect your ability to produce sex hormones, and if you don't have enough sex hormones, that can affect your menstrual cycle. Many girls diagnosed with Crohn's or colitis before or during puberty have a delay in getting their first period. And many women with active disease can have irregular periods. The good news (or bad news, depending on your perspective): When the disease goes into remission, regular periods usually return.

Just before and during your periods, you may feel worse. Your diarrhea, abdominal pain, or other symptoms may become severe. Some women call these "mini-flares."

Keep track of any monthly changes in symptoms. A record of what you're going through every month will prevent your doctor from overtreating the disease.

During your period, taking over-the-counter pain medications — for cramps or other period symptoms — can worsen your Crohn's or colitis symptoms. These medications may contain non-steroidal anti-inflammatory drugs (NSAIDs), such as ibuprofen or aspirin, which can cause more inflammation in your intestines. Before taking anything to relieve period-related symptoms, talk with your doctor. Small doses of NSAIDs are usually okay, especially when your disease is under control.

Some women may experience extreme worsening of their Crohn's or colitis during their periods — so much so that symptoms become debilitating. Stopping menstruation with medications, such as injectable contraceptives or hormones, is usually helpful in these situations.

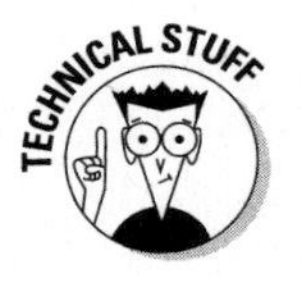

Some studies show that women with Crohn's disease may enter menopause early, but scientists aren't sure why this may happen. One study showed that post-menopausal women with Crohn's and colitis are just as likely to have a flare as women who are premenopausal. Scientists have found that hormone replacement therapy (HRT) has a protective effect on disease activity. However, doctors are still waiting for more research in this area before HRT can be recommended to all menopausal women with Crohn's and colitis.

Fertility

If you and your partner are having trouble conceiving, don't rush to blame your disease — in the United States, 7 percent of couples are infertile. Most studies have shown that Crohn's and colitis themselves don't decrease the fertility rate as compared to the general population.

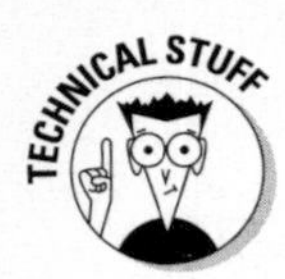

The cause of low birth rates among Crohn's and colitis patients is attributed to people choosing not to get pregnant.

When it comes to getting pregnant, the most important factor is your disease activity state. If you have actively flaring Crohn's or colitis, you may have a decreased chance of getting pregnant. Think of this as Mother Nature protecting you and your future baby from complications. Active disease at the time of conception is associated with a poor outcome. If your disease is in remission, not only do you have a better chance of getting pregnant, but you'll also be more likely to have a healthy pregnancy.

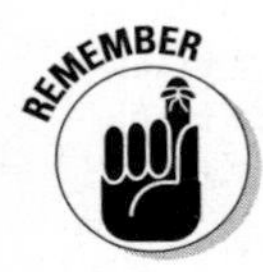

There is generally a rule of three for female patients with active Crohn's and colitis when they get pregnant: One-third get worse, one-third remain the same, and one-third actually get better when they get pregnant.

Sulfasalazine, which is sometimes used to treat colitis, may cause temporary infertility in about half of the men taking it. Your doctor may advise you to stop taking the drug or switch to another drug for at least six weeks before trying to conceive.

Nearly half of women who undergo surgery for their colitis and get a J-pouch may experience problems getting pregnant. We still don't know the exact reason for this infertility. Scientists believe that it may be related to scarring in the female reproductive system after the surgery. If you're hoping to get pregnant in the future, be sure to discuss this with your doctor and your surgeon before undergoing a J-pouch procedure. You may be able to opt for an alternative, like having a temporary ileostomy and waiting until you're done having babies before you get a J-pouch.

Pregnancy

Pregnancy is life changing for everyone involved, regardless of whether the mother has Crohn's or colitis. But if you do have one of these diseases, you need to put a little extra care into planning and thinking about getting pregnant. As I mention earlier in this chapter, except in the case of women who've had J-pouch surgeries, there isn't any increase in the incidence of infertility among Crohn's and colitis patients. That's great news! But it doesn't mean you can run out and get pregnant next time you and your partner are feeling frisky. Pregnancy can affect your Crohn's and colitis, and vice versa, and it's important to know how so that you can time your pregnancy to give you and your baby the best possible outcome.

Pregnancy planning

Planning before you get pregnant is very important. Simply put, the healthier you are as you're trying to get pregnant, the more likely you are to have a healthy baby. Planning your pregnancy may help you to conceive more easily, have a healthier pregnancy, give birth to a healthier baby, and have a more pleasant postpartum experience. It will also help minimize your child's risk of health problems in adulthood.

You may be emotionally prepared to have a baby, but is your body ready for the task ahead? You need to make sure your disease is under control and in complete remission before getting pregnant. Also, you need to discuss the effects of your current medications on an upcoming pregnancy *before* conceiving.

You also want to get screened for other infections, such as hepatitis B, and get vaccinated as indicated. Hepatitis B can be given even if you become pregnant. Certain vaccines such as live influenza, varicella, and measles vaccines cannot be given during pregnancy. If you have received these live vaccines, you need to wait about four weeks before getting pregnant. Discuss vaccination issues with your doctor before becoming pregnant.

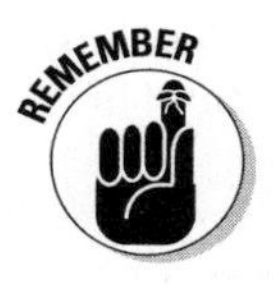

If you've been on birth control pills, ovulation is possible as soon as two weeks after stopping the medications; in some cases, it may take longer.

How Crohn's or colitis may affect your pregnancy

Pregnancy isn't a cakewalk even if you *don't* have Crohn's or colitis. Many women experience nausea, vomiting, and other not-so-fun symptoms. But if you have active Crohn's or colitis while you're pregnant, you're adding on top of that frequent trips to the bathroom, abdominal pain, and even more nausea and vomiting.

Not only does active disease make pregnancy more stressful, but it can also hurt the baby. Medical research has shown that patients with active disease have a 35 percent greater chance of miscarriage than those who are in remission. Studies have shown that active disease in pregnancy can also lead to low birth weight, premature birth, and even loss of the baby.

How your pregnancy may affect your Crohn's and colitis

The good news is that pregnancy itself doesn't cause flares of Crohn's or colitis.

Will I pass my Crohn's and colitis on to my kids?

The fear of passing this illness on to your kids can be very disturbing. But keep in mind that there are many causes of Crohn's and colitis (see Chapter 4). Genetic mutations have been shown to be involved in these diseases, so it isn't unusual to see more than one family member affected with Crohn's or colitis.

If one parent has the disease, the risk of a child getting Crohn's or colitis is about 2 percent to 5 percent. This risk increases to 33 percent to 52 percent if both parents have the disease. As compared to other genetic disorders, this risk is still very small.

Some earlier studies showed that disease activity increases during the first trimester, but subsequent larger studies failed to show this phenomenon. Increased chances of flare seen in earlier studies were more likely because of discontinuation of the Crohn's or colitis medication, which was a common practice in the past.

Disease flares during pregnancy are dictated by whether you have active or inactive disease at the time of conception. If your disease is in remission when you conceive, there is a 70 percent to 80 percent chance that you'll remain in remission throughout your pregnancy.

Colitis patients who have J-pouches may have problems during pregnancy. The uterus can put pressure on the J-pouch, which may not be able to hold the waste matter properly, and you may have more frequent bowel movements.

While you're pregnant

While you're pregnant, you can continue to take many medications used to treat Crohn's or colitis — but some are off-limits. Paying attention to what you eat when you have Crohn's or colitis is always important, but it's especially so during pregnancy. Finally, if you're pregnant and surgery becomes a necessity, it helps to know what to expect. I cover all these topics in this section.

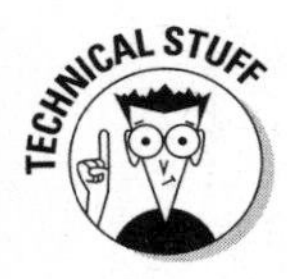

A recent European study of women with Crohn's and colitis found that the rate of future flares decreases in the years following pregnancy. This suggests that pregnancy may sometimes have a positive effect on the disease process. In addition, if Crohn's or colitis becomes active during pregnancy, there is no evidence to suggest that it will do so again in future pregnancies; similarly, if a pregnancy occurs without an episode of flare, there is no assurance that the disease will remain inactive in subsequent pregnancies.

Medications: What you can take and what you can't

Some medications are safe to take during pregnancy. Others aren't, or their effects on your baby may not be known. Luckily, most of the medications taken for Crohn's and colitis are safe during pregnancy.

Let's start with the good news. The following medications are generally okay to take during pregnancy:

- **Sulfasalazine (Azulfidine):** This medication is generally considered safe during pregnancy. ***Note:*** If you take sulfasalazine you also need to take a high-dose folic acid supplement (2 mg daily). Sulfasalazine blocks absorption of folic acid, which is very important for the growth of the baby's brain and spinal cord.
- **Metronidazole (Flagyl):** Metronidazole is an antibiotic used to treat Crohn's and colitis. It appears to be low risk and can be used during pregnancy.
- **Mesalamine (Apriso, Asacol, Lialda, Pentasa):** Mesalamine is safe during pregnancy.
- **Steroids:** Steroids are considered low risk during pregnancy if you need them to control active disease. However, there is an increased risk of gestational diabetes and large-birth-weight babies with steroid use. In addition, cleft palate has been associated with steroid use during pregnancy, but it usually happens in asthmatic mothers, not in those with Crohn's and colitis.
- **Azathioprine (Azasan, Imuran) and 6-MP (Purinethol):** The use of azathioprine and 6-MP has been a bit controversial. Most of the recent data show that these drugs are safe during pregnancy. The majority of doctors recommend continuing this drug during pregnancy because the risk of stopping the medications and having flares is greater than the risk of the drug itself. If you still want to stop these drugs while pregnant, talk with you doctor well before trying to conceive. These drugs stay in your system for several weeks.
- **Biologics:** All three biologics — infliximab (Remicade), adalimumab (Humira), and certolizumab (Cimzia) — appear safe during pregnancy. Recent studies of hundreds of babies born to mothers taking biologics have not shown any increased risk of birth defects.

  Your newborn baby should not receive any live vaccines such as rotavirus during the first six months if you were on biologics while pregnant.
- **Cyclosporine (Gengraf, Neoral, Sandimmune, Sangcya):** This drug is sometimes used in severe ulcerative colitis patients and has been shown to be an effective medication in controlling symptoms and preventing surgery. With the development of biologics that have somewhat similar efficacy, this drug is not commonly used. There are many side effects associated with this drug, such as increase in blood pressure and kidney

toxicity. This drug has been used by some experts in pregnant patients with severe colitis when other medications have failed and surgery had to be avoided. No serious harm to mother and baby has been reported with its use.

The following medications should be avoided:

- **Ciprofloxacin (Cipro, Proquin):** Ciprofloxacin is a commonly used antibiotic in Crohn's and colitis. Doctors usually avoid ciprofloxacin during pregnancy because of some risks to the baby's bones and cartilage.
- **Thalidomide (Thalomid):** Never take thalidomide during pregnancy. It can cause serious birth defects. Doctors usually recommend stopping this medication at least three to six months before trying to get pregnant. If you're taking this medication, you should use at least two different methods of contraception to prevent pregnancy.
- **Methotrexate (Rheumatrex, Trexall):** Never take methotrexate during pregnancy. It can cause serious birth defects. Doctors usually recommend stopping this medication at least three to six months before trying to get pregnant. If you're taking this medication, you should use at least two different methods of contraception to prevent pregnancy.
- **Diphenoxylate (Lomotil):** This antidiarrheal medication should be avoided during pregnancy.
- **Some supplements:** You may be using alternative therapies such as herbal products to treat your Crohn's and colitis. If so, you should avoid the following supplements while pregnant:
    - Black cohosh
    - Cascara
    - Chaste tress berry
    - Ginseng
    - Juniper
    - Kava kava
    - Meadow saffron
    - Senna
    - Wormwood
    - High doses of vitamin A

Talk to your doctor about all supplements you take. Just because something is "natural," doesn't mean it's healthy to you or your unborn baby.

Nutritional considerations

For any pregnant woman, a balanced diet with enough calories, vitamins, and minerals is very important for the growth of the baby. If you have Crohn's or colitis, though, your nutritional demands will increase, particularly if you have active disease or are underweight.

Seek the advice of a dietitian to help you map out a well-balanced dietary plan. Your doctor should be able to recommend someone.

Getting enough fruits, vegetables, fortified cereals, meat, and dairy may be easier said than done. Morning sickness alone could make you swear off many of these foods. For many women with Crohn's or colitis, some of the healthiest foods also may be symptom triggers. Adjust your diet according to how you feel, but be careful not to avoid nutritious foods you really need.

You may have to get creative to make sure you're getting the nutrients you need. For example:

- If fruits and vegetables bother you, try drinking fruit or vegetable juice instead. Just make sure its 100 percent juice with no sugar added. (Sugars may cause a flare.)
- Fish, which contains omega-3 fatty acids, is good for healing inflammation, but especially when you're pregnant, you want to make sure you consume low-mercury fish such as salmon, pollock, catfish, and shrimp.
- Taking a daily prenatal multivitamin helps replenish vitamins and minerals that you may lose through diarrhea. Plus, prenatal vitamins are recommended for pregnant women in general — not just those with Crohn's or colitis.

Here are some special nutrients you need to pay particular attention to when you're pregnant:

- **Calcium and vitamin D:** Calcium and vitamin D are important to build your baby's bones and teeth. Vitamin D deficiency also puts you at risk for certain pregnancy-related complications such as gestational diabetes and *pre-eclampsia* (a potentially dangerous condition in which your blood pressure goes up). You're at a higher risk for calcium and vitamin D deficiency if you're taking steroids. Getting enough calcium and vitamin D will help prevent these complications.

  Newer studies have found that taking higher doses of vitamin D (for example, 4,000 IU per day) is really helpful in preventing complications during pregnancy. Talk to your doctor about the dosage that's right for you.

- **Vitamin B12:** If you have Crohn's disease and part of your small intestine is removed (especially the terminal ileum), you may need regular injections of vitamin B12 to prevent anemia during pregnancy.
- **Iron:** Iron deficiency is quite common is Crohn's and colitis. This becomes even more important during pregnancy, because pregnancy increases your body's iron demands. Iron supplements are often required to meet the increased demands.
- **Folic acid:** Take a folic acid supplement before conception and for the first 12 weeks of your pregnancy to reduce the risk of your baby having neurologic problems. The usual recommendation is 400 mcg per day. This applies to all women, not just those with Crohn's or colitis, but it's particularly important in patients with Crohn's disease of the small intestine because absorbing folic acid may be more difficult. If you take sulfasalazine (Azulfidine) or have had surgery to remove part of the small intestine, the recommendation is usually to increase your folic acid to 2 mg (2,000 mcg) per day. Again, talk with your doctor about what's right for you.

If you need surgery

Sometimes surgery is required in people with Crohn's or colitis — for example, if you have an obstruction, perforation, abscess, or bleeding. Obviously, surgery during pregnancy is always high risk, so your doctors will do everything they can to manage your disease nonsurgically and defer any surgical procedure until late in pregnancy or after you give birth.

Endoscopy procedures are usually avoided during pregnancy. If it's absolutely necessary (such as to rule out infection or to assess the disease severity), flexible sigmoidoscopy can be safely performed with minimal sedation. Studies have also shown that colonoscopy can be safely performed during pregnancy. Discuss the risks and benefits of the procedure with your doctor. Sometimes, performing endoscopy and finding that disease is mild or inactive and symptoms are more likely secondary to pregnancy may save you and your baby from unnecessary drugs.

The big day and beyond

Being sick is bad; being sick with a baby is worse. So, just as planning for pregnancy is important, planning your childbirth and life after you give birth are important.

Childbirth options

When your pregnancy has come to term, your next fear may be about how the baby will come out. Choosing a childbirth option — vaginal or cesarean section — can be overwhelming. In most cases, you can have a vaginal delivery without any problem unless there are some other obstetric or personal reasons for going with a C-section.

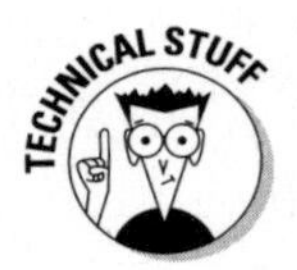

The indications for caesarean section mostly do not differ in women with Crohn's and colitis, but studies have shown that they do undergo elective caesarean sections more frequently than women who don't have Crohn's or colitis, probably because of fear and lack of education.

Your doctor will suggest a C-section if you have

- **Perianal disease at the time of delivery:** The trauma of the birthing process may worsen perianal disease.
- **A J-pouch:** The anal sphincter may be damaged during vaginal delivery and can compromise a J-pouch's functioning.

Breastfeeding

No one can argue the benefits of breastfeeding. It's natural and safer, not to mention cheaper! Breastfeeding protects mothers from breast cancer and improves babies' immune health. There are even some studies showing that breastfed children have a lower chance of getting Crohn's or colitis.

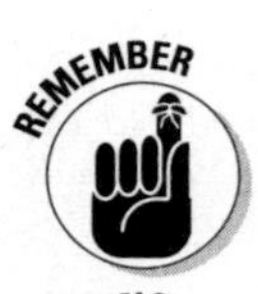

Despite all these benefits, whether to breastfeed is still your personal decision and no one can make the decision for you.

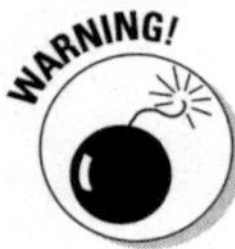

Many drugs that you take for your disease may actually be secreted in the breast milk. These drugs may not be safe for your baby. Following is information on common drugs and whether they're safe while you're breastfeeding:

- **Mesalamine (Apriso, Asacol, Lialda, Pentasa):** Very low levels of mesalamine are secreted in breast milk, and most studies consider it to be a safe drug.
- **Azathioprine (Azasan, Imuran) and 6-MP (Purinethol):** Very low levels are secreted in breast milk. Newer studies consider it be a safe drug during breastfeeding. Some physicians may still suggest taking your pills at night and dumping the first milk of the morning.
- **Biologics:** All three biologics — infliximab (Remicade), adalimumab (Humira), and certolizumab (Cimzia) — are secreted in small amounts in breast milk, but they usually aren't absorbed by the baby's gut. Most experts generally consider them to be safe while breastfeeding.
- **Steroids:** Most experts allow steroids during breastfeeding.
- **Methotrexate (Rheumatrex, Trexall):** Do not take while breastfeeding.
- **Thalidomide (Thalomid):** Do not take while breastfeeding.
- **Cyclosporine (Gengraf, Neoral, Sandimmune, Sangcya):** Do not take while breastfeeding.

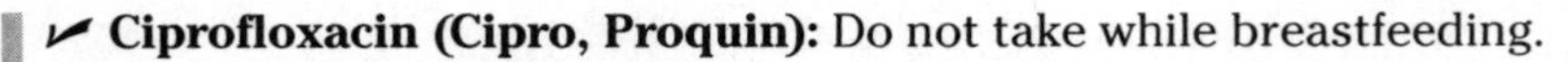

- **Ciprofloxacin (Cipro, Proquin):** Do not take while breastfeeding.
- **Metronidazole (Flagyl):** Do not take while breastfeeding.

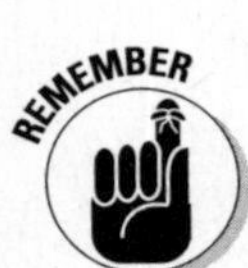

Be sure to talk with your doctor about what's safe for you to take while breastfeeding.

Some lactation experts recommend an herbal supplement called fenugreek to enhance milk production. However, this supplement causes rectal bleeding and can worsen colitis.

Life after pregnancy

The most important thing you can do for yourself after you come home from the hospital with your little bundle of joy is to make sure you get enough rest. A rested body can withstand the stress of Crohn's or colitis — and especially new parenthood — better than an exhausted one.

Get help from friends and family members so that it isn't all on you. Don't try to be a hero.

Part VI

The Part of Tens

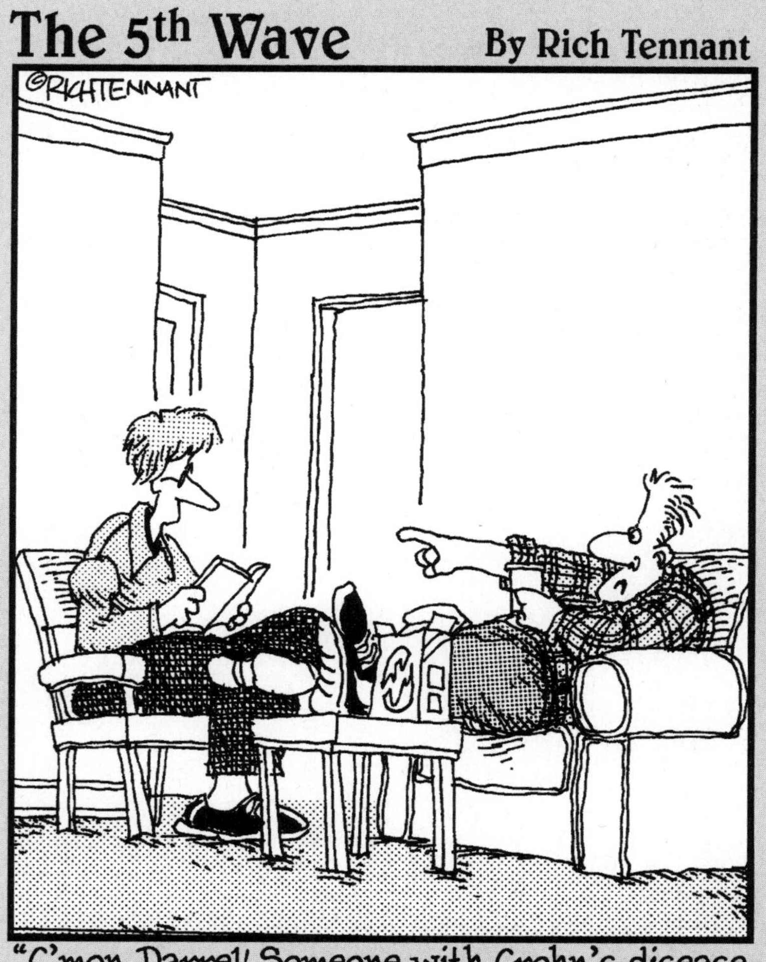

"C'mon, Darrel! Someone with Crohn's disease shouldn't be lying around all day. Whereas someone with no life, like myself, has a very good reason."

In this part . . .

This part gives you loads of valuable information in a small amount of space. Here, I debunk ten myths about Crohn's and colitis and provide ten great resources for more information on these diseases.

Chapter 17

Ten Myths about Inflammatory Bowel Disease

In This Chapter

- Getting clear on the facts
- Setting aside the myths

Today, endless information is as close as your computer. You can Google your symptoms and practically self-diagnose your disease. Although there's no lack of information online, not all the information you find is accurate. Blogs and message boards are loaded with people's personal anecdotes, but what applies to one person doesn't necessarily apply to you. News headlines about drugs or treatments may create more confusion than clarity, because the stories don't always put the information in the proper context.

People are gradually replacing the folklore, old wives' tales, and rumors about the causes and treatment of Crohn's and colitis with accurate and up-to-date information. But misunderstandings still exist among patients and their family members. Some of these myths are harmless; others can be dangerous. Knowledge about the disease is important, but inaccurate information can lead to mismanagement of the disease. In this chapter, I debunk ten common myths about inflammatory bowel disease (IBD).

Diet Is the Cure

Diet plays an important role in the management of Crohn's and colitis. The wrong diet, especially during active disease, will produce symptoms. When you have Crohn's or colitis, you're also at risk for nutritional deficiencies because active inflammation prevents absorption of important nutrients such as vitamins and minerals. Eating right and making sure you're getting enough of these nutrients will help you feel healthier and more energetic (see Chapter 9 for more on diet).

Although diet can certainly help improve your symptoms, it isn't a cure for the disease. We still don't know exactly how much of each nutrient is needed to provide complete remission and suppress inflammation. The drugs used to treat Crohn's and colitis, on the other hand, have been carefully studied in clinical trials, and their correct and safe doses are identified before they're approved for use in humans.

Until large and well-designed clinical trials are performed, I don't recommend using diet as the main therapy for Crohn's and colitis. Diet's role as curative therapy is far from reality. Until we prove its effectiveness, diet should be thought of as a supplement to regular drug therapy.

Sometimes, dietary components can have unknown side effects or even drug interactions that may be harmful to you, so be sure to discuss your diet and any supplements you take with your doctor.

Kids Get It from Their Parents

If one of your family members (particularly a first-degree relative, such as a sibling or parent) has Crohn's or colitis, you may be at risk for developing the illness yourself. If you have Crohn's disease, there is a 5 percent chance that one of your kids will have the disease; if you have colitis, there is a 2 percent chance that one of your kids will have the disease. The risk of your child developing Crohn's or colitis increases to 45 percent if both parents have the disease.

Although there is some genetic connection with Crohn's and colitis, unlike some other hereditary diseases, Crohn's and colitis are not transmitted to kids from their parents. Scientists are still learning about the causes of these illnesses. They believe that it's usually a *combination* of the different environmental, immune, and genetic factors that bring about this illness in someone.

You may have inherited some mutated genes from your parents but still not get Crohn's or colitis. In order to develop the disease, you also need some sort of other trigger, such as change in diet or exposure to certain chemicals or drugs that cause damage to the inner layer of the intestines. In many people, this trigger may never occur. So, despite having mutated genes, they may not develop Crohn's or colitis.

It's Caused by Stress

Stress reduces the ability of the immune system to fight infections and other invaders. Studies have shown that stress may play a role in Crohn's and colitis flares. However, stress has not been confirmed as the *cause* of Crohn's or colitis. Some older studies showed that stress could play a role in the development of Crohn's and colitis, but the medical community in general believes that stress does *not* cause these illnesses.

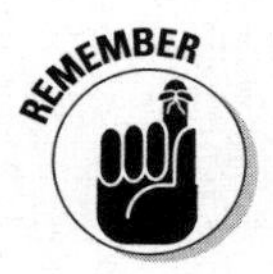

Even though stress isn't the cause of Crohn's and colitis, it does play an important role. Having a lifelong disease is no fun, and knowing that your symptoms are going to wax and wane for the rest of your life can create stress, which can manifest itself as irritability, depression, or even panic attacks. This, in turn, can cause worsening of symptoms and more stress, perpetuating a vicious cycle.

You Can't Get Pregnant if You Have It

Most studies have shown that Crohn's and colitis don't decrease the fertility rate as compared to the general population (about 7 percent of couples experience infertility). So, generally speaking, you can get pregnant and have healthy babies even if you have Crohn's or colitis. (I say "generally speaking" because each person is different, and you may have fertility issues that have nothing to do with your disease.)

When it comes to getting pregnant, the key is your disease activity state. Active disease may lower your chances of getting pregnant, and if you do get pregnant during active disease, it can put you and your baby at risk. If your disease is in remission, you have a better chance of getting pregnant and carrying a healthy baby to term.

Some Crohn's and colitis medications — such as methotrexate or thalidomide — are associated with birth defects. You should not become pregnant while taking these medications. If you're considering getting pregnant, be sure to talk with your doctor about your medications beforehand.

Women who've undergone surgery for colitis and gotten a J-pouch may experience problems getting pregnant. This difficulty may be related to scarring in the female reproductive system after surgery. If you're considering having J-pouch surgery and you think you may want to get pregnant down the road, you may want to consider alternatives, such as having a temporary ileostomy and waiting until you no longer want to get pregnant to have J-pouch surgery.

Surgery Is Required

Most Crohn's patients will ultimately have surgery, but surgery isn't right for everyone. Some people have a very mild form of Crohn's disease that never progresses to surgery; others have a very aggressive form that may require surgery at the time of diagnosis or multiple surgeries over their lives.

When it comes to Crohn's disease, surgery may be required because medical therapy has failed or because the patient has developed complications such as an abscess, fistula, or cancer. The thing is, we don't know which patients will develop complications. You and your doctor should work together to prevent complications that may lead to surgery. You can do that by suppressing inflammation with medication — and being sure to take your prescribed medications even when you're feeling better.

For people with colitis, surgery is a cure — you don't have to have repeated surgeries the way people with Crohn's might. Common reasons for surgery include failure of medical therapy, severe bleeding, colon perforation, or development of precancerous or cancerous lesions in the colon. Your chances of needing surgery may increase with time, but taking medications regularly and suppressing inflammation will decrease your chance of having surgery in the near future.

Crohn's and colitis are very personal diseases. Your disease hasn't read the textbooks or research papers. It'll behave differently from Crohn's and colitis in other people (because *you're* different from other people).

If You Have It, You're Guaranteed to Get Cancer

The risk of small bowel cancer is very low in Crohn's disease — in fact, small bowel cancer is downright rare.

The risk of colon cancer in Crohn's and colitis depends on how long you've had the disease and how much of your colon is affected by inflammation. The risk doesn't start to increase until you've had Crohn's or colitis for eight to ten years. If your disease affects the entire colon, you have a greater risk of getting colon cancer than if you have inflammation only in the rectum (where the risk is lowest).

Other risk factors include the following:

- **Family history:** If you have a family member with colon cancer, you're at greater risk of developing colon cancer yourself.
- **Diet:** A diet high in red meat, refined foods, and unhealthy fats has been linked to an increased risk of colon cancer. The good news is that diets high in fruits and vegetables have been linked to a decreased risk of colon cancer.
- **Exercise:** Studies have shown that people who engage in regular, moderate exercise (such as brisk walking) have a lower risk of developing colon cancer.

Getting regular colonoscopies is the best way to prevent colon cancer. Talk to your doctor about whether a colonoscopy is a good idea for you and, if so, how often you should have one. (Chapter 6 provides more information on colonoscopies.)

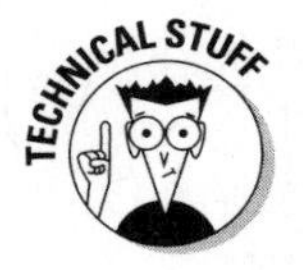

Newer studies are showing even lower risk of colon cancer after eight to ten years of colitis than previously thought. This may be because of better control of inflammation with medications. Persistent inflammation is one of the important risk factors of developing cancer, and taking effective medications can reduce this risk. Scientists believe that previously quoted 18 percent risk of colon cancer after 30 years of colitis is actually now 7 percent.

You're Responsible for Your Flares

There are many reasons people with Crohn's and colitis get flares (see Chapter 13). You can control some triggers, such as certain drugs and foods. Good sleep and avoiding stress are also important in keeping flares at a bay. Sometimes, however, unavoidable circumstances may lead to a flare. For example, sleep disturbances, unanticipated travel, and seasonal changes (including allergies) all can cause flares — and you can't control these things. If you're on immunosuppressive drugs, you can try your best to avoid infections, but you may get an infection anyway, and certain infections, such as viral infections, can trigger inflammation.

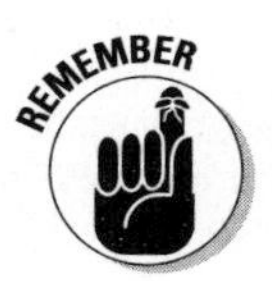

It's important to know the triggers that can lead to flares and do your best to avoid them, but if you experience a flare, don't beat yourself up about it. That'll only add to your stress and anxiety, which won't help you heal or feel better.

Surgery Cures It

If you have colitis, when you get to the point where you need surgery, your entire large intestine (colon and rectum) is removed. Because colitis only involves the colon, the disease doesn't recur after the surgery. So, surgery does cure the disease.

Crohn's disease is different: It's lifelong, and it has no cure. You may end up needing surgery when medical therapy fails, but that's not the end of the story. Crohn's disease will come back. It can come back as early as a few months after surgery, or it may take several years to recur.

Medical research has shown that Crohn's disease can recur after the surgery earlier than previously thought. Putting patients on medical therapy right after the surgery to prevent it from coming back or progressing more can be a useful strategy. Most Crohn's patients get started on medical therapy if they undergo surgery at a very early age or earlier in their disease course. They also get put on the medical therapy if their disease is complicated and involves a larger portion of the small and large intestines or if this is their second or third surgery.

You Can Stop Taking Your Medications if You Feel Better

The current goals of drug therapy are to keep you in remission without the use of steroids, to prevent hospitalization, and to delay or prevent surgery. These goals can only be met if you take your medications regularly.

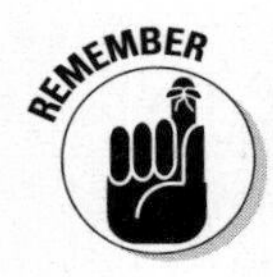

There are two stages of medical therapy: In the first stage, your doctor brings your disease under control with the help of medications. In the second stage, you take medications to keep your symptoms under control. Taking medications is not a guarantee that you'll avoid surgery, but taking them on a regular basis can help lessen the inflammation and, thus, your symptoms. You'll get a better quality of life and be more productive. And you'll have less frequent trips to the emergency room or urgent-care clinics.

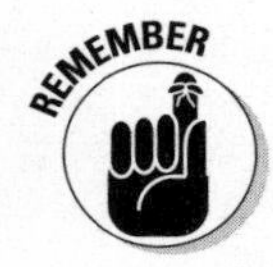

Patients who adhere to their medications have less chance of flares over time.

Taking medications every day is hard for some people, but it truly is for your own good. If you stop taking your medications, you're more likely to have a flare that may end up requiring steroid prescriptions or hospitalization if the flare is severe.

With certain medications, such as Remicade and Humira, not taking them on a regular basis can lead to antibody formations — you develop resistance or even drug reactions to these medications. If this happens, not only do you lose that drug forever, but it could be dangerous to your health.

Discuss with your doctor why you're taking medication, what it will do for your Crohn's or colitis, and what the potential benefits and risks of the medication are.

You Have to Stop Taking Your Medications during Pregnancy

Most of the medications prescribed for Crohn's and colitis are safe to take during pregnancy. For a complete rundown on what's safe and what isn't, check out Chapter 16.

Active Crohn's disease and ulcerative colitis can bring more serious problems to mother and baby than some medications may bring. Be sure to work with your doctor to ensure that you get the proper treatment for your Crohn's or colitis while you're pregnant.

Chapter 18

Ten Reliable Resources

In This Chapter

- Finding more information about Crohn's or colitis
- Knowing which sources you can trust

Today, information is all around — from books, magazines, and journals, to websites, blogs, social media, and more. If you want more information on Crohn's and colitis, you won't have trouble finding it. What you may have trouble with, though, is finding *accurate* information. As you know, you can't always trust what you read. So, the key is to make sure you're getting your information from sources you can trust.

In this chapter, I point you to ten reliable resources where you can turn for more information.

I regularly provide information on my Twitter account (`www.twitter.com/ibdtweets`) for patients suffering from Crohn's and colitis. Follow me on Twitter to keep in touch!

The Crohn's and Colitis Foundation of America

The Crohn's and Colitis Foundation of America (CCFA; `www.ccfa.org`) is a nonprofit organization dedicated to patients with Crohn's and colitis. It was founded in 1967 and today has more than 50,000 members and more than 40 chapters nationwide.

The CCFA provides information and education for patients and their families through a variety of periodicals, books, awareness campaigns, local chapter events, and webcasts. Its "Take Steps for Crohn's & Colitis" campaign (`http://shar.es/GWku4`), a fundraising event consisting of community walks throughout the United States, has raised more than $32 million to date.

Finding Crohn's and colitis foundations around the world

Many other countries have national Crohn's and colitis foundations. Here are the foundations in other major English-speaking countries:

- **Australia:** Crohn's & Colitis Australia (www.acca.net.au)
- **Canada:** Crohn's and Colitis Foundation of Canada (www.ccfc.ca)
- **New Zealand:** Crohn's & Colitis New Zealand (www.crohnsandcolitis.org.nz)
- **United Kingdom:** Crohn's and Colitis UK (www.nacc.org.uk)

If your country isn't listed here, just Google your country's name and the words *Crohn's colitis foundation.*

The CCFA's Information Resource Center (available at 888-694-8872) provides accurate, disease-related information to the public, healthcare professionals, patients, and their families. It helps people understand diagnosis, treatment, and living with Crohn's and colitis. The Information Resources Center is staffed by master's-degree-level health professionals. They're available from 9 a.m. to 5 p.m. Eastern time Monday through Friday.

You can get involved with the CCFA by following it on Twitter (www.twitter.com/ccfa) and Facebook (www.facebook.com/ccfafb). You can also join a local CCFA support group in the United States; to find a support group near you, go to www.ccfa.org/chapters. If you don't live near one of the 40 local chapters, check out the CCFA Online Support Group at www.ccfacommunity.org/ChatSeries.aspx.

Finally, if you're a college student with Crohn's or colitis, be sure to check out CCFA Campus Connection (www.ccfa.org/campus-connection).

The United Ostomy Associations of America

The United Ostomy Associations of America (UOAA; www.ostomy.org) is a national network for ostomy support groups in the United States. The primary goal of the organization is to provide support, information, and advocacy to people with ostomies and their caregivers. The UOAA offers information both on the web and through local chapters. The UOAA website offers a wealth of information on different types of ostomies, diet, and nutrition. It also covers difficult but important topics, such as intimacy issues with ostomy.

You can find a UOAA support group in your area, as well as online support groups, at www.ostomy.org/supportgroups.shtml. Chat with other people with ostomies at the UOAA Discussion Board: www.ostomy.org/forum/index.php. You can follow the UOAA on Twitter at www.twitter.com/uoaa and on Facebook at www.facebook.com/UOAAinc.

If you're looking for more information, you may want to subscribe to the UOAA's quarterly magazine, *The Phoenix*. You can find more information at www.phoenixuoaa.org. The magazine covers everything from advice from medical professionals to new ostomy products to skin care and odor control. It also publishes personal stories of people undergoing ostomy surgeries and living with ostomies.

You and IBD

You and IBD (www.youandibd.com) is one of my favorite websites, and I recommend it to my patients all the time. This highly informative website, designed specifically for Crohn's and colitis patients, is an excellent resource for individuals who've just been diagnosed or those who want to become more informed about the disease. You can find the latest information and receive advice about Crohn's and colitis from the leading medical experts in the United States. The website has video discussions between these experts, as well as interviews with IBD patients.

You and IBD also includes many slideshows, downloads, and some really cool animations. It covers a variety of topics, such as understanding Crohn's and colitis and the differences between the two illnesses. There are videos on the role of diet, stress, smoking, and alcohol in Crohn's and colitis. The site also provides information on medications, vaccinations, alternative methods of treatments, and surgical options. The videos providing information about getting pregnant and breastfeeding with Crohn's and colitis are particularly worthwhile.

MyIBD.org

MyIBD.org (www.myibd.org), published by the Foundation for Clinical Research in Inflammatory Bowel Disease, offers lots of information on IBD, including guidance for people who've recently been diagnosed. On this website, you can find basic information on the disease, as well as info on medications, advances in IBD treatment, and clinical trials. Finally, you can get links to other great sources of information on IBD.

WebMD

WebMD (www.webmd.com) is geared toward patients and offers a wide variety of information about specific diseases, medications, and healthy living. A separate section dedicated to Crohn's and colitis, the Inflammatory Bowel Disease Health Center (www.webmd.com/ibd-crohns-disease), provides very detailed information about the two illnesses.

The WebMD Q&A section (http://answers.webmd.com/explore-topics/inflammatory-bowel-disease-questions) provides answers to some commonly asked questions about Crohn's and colitis.

The information about different medications is also very useful, especially when your healthcare provider wants you to start a new medication — you can find out how the medication works and what side effects may be common.

The site also posts the latest headlines and top stories related to Crohn's and colitis. This is a great way to stay in the loop. I always learn something new from it.

Mayo Clinic

Mayo Clinic is a highly respected hospital in Minnesota, but you don't need to live in the snowy upper Midwest to take advantage of the Mayo Clinic's information. Go to www.mayoclinic.com/health-information and select your disease (either Crohn's disease or ulcerative colitis) from the alphabetical index. (Or just go to www.mayoclinic.com/health/crohns-disease/DS00104 or www.mayoclinic.com/health/ulcerative-colitis/DS00598.) You'll find information on symptoms, causes, risk factors, complications, how to prepare for a doctor's appointment, tests and diagnosis, treatment and drugs, lifestyle and home remedies, alternative medicine, and coping and support.

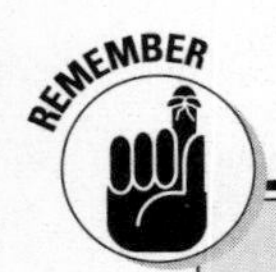

Questions to ask about any website

Before you trust what you read on the Internet, ask yourself the following questions:

- **Who runs the website?** Credible health-related websites should clearly state who's responsible for the information provided.
- **Who pays for the website?** If the site is being paid for by a drug company or other medical company, the information on the site may skew toward promoting the company's product. Web addresses that end

in .gov are sponsored by the U.S. federal government or a state government; those that end in .edu are educational institutions. Sites that end in .org are typically nonprofit organizations, and sites that end in .com typically are commercial in nature.

- **What is the purpose of the website?** Most websites have an About page or an Our Mission page. These pages can help you figure out if the website is credible.
- **What are the sources of the health information provided? Are the sources even offered?** If the people or organization behind the website didn't come up with the information they're providing on their own (for example, through their own research), the source of the information should be clearly listed.
- **How did the people or organization behind the website choose what information they provide?** Before a website decides that something is credible enough to share with the public, it should have a way to review the information and make sure it's reliable. If the site mentions an editorial board, this is a good indication that the information was reviewed (as opposed to being thrown onto a website by one guy sitting alone in his apartment).
- **Is the information up to date?** Information provided on credible websites should be reviewed and updated regularly. Outdated information is dangerous and may be misleading.
- **Are links to other websites available on the site? What websites has the site linked to?** This may help answer questions about who's funding the website as well.
- **Did the website ask you to "subscribe" or "become a member"?** Credible sites may ask you to do this, but they should clearly state what you get as a subscriber or member and what they will and won't do with the information you provide for them. You should be able to find the latter on the site's Privacy page; usually, you'll see a link to this page on the home page.

The Culinary Couple's Creative Colitis Cookbook

During active Crohn's and colitis, your doctor may recommend that you eat a low-fiber or low-residue diet. A variety of websites can tell you what foods to eat and what foods to avoid, but many of my patients complain that they don't know how to cook food that's low fiber or low residue. They're frustrated by a lack of recipes for low-fiber and low-residue food. Well, here's the good news: *The Culinary Couple's Creative Colitis Cookbook,* by Denise and Ross Weale (Front Burner Publishing), has solved the problem and put many patients with active disease at ease.

Both authors graduated from Johnson and Wales Culinary School in Providence, Rhode Island. In 1990, Ross was diagnosed with colitis. Because Ross needed to stick to a low-residue diet, he and Denise collaborated to write this book, which contains 100 easy-to-prepare, low-fiber, non-dairy recipes for everything from breakfast, bread, soup, and side dishes to main courses and desserts.

You can buy the book from your favorite book seller or from `www.colitiscookbook.com`. The website gives access to about a dozen free recipes. My favorites are Carol's Coffee Cake and Raspberry Souvaroff Cookies.

The International Association for Medical Assistance to Travelers

Traveling can be stressful when you have Crohn's or colitis. The International Association for Medical Assistance to Travelers (IAMAT; `www.iamat.org`) can help you plan a healthy trip and provides access to trusted medical and mental health practitioners around the world. It coordinates an international network of qualified doctors and mental health practitioners specially trained to provide medical care to travelers. It also provides information for travelers on vaccinations, health risks, and food and water safety advice for more than 90 countries.

KidsHealth

KidsHealth (`www.kidshealth.org`) is sponsored by Nemours Foundation, a nonprofit children's health organization. It's geared toward kids, teens, parents, and educators, and has comprehensive information on kids' general health, behavior, and development.

The site covers a wide range of physical, emotional, and behavioral issues that affect children and teens. The medical information is provided in a very easy-to-understand way. The site claims that all articles, animations, and other medical content go through a rigorous medical review by physicians and medical experts. The information is reviewed regularly to ensure that it's up to date. This website has won the Parents' Choice Gold Award, the Teachers' Choice Award for the Family, and the International Pirelli Award for best educational media for students.

I really like its recipes for lactose intolerance, a problem that 15 percent to 20 percent of Crohn's and colitis patients have.

IBD U

This is one of my favorite resources for teens and young adults. IBD U (short for University) was initiated as a collaborative effort of the Starlight Children's Foundation and the Children's Digestive Health Nutrition Foundation (CDHNF). IBD U (`www.ibdu.org`) is a great resource for young adults with Crohn's and colitis who are graduating and transitioning into adult healthcare. The website includes information to support and guide teens, as well as their parents, friends, teachers, and employers during this important transitional period. The website offers the following sections:

- **Education:** Offers information about the causes of IBD and the different medical therapies that are available to individuals. This section does a great job of explaining everything in terms that are easy to understand. The information and format are beneficial for anyone trying to learn about Crohn's or colitis, but especially for those who are younger.
- **Healthcare:** Offers tips to help you prepare for school and work. Shifting to college and adult life is hard for everyone, but it can be especially stressful for those with IBD. Not only are they dealing with their disease, but they're also dealing with leaving home and making decisions on their own. This section helps with those decisions.
- **Lifestyle:** Addresses good health habits when it comes to issues like sleep, exercise, and sex.
- **Self-Help:** Offers tips to succeed in college, at work, and in your everyday life. The YouTube channel of IBD U offers lots of video stories related to Crohn's and colitis and coping skills.
- **Community:** Offers access to Starbright World, "an online social network for teens with a serious illness or life-threatening condition, including teens with IBD."
- **Resources:** Here you can find links to a variety of web resources, as well as to the IBD U YouTube channel.

Glossary

abscess: A collection of pus caused by infection. Abscesses can occur in any part of the body.

adaptive immunity: An active immunity that develops throughout your life. It involves the white blood cells and develops as people are exposed to diseases and develop immunization against a disease with vaccines.

albumin: A protein produced in the liver that circulates in the blood. Low albumin levels may indicate low protein reserves in the body or liver problems. Low albumin levels are also seen during active inflammation of Crohn's or colitis.

aminosalicylates: A group of drugs used in the treatment of ulcerative colitis and less commonly in Crohn's disease. Aminosalicylates have anti-inflammatory properties and act on the mucosa of the intestine. They're further divided into sulfasalazine and mesalamine; different types of mesalamines are available to treat Crohn's and colitis.

anal fissure: A small tear in the lining of the lower rectum called the anus. Although anal fissures can happen in both Crohn's disease and ulcerative colitis, they're more common in Crohn's disease. Anal fissures are usually caused by inflammation of the anal canal and persistent diarrhea. They cause painful bowel movements and rectal bleeding. They may produce severe pain such as passing what feels like razor blades or cut glass.

anastomosis: The process that rejoins the two parts of the intestines after *resection* (removal). *See also* enterectomy.

antibody: A special type of large, sticky protein made by B cells. Also called *immunoglobulin* (Ig).

anti-TNF agent: A drug that attaches to TNF-α to prevent it from causing inflammation. *See also* tumor necrosis factor–alpha (TNF-α).

arthralgia: Pain in a joint. *See also* arthritis.

arthritis: Inflammation of the joint that causes the joint to swell and become red, warm, and painful. *See also* arthralgia.

barium: A white, chalky substance that coats the internal lining of the intestinal tract. You may drink a barium solution before having an X-ray to help the radiologist see any abnormalities like strictures or obstructions.

biologics: Drugs manufactured through a biological process using human, animal, or microorganism sources. This is in contrast to pharmaceutical drugs, which are manufactured through chemical processes. Vaccines, insulin, and different blood products used from transfusions are examples of biologics.

biopsy: A small piece of tissue taken from any area of the body and checked under the microscope.

bisphosphonates: Bisphosphonates are the most widely used medications for treating osteoporosis. They slow down the breakdown of the bones.

bone mineral density: A measurement of the minerals in the bones, indicating how strong the bones are. *See also* osteoporosis *and* osteopenia.

bowel urgency: A sudden, compelling need to have a bowel movement. Also called *fecal urgency.*

budesonide: A non-systemic steroid. Its effects are limited to the gut, so it can be great for gut-specific diseases like Crohn's and colitis. This local action provides many of the benefits of systemic steroids without the side effects that are caused by their action on organs outside the gastrointestinal tract.

CAT scan: *See* CT scan.

celiac disease: Inflammation of the small intestines, usually the first part of the intestines known as the *duodenum.* Celiac disease is a disease caused by a problem in the immune system that makes you allergic to gluten.
See gluten.

colectomy: Surgical removal of the colon. Colectomy can be partial (where only part of the colon is removed) or total (where the entire colon is removed). *See also* proctocolectomy.

colitis: Inflammation of the lining of the colon.

colon: The large intestine. The colon connects the small intestine (terminal ileum) to the rectum. The colon has different parts, starting with the cecum (where the appendix is attached) and moving to the ascending colon (on the right side), the transverse colon, the descending colon (on the left side), and the sigmoid colon. The sigmoid colon attaches to rectum, the last part of intestinal tract.

colonoscopy: A procedure that enables a physician to see the inside the rectum and colon with the help of a lighted, flexible tube called a *colonoscope.* The colonoscope is introduced through the anus and advanced through the rectum, sigmoid colon, descending colon, transverse colon, ascending colon, and cecum. Frequently, physicians also peek into the last part of the small intestine, called the *terminal ileum,* with the colonoscope.

C-reactive protein (CRP): C-reactive protein is a special protein made in the liver that circulates in the bloodstream during inflammation. Testing for CRP can be helpful in detecting the presence of inflammation.

Crohn's disease: A chronic disease that causes inflammation of the intestinal tract, anywhere from the mouth to the anus.

CT scan: An imaging method that uses X-rays to create cross-sectional pictures of part of the body. Also known as *CAT scan.*

DEXA scan: An imaging method that indicates whether a person has weak bones. *See also* osteoporosis *and* osteopenia.

diarrhea: The frequent passage of watery or semi-formed stools. Diarrhea is one of the most common symptoms of Crohn's disease and ulcerative colitis.

digestion: The mechanical and chemical process in which food is broken down into smaller pieces.

diverticulitis: Inflammation of the *diverticula* (small pockets in the colon).

diverticulosis: Small pockets or pouches in the inner lining of the colon. A single pocket is a *diverticulum;* more than one pocket are *diverticula. See also* diverticulitis.

duodenum: The first part of the small intestine. The duodenum is immediately after the stomach in the gastrointestinal tract.

dysplasia: A precancerous stage of the cells.

elemental diet: A liquid diet that contains all the nutrients your body needs. The nutrients are usually in digested form, so they put no stress on the digestive system. Elemental diets supply all your nutritional needs while giving your digestive system a rest.

endoscopy: A medical procedure that uses a tubelike instrument called an *endoscope.* The endoscope is put into the body to look inside and perform certain surgical procedures such as taking a biopsy from the internal lining of the intestines. *See also* colonoscopy.

enteral feeding: A way to deliver nutrients through a tube if you can't take food or drink through your mouth. The tube can be passed through the nose or directly into the stomach through the abdomen. Also known as *tube feeding.*

enterectomy: Surgical *resection* (removal) of the small intestine. *See also* anastomosis.

enteritis: Inflammation of the small intestine. Depending on the location, enteritis is also known as *duodenitis* (inflammation of the duodenum), *jejunitis* (inflammation of the jejunum), or *ileitis* (inflammation of the ileum).

erythema nodosum: Small, red, round, painful skin nodules, most commonly present on the shins and ankles. These nodules appear with increased inflammation of the intestines and disappear with treatment of the disease.

esophagus: The food pipe that connects the oral cavity to the stomach.

fissure: *See* anal fissure.

fistula: A tunnel connecting the intestine to another loop of intestine, to an adjacent organ, to the skin, or blindly into the abdominal cavity.

flare: The active state of inflammatory bowel disease, including ulcerative colitis and Crohn's disease. The duration and severity of the flare varies widely from person to person. During a flare, patients have symptoms of abdominal pain, diarrhea, fever, or blood in the stool, depending upon the type and location of inflammatory bowel disease. *See also* remission.

gastroenterologist: A physician certified to diagnose and treat gastrointestinal and liver diseases.

gluten: A type protein found in foods processed from wheat and related grain species, including barley and rye. *See also* celiac disease.

hematochezia: Passage of fresh blood from the anus, usually with or in the stool. It's a common symptom in ulcerative colitis.

hygiene hypothesis: A scientist named David Strachan proposed the hygiene hypothesis in 1989 when he observed that children from larger families have lower chances of having allergic diseases, such as hay fever or eczema. The hygiene hypothesis is based on the possibility that a child could be overprotected from the exposure to common germs because of improved hygiene. In these cases, the body fails to make the standard immune response when exposed to germs. This puts you at risk for many diseases such as Crohn's and colitis.

ileocecal valve: A narrow valve at the junction of the small intestine (ileum) and large intestine (colon). The ileocecal valve is the most common part involved in Crohn's disease.

ileostomy: A surgical procedure in which part of the small intestine is brought out to the skin of the abdomen. It can be permanent or temporary.

immune system: The body's defense against invaders such as infectious organisms. The immune system is made up of a network of cells and organs that work together to protect the body.

immunity: Protection from disease. All the specialized cells and proteins of the immune system offer the body immunity. *See also* adaptive immunity, passive immunity, *and* innate immunity.

immunoglobulin (Ig): *See* antibody.

immunomodulator: A drug that decreases the number of inflammatory cells in the body. Immunomodulators are used to treat many autoimmune diseases, to prevent the rejection of transplanted organs, and to treat some types of cancer. Common examples of such drugs include azathioprine and 6-mercaptopurine.

indeterminate colitis: A condition in which doctors are unable to differentiate between Crohn's colitis and ulcerative colitis.

innate immunity: The type of general protection that people are born with.

irritable bowel syndrome (IBS): A condition of the intestines in which nerve and muscle function is affected. Patients typically present with abdominal pain and altered bowel movements. Sometimes, IBS is confused with Crohn's or colitis. In addition, up to 30 percent of patients with Crohn's and colitis also have IBS.

J-pouch: A surgical technique in which the surgeon creates a J-shaped ileum and connects it to the anal canal. This procedure is done after colectomy. *See also* colectomy.

leukocytosis: White blood cell count above the normal range. Leukocytosis is frequently a sign of inflammation or infection.

lymphoma: A type of cancer that begins in immune system cells called *lymphocytes,* also known as white blood cells. Lymphoma may develop in many parts of the body, including the lymph nodes, spleen, bone marrow, blood, or other organs.

macronutrients: Larger molecules that form the majority of your diet. Examples include proteins, fats, and carbohydrates. *See also* micronutrients.

melanoma: Skin cancer that arises from pigment-making cells of the skin called *melanocytes.*

melena: Passage of dark, tarry stools. Melena usually indicates bleeding from the upper gastrointestinal tract, such as the stomach or small intestine.

micronutrients: Smaller molecules that are important for nutrition. Examples include vitamins and minerals. *See also* macronutrients.

microscopic colitis: The microscopic inflammation of the colon that causes you to have watery diarrhea. It is called microscopic because inflammation is not visible to the eyes and is seen only on biopsy of the intestine. It usually affects middle-aged and older adults.

mucosa: The innermost lining of the intestinal tract. It helps in the absorption of food and secretes digestive enzymes.

mucus: A slippery secretion produced by the cells lining the inner layer of intestines and covering the mucus membrane or mucosa. Mucous fluid is typically produced from mucous cells found in mucous glands.

NOD-2 gene: One of the first genes discovered in Crohn's disease patients, confirming the fact that genes are involved in causing this disease. In early 2000, scientists from the University of Chicago discovered that patients with Crohn's disease have mutation in this gene.

non-steroidal anti-inflammatory drugs: *See* NSAIDS.

NSAIDs: NSAIDs are used to treat inflammation such as joint and muscle aches. Their use in Crohn's and colitis may be associated with worsening of symptoms because one of their side effects is formation of ulcers in the intestinal tract.

osteopenia: Bone mineral density that is lower than normal but not low enough to be called osteoporosis. *See also* bone mineral density *and* osteoporosis.

osteoporosis: Weakening of the bones, leading to increased risk of fractures. *See also* bone mineral density *and* osteopenia.

ostomy: An opening on the skin of the belly that the surgeon creates for the discharge of waste matter.

pancolitis: Inflammation of the entire colon. *See also* colitis.

passive immunity: Immunity that you get from sources other than your body. Passive immunity lasts for a short time. For example, antibodies in a mother's breast milk provide a baby with temporary immunity until the baby develops its own immune system.

pouchitis: Inflammation of the J-pouch. *See also* J-pouch.

prebiotics: Food for good bacteria. Most types of grains contain prebiotics, as do many vegetables (like onions and beans) and fruits (like kiwi and banana).

primary sclerosing cholangitis (PSC): Inflammation of the bile duct. This type of inflammation can happen to the bile ducts that are inside the liver as well as outside the liver. It causes narrowing and blockage of the ducts. After a long period of time, PSC causes scarring of the liver called *liver cirrhosis.* It happens more with ulcerative colitis than Crohn's disease. PSC does not produce any symptoms in the beginning; it's usually detected by blood tests that show abnormalities in liver enzymes. Later on, it can cause obstruction and infection of the ducts leading to pain and fever.

probiotics: Live bacteria that provide various health benefits.

proctitis: Inflammation of the lining of the rectum. It commonly occurs in ulcerative colitis where the rectum is the starting point of the inflammation.

proctocolectomy: A surgical procedure in which the entire colon and rectum are removed. After a proctocolectomy, most patients have ileostomies. This is typical surgery for ulcerative colitis. *See also* ileostomy *and* J-pouch.

pyoderma gangrenosum: A skin problem that starts as a small blister and then becomes large and develops into an ulcer. Sometimes you have to apply local medical therapy to treat the ulcer. When it heals, it usually leaves behind a scar. This condition occurs more commonly in ulcerative colitis than in Crohn's disease.

regional enteritis: Another name for Crohn's disease. *See also* Crohn's disease.

remission: Remission is the opposite of a flare and is generally used to refer to an inactive state of inflammatory bowel disease, including ulcerative colitis and Crohn's disease. During remission, you feel better and have no or minimal symptoms. One of the goals of treatment is to bring your disease under remission. *See also* flare.

small bowel follow-through (SBFT): A special type of X-ray performed after you drink a contrast solution, such as barium. SBFT is done to rule out strictures, fistulas, narrowing, or obstruction. *See also* upper GI series *and* barium.

steroids: The name commonly used to refer to *glucocorticoids,* a class of drugs related to the natural hormone hydrocortisone or simply cortisol. Their anti-inflammatory properties are used to treat many medical conditions like asthma, certain rashes, arthritis, and many autoimmune diseases.

stoma: The actual end of the small or large intestine you see protruding through the abdominal wall after the surgeon removes the diseased part of the intestine.

stricture: Narrowed lumen of the intestine. When inflammation of the intestines is present for a long time, it can cause scarring. Scar tissue is not as flexible as healthy tissue and it can cause stricture.

stricturoplasty: A surgical procedure to repair stricture.

suppository: A drug that is inserted into the rectum where it dissolves or melts. Suppositories are usually given for some local action or when you're unable to take anything by mouth.

tenesmus: A constant sensation of fullness and incomplete relief during bowel movement. Patients feel an urgent desire to defecate without significant production of feces. It can also produce abdominal or rectal pain.

terminal ileum: The last part of the small intestine. It's connected to the large intestine by the *ileocecal valve.* The terminal ileum is the most common part of the intestinal tract involved in Crohn's disease.

total parenteral nutrition (TPN): A method of feeding a person solely through the veins.

toxic megacolon: Severe inflammation of the colon, leading to dilation of the colon and making the patient acutely ill with high fever, abdominal distension, and severe pain. It happens in about 5 percent of patients suffering from severe colitis.

tube feeding: *See* enteral feeding.

tumor necrosis factor–alpha (TNF-α): A protein manufactured in the liver that is a powerful component in the inflammatory process and plays a large role in the disease process of Crohn's and colitis.

ulcerative colitis: Chronic inflammatory bowel disease of the large intestine that usually starts with the rectum and can involve the sigmoid colon, ascending colon, transverse colon, ascending colon, or cecum. Unlike Crohn's disease of the colon, the inflammation in ulcerative colitis is almost always continuous, starting from rectum and moving its way upward.

upper GI series: An X-ray examination performed after you drink a contrast solution, such as barium, to look for any obstruction, narrowing, or inflammation. *See also* small bowel follow-through *and* barium.

urgency: *See* bowel urgency.

vaccine: A biological preparation that resembles a disease-causing microorganism and is often made from weakened or killed forms of the microbe, its toxins, or one of its surface proteins. A vaccine stimulates the immune system and protects the body against a specific disease.

Index

• B •

• C •

• D •

• E •

• F •

• I •

• J •

• K •

• Q •

• R •

• S •

• T •

• U •

• V •